Essentials
of Hospital
Neurology

ESSENTIALS OF HOSPITAL NEUROLOGY

Edited By

Karl E. Misulis, MD, PhD

Clinical Professor of Neurology & Biomedical Informatics

Vanderbilt University School of Medicine

Nashville, TN

E. Lee Murray, MD

Clinical Assistant Professor of Neurology

University of Tennessee Health Science Center

Memphis, TN

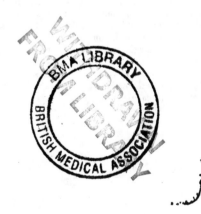

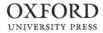

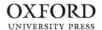

OXFORD
UNIVERSITY PRESS

Oxford University Press is a department of the University of Oxford. It furthers
the University's objective of excellence in research, scholarship, and education
by publishing worldwide. Oxford is a registered trade mark of Oxford University
Press in the UK and certain other countries.

Published in the United States of America by Oxford University Press
198 Madison Avenue, New York, NY 10016, United States of America.

© Oxford University Press 2017

Library of Congress Cataloging-in-Publication Data
Names: Misulis, Karl E., author. | Murray, E. Lee (Earnest Lee), author.
Title: Essentials of hospital neurology / Karl E. Misulis, E. Lee Murray.
Description: New York, NY : Oxford University Press, [2017] | Includes
bibliographical references and index.
Identifiers: LCCN 2016034960 | ISBN 9780190259419 (alk. paper)
Subjects: | MESH: Nervous System Diseases—diagnosis | Diagnostic Techniques,
Neurological | Diagnosis, Differential | Neurology—methods |
Hospitalists—methods | Hospital Medicine—trends
Classification: LCC RC346 | NLM WL 141 | DDC 616.8—dc23 LC record available at
https://lccn.loc.gov/2016034960

9 8 7 6 5 4 3 2 1
Printed by Webcom Inc., Canada

I would like to thank God for all His blessings, my friend and colleague Karl Misulis for allowing me to keep my academic flame alive, all my teachers and mentors who have taught me the art of neurology, my patients who remind me what my calling is, and my parents and family for all their love and support. I dedicate this work to my wife Carmen, son Bennett, and future daughter for the joy they bring each and every day and the sacrifices they make way too often.

—E. Lee Murray

I dedicate my part in this work to all those who have traveled with me through my long career, from family and friends to colleagues and to those who have read or listened to my works. I want to express special gratitude to the many thousands of patients who have trusted me with their health and often with their lives. It has been an honor and a privilege to serve.

—Karl E. Misulis

Contents

Preface   xi

Contributor List   xiii

Abbreviations   xv

Section I Introduction

1. Overview of Hospital Neurology, *Karl E. Misulis, MD, PhD, E. Lee Murray, MD,
    and Monico Peter Bañez, MD, MBA, FACP, SFHM*   3

2. Interface Between Hospital and Outpatient Neurology, *Karl E. Misulis, MD, PhD
    and Monico Peter Bañez, MD, MBA, FACP, SFHM*   7

3. Business of Hospital Neurology, *Karl E. Misulis, MD, PhD and
    Monico Peter Bañez, MD, MBA, FACP, SFHM*   11

Section II Approach to Neurologic Problems

4. Motor and Sensory Disturbance, *E. Lee Murray, MD and
    Veda V. Vedanarayanan, MD, FRCPC*   17

5. Mental Status Change, *Karl E. Misulis, MD, PhD
    and E. Lee Murray, MD*   29

6. Approach to Visual Deficits, *Karl E. Misulis, MD, PhD and
    E. Lee Murray, MD*   41

7. Language and Hearing Deficits, *Howard S. Kirshner, MD and
    Karl E. Misulis, MD, PhD*   49

8. Cranial Neuropathies, *Karl E. Misulis, MD, PhD
    and E. Lee Murray, MD*   55

9. Dizziness, Vertigo, and Imbalance, *Karl E. Misulis, MD, PhD and
    E. Lee Murray, MD*   59

10. Pain and Headache, *E. Lee Murray, MD and Karl E. Misulis, MD, PhD*   67

Section III Neurologic Diagnoses

11. Neurologic Complications in Medical Patients, *Karl E. Misulis, MD, PhD and
    E. Lee Murray, MD*   81

12. Neurologic Complications in Surgical Patients, *E. Lee Murray, MD and Karl E. Misulis, MD, PhD*   97

13. Neurologic Manifestations of Systemic Disease, *Karl E. Misulis, MD, PhD and E. Lee Murray, MD*   103

14. Hypoxic-Ischemic Encephalopathy, *Karl E. Misulis, MD, PhD and E. Lee Murray, MD*   117

15. Brain Death and Persistent Vegetative State, *Karl E. Misulis, MD, PhD and E. Lee Murray, MD*   121

16. Vascular Disease, *E. Lee Murray, MD and William C. Barrow, MD*   125

17. Infectious Diseases, *Karl E. Misulis, MD, PhD and E. Lee Murray, MD*   147

18. Cognitive Disorders, *Howard S. Kirshner, MD and Karl E. Misulis, MD, PhD*   163

19. Seizures and Epilepsy, *Bassel W. Abou-Khalil, MD and Karl E. Misulis, MD, PhD*   173

20. Headache, *E. Lee Murray, MD and Karl E. Misulis, MD, PhD*   189

21. Neuromuscular Disorders, *E. Lee Murray, MD and Veda V. Vedanarayanan, MD, FRCPC*   197

22. Demyelinating Diseases, *Karl E. Misulis, MD, PhD and E. Lee Murray, MD*   215

23. Movement Disorders, *John Y. Fang, MD and David A. Isaacs, MD*   223

24. Spinal Cord Disorders, *Karl E. Misulis, MD, PhD and E. Lee Murray, MD*   243

25. Neuro-Oncology, *Mark D. Anderson, MD and Karl E. Misulis, MD, PhD*   251

26. CSF Circulation Disorders, *Karl E. Misulis, MD, PhD and E. Lee Murray, MD*   261

27. Pregnancy and Neurology, *Georgia Montouris, MD and Maria Stefanidou, MD, MSc*   267

28. Endocrine Disorders, *Karl E. Misulis, MD, PhD and E. Lee Murray, MD*   277

29. Nutritional Deficiencies and Toxicities, *Karl E. Misulis, MD, PhD and E. Lee Murray, MD*   285

30. Neurotoxicology, *Karl E. Misulis, MD, PhD and E. Lee Murray, MD*   289

31. Neuro-Ophthalmology, *Karl E. Misulis, MD, PhD and E. Lee Murray, MD*   297

32. Neuro-Otology, *Karl E. Misulis, MD, PhD and E. Lee Murray, MD*   301

33. Cranial Nerve Disorders, *Karl E. Misulis, MD, PhD and E. Lee Murray, MD*   307

34. Autonomic Disorders, *Karl E. Misulis, MD, PhD and E. Lee Murray, MD*   313

35. Traumatic Brain Injury, *Karl E. Misulis, MD, PhD and E. Lee Murray, MD* 317

36. Sleep Disorders, *Karl E. Misulis, MD, PhD and E. Lee Murray, MD* 323

37. Developmental and Genetic Disorders, *Karl E. Misulis, MD, PhD and E. Lee Murray, MD* 327

38. Psychiatric Disorders, *Karl E. Misulis, MD, PhD and E. Lee Murray, MD* 333

Section IV Neurology Toolkit

39. Toolkit—Assessments, *Karl E. Misulis, MD, PhD and E. Lee Murray, MD* 341

40. Toolkit—Studies, *Karl E. Misulis, MD, PhD and E. Lee Murray, MD* 347

41. Toolkit—Neurologic Management, *Karl E. Misulis, MD, PhD and E. Lee Murray, MD* 357

42. Toolkit—Difficult Encounters, *Karl E. Misulis, MD, PhD and E. Lee Murray, MD* 365

References 371
Index 387

Preface

Hospital neurology is a growing subspecialty. Advances in diagnostics and therapeutics have added to the complexity of hospital care of neurologic disorders, and hence a need for increasing hospital presence of neurologists. Just as a single individual can no longer be expert in neuromuscular, epilepsy, and movement disorders, no longer can a single individual easily cover both a busy office practice and a busy hospital practice.

This book discusses the spectrum of neurologic diseases likely to be encountered in hospital practice. The focus is on hospital management, so details of disorders usually treated in the outpatient arena are left to other texts.

Our intent is to make this book concise yet comprehensive, emphasizing practical diagnostic and therapeutic topics. Details of historical or pathophysiological interest are not included unless important for patient care.

Our goal is to advance the quality and efficiency of neurologic care in the hospital setting. The authors would like to express their great appreciation to the contributors for their expert and exemplary work.

Karl Misulis
Lee Murray
January 2017

Contributor List

Bassel W. Abou-Khalil, MD
Director, Epilepsy Center
Department of Neurology
Vanderbilt University Medical Center
Nashville, TN

Mark D. Anderson, MD
Neuro-Oncology
Department of Neurology
The University of Mississippi
Jackson, MS

William C. Barrow, MD
Neurohospitalist/Vascular Neurology
Jackson-Madison County General
    Hospital
West Tennessee Neuroscience
Jackson, TN

Monico Peter Bañez, MD, MBA,
    FACP, SFHM
Internal Medicine, Jackson General
    Hospitalists
West Tennessee Healthcare
Jackson, TN

John Y. Fang, MD
Department of Neurology
Division of Movement Disorders
Vanderbilt University Medical Center
Nashville, TN

David A. Isaacs, MD
Department of Neurology
Division of Movement Disorders
Vanderbilt University Medical Center
Nashville, TN

Howard S. Kirshner, MD
Vice-Chairman, Department of
    Neurology
Director, Vanderbilt Stroke Center
Stroke, Behavioral Neurology
Vanderbilt University Medical Center
Nashville, TN

Georgia D. Montouris, MD
Clinical Associate Professor of
    Neurology
Boston University School of Medicine
Director of Epilepsy Services
Boston Medical Center
Boston, MA

Maria Stefanidou, MD, MSc
Department of Neurology
Boston University School of Medicine
Boston Medical Center
Boston, MA

Veda V. Vedanarayanan, MD, FRCPC
Director, Division of Neuromuscular
    Medicine
Professor Neurology, Pediatrics and
    Pathology
University of Mississippi Medical
    Center
Jackson, MS

Abbreviations

AAN	American Academy of Neurology
ABG	arterial blood gasses
ABMS	American Board of Medical Specialties
ABPMR	American Board of Physical Medicine and Rehabilitation
ABPN	American Board of Psychiatry and Neurology
ACA	Anterior cerebral artery
ACE	Angiotensin converting enzyme
AChR	Acetylcholine receptor
ACTH	Adrenocorticotropic hormone
AD	Alzheimer disease
ADEM	Acute disseminated encephalomyelitis
AED	Anti-epileptic drug
AICA	Anterior inferior cerebellar artery
AIDP	Acute inflammatory demyelinating polyneuropathy
AION	Anterior ischemic optic neuropathy
AIS	Acute ischemic stroke
ALS	Amyotrophic lateral sclerosis
AMAN	Acute motor axonal neuropathy
AMSAN	Acute motor and sensory axonal neuropathy
APS	Antiphospholipid antibody syndrome
ARDS	Acute respiratory distress syndrome
ASRH	Acute stroke ready hospital
AVM	Arteriovenous malformation
BBB	Blood-brain barrier
BMI	Body mass index
BP	Blood pressure
BPPV	Benign paroxysmal positional vertigo
CADASIL	Cerebral Autosomal-Dominant Arteriopathy with Subcortical Infarcts and Leukoencephalopathy
CBC	Complete blood count
CBS	Corticobasal syndrome
CDC	Centers for disease control
CDS	Carotid duplex sonography
CEA	Carotid endarterectomy
ChEI	Cholinesterase inhibitor
CHF	Congestive heart failure

CIDP	Chronic inflammatory demyelinating polyneuropathy
CIN	Critical illness neuromyopathy
CJD	Creutzfeldt-Jakob disease
CMAP	Compound motor action potential
CMV	Cytomegalovirus
CN-x	Cranial nerve, where "x" indicates the number
CNS	Central nervous system
Coags	Coagulation studies, esp. PT, PTT
COPD	Chronic obstructive pulmonary disease
CPA	Cerebellopontine angle
CPK	Creatine phosphokinase
CPM	Central pontine myelinolysis
CADISS	Cervical Artery Dissection in Stroke Study
CPR	Cardio-pulmonary resuscitation
CRP	C-reactive protein
CRVO	Central retinal vein occlusion
CRYSTAL AF	Cryptogenic Stroke and Underlying Atrial Fibrillation trial
CSC	Comprehensive stroke center
CSF	Cerebrospinal fluid
CSH	Carotid sinus hypersensitivity
CT	Computed tomography
CTA	CT Angiography
CTE	Chronic traumatic encephalopathy
CTV	CT Venography
CVA	Cerebrovascular accident.
CVT	Cerebral venous thrombosis
DAI	Diffuse axonal injury
DDx	Differential diagnosis
DHE	Dihydroergotamine
DIP	Drug-induced parkinsonism
DKA	Diabetic ketoacidosis
DLB	Dementia with Lewy bodies
DM	Diabetes mellitus
DNR	Do not resuscitate
DTs	Delirium tremens
DVT	Deep vein thrombosis
EBV	Epstein-Barr virus
Echo	Echocardiogram
ED	Emergency department
EDH	Epidural hematoma
EDS	Excessive daytime sleepiness
EEG	Electroencephalogram
EKG	Electrocardiogram
EMG	Electromyogram
EMR	Electronic medical record
EMS	Emergency medical services
ENT	Earn, nose, and throat

Esp	Especially
ESR	Erythrocyte sedimentation rate
FA	Friedreich ataxia
FDA	Food and Drug Administration
FTD	Frontotemporal dementia
GCA	Giant cell arteritis
GI	Gastrointestinal
HD	Huntington disease
HHS	Hyperosmolar hyperglycemic state
HIE	Hypoxic ischemic encephalopathy
HIV	Human immunodeficiency virus
HSP	Hereditary spastic paraparesis
HSV	Herpes simplex virus
ICH	Intracerebral hemorrhage
ICP	Intracranial pressure
ICU	Intensive care unit
ILR	Implantable loop recorder
IM	Intramuscular
INR	International normalized ratio
IOH	Idiopathic orthostatic hypotension
IOIS	Idiopathic Orbital Inflammatory Syndrome.
ION	Ischemic optic neuropathy
IOP	Intraocular pressure
IS	Information systems
IV	Intravenous
IVIg	Intravenous immunoglobulin
LDL	Low-density lipoprotein
LEMS	Lambert Eaton Myasthenic Syndrome
LFT	Liver function tests
LP	Lumbar puncture
MAOI	Monoamine oxidase inhibitor
MAP	Mean arterial pressure
MCA	Middle cerebral artery
MCT	Mobile cardiac telemetry
MD	Muscular dystrophies
Med	Medication
MELAS	Mitochondrial Encephalopathy and Lactic Acid Stroke-like episodes
MG	Myasthenia gravis
MI	Myocardial infarction
MMA	Methylmalonic acid
MMN	Multifocal motor neuropathy
MRA	Magnetic resonance angiography
MRI	Magnetic resonance imaging
MRV	Magnetic resonance venography
MS	Multiple sclerosis
MSA	Multiple system atrophy
NASCET	North American Symptomatic Carotid Endarterectomy Trial

NBTE	Nonbacterial thrombotic endocarditis
NCS	Nerve Conduction Study
NCSE	Nonconvulsive status epilepticus
NCV	Nerve conduction velocity
NF	Neurofibromatosis
NIF	Net inspiratory force
NIH	National Institutes of Health
NIHSS	NIH Stroke Scale
NMDA	N-methyl-D-aspartate
NMJ	Neuromuscular junction
NMO	Neuromyelitis Optica
NMS	Neuroleptic malignant syndrome
NPH	Normal pressure hydrocephalus
NSAID	Non-steroidal anti-inflammatory drug
ON	Optic neuritis
OP	Opening pressure
OSA	Obstructive sleep apnea
PAN	Polyarteritis nodosa
PCA	Posterior cerebral artery
PCD	Paraneoplastic cerebellar degeneration
PCP	Primary care provider
PD	Parkinson disease
PDD	Parkinson disease with dementia
PET	Positron emission tomography
PFO	Patent foramen ovale
PICA	Posterior inferior cerebellar artery
PLED	Periodic lateralized epileptiform discharge
PLMD	Periodic limb movement disorder
PMC	PubMed central
PML	Progressive multifocal leukoencephalopathy
PNES	Psychogenic non-epileptic seizure
PO	Per os (i.e., Oral)
PPA	Primary progressive aphasia
PPM	Permanent pacemaker
PRES	Posterior Reversible Encephalopathy Syndrome
PSC	Primary stroke center
PSG	Polysomnography
PSP	Progressive supranuclear palsy
PVS	Persistent vegetative state
QOL	Quality of life
RA	Rheumatoid arthritis
RCVS	Reversible Cerebral Vasoconstriction Syndrome
RLS	Restless legs syndrome
RNS	Repetitive nerve stimulation
SAH	Subarachnoid hemorrhage
SBE	Subacute bacterial endocarditis
SDH	Subdural hematoma

SIADH	Syndrome of inappropriate anti-diuretic hormone
SIRS	Systemic inflammatory response syndrome
SLE	Systemic lupus erythematosus
SNAP	Sensory nerve action potential
SNRI	Serotonin norepinephrine reuptake inhibitor
SPEP	Serum protein electrophoresis
SSRI	Selective serotonin reuptake inhibitor
SUNCT	Short-lasting unilateral neuralgiform headache with conjunctival injection and tearing
TBI	Traumatic brain injury
TCA	Tricyclic antidepressant
TD	Tardive dyskinesia
TED	Thyroid eye disease
TEE	Transesophageal echocardiogram
TGA	Transient global amnesia
TH	Therapeutic hypothermia
TIA	Transient ischemic attack
TJC	The Joint Commission
TLOC	Transient loss of consciousness
TOAST	Trial of Org 10172 in Acute Stroke Treatment
tPA	Tissue plasminogen activator
TSH	Thyroid stimulating hormone
TTE	Transthoracic echocardiogram
TTM	Targeted temperature management
UCNS	United Council for Neurologic Subspecialties
US	United States
UTI	Urinary tract infection
VaD	Vascular dementia
VGCC	Voltage gated calcium channel
VOR	Vestibulo-ocular reflex
VZV	Varicella zoster virus
WBC	White blood count
WNV	West Nile virus

SECTION I
INTRODUCTION

SECTION CONTENTS

1 Overview of Hospital Neurology
2 Interface Between Hospital and Inpatient Neurology
3 Business of Hospital Neurology

1 Overview of Hospital Neurology

Karl E. Misulis,MD, PhD,
E. Lee Murray, MD, and
Monico Peter Bañez, MD, MBA, FACP, SFHM

CHAPTER CONTENTS

- Overview
- Models of a Hospital Neurology Service
- Training and Subspecialties in Hospital Neurology
- Neurology Midlevel Providers
- Organizational Issues in Hospital Neurology

OVERVIEW

Hospital neurology is a rapidly growing subspecialty. In addition to hospital-based general neurologists, there has also been an expansion of hospital-based specialty care services, including stroke centers, epilepsy centers, and neuro-critical care services.

There is a clear need for more neurologists of all types, but particularly hospital neurologists. Neurologic diagnoses make up between 10% and 20% of admissions to hospitals,[1] and a disproportionate number of delayed discharges have primary neurologic diagnoses.[2] Hospital neurology services can help to improve the quality and efficiency of care.

Where will the hospital neurologists come from? A diverse group is a product of diverse pathways. A few will do defined hospital neurology fellowships, some will have completed stroke or neuro-critical care fellowships, whereas others will be general neurologists.

In this book, we use the term *hospital neurologist*. An equivalent term is *neurohospitalist*. Other predominately hospital-based neurologists include stroke neurologists and neurointensivists.

MODELS OF A HOSPITAL NEUROLOGY SERVICE

The organization of a hospital neurology service depends greatly on the features of the practice, including institution size, patient volume, referral patterns, and community culture (see Table 1.1).

Table 1.1 Models of a hospital neurology practice

Practice type	Features	Advantages	Disadvantages
Hospital neurologist	Neurologist who spends most or all practice time in hospital. Can be admitting or purely consultative practice, especially in larger hospitals.	No conflict of divided time with clinic duties. Usually shift-work. Compensation usually better than most clinic work.	Reduced control over patient load. More weekend and holiday work. Reduced control over who is sharing care responsibilities.
Teleneurology	Phone and/or Internet-based communication between a neurologist and provider at a remote location.	Hospital can be covered 24/7 even if it does not have sufficient on-call neurologists. Transfers can be facilitated or obviated.	Acceptance by some providers and patients is incomplete. Reimbursement is complex and dependent on facility, location, and service provided.
Mixed office and hospital	Traditional office practice with hospital call.	Mix of inpatient and outpatient care is interesting for many neurologists. Ease of scheduling of hospital follow-ups to the provider's own clinic.	Pull between clinic and hospital(s) can stress the capabilities of the provider.

TRAINING AND SUBSPECIALTIES IN HOSPITAL NEUROLOGY

Presently, most hospital neurologists are residency-trained in general neurology with substantial experience in inpatient care. Depending on the size and mission of the hospital, additional training and/or experience may be needed; a stroke fellowship is particularly valuable. Large centers that are specifically designated as stroke centers may require stroke fellowship training for at least some of the hospital neurology staff.

Most trauma is best cared for by comprehensive trauma centers with neurosurgical coverage. A small subset of neurologists is involved in emergency evaluation and management of neurologic trauma.

A summary of training for specific practice concentrations is presented in Table 1.2.

Table 1.2 Practice concentrations for neurology

Specialty	Training	Certification
Hospital neurology	Most hospital neurologists obtain training solely during residency. Hospital neurology fellowships are available.	No ABMS/ABPN or UCNS certification currently available.
Vascular neurology	Fellowships are available. Many residencies provide extensive vascular neurology experience.	ABPN certification available. Certification without fellowship (grandfather) no longer available.
Brain injury medicine	Fellowships are available. Most neurology residencies do not provide extensive brain injury experience.	Certification available for neurologists through ABPN. For physiatrists through ABPMR.
Neuro-critical care	Fellowships available for neurologists and other specialties.	No ABPN certification presently. UCNS certification available.

ABMS, American Board of Medical Specialties; ABPN, American Board of Psychiatry and Neurology; ABPMR, American Board of Physical Medicine and Rehabilitation; UCNS, United Council for Neurologic Subspecialties.

NEUROLOGY MIDLEVEL PROVIDERS

Neurology nurse-practitioners and physician assistants have been used in clinics to help especially with follow-up visits, but there are increasing numbers of midlevel providers who are trained and skilled in hospital neurology and neuro-critical care. These providers are a valuable part of the neurology team, not as a substitute for neurology physicians but rather as colleagues who share in the care of hospitalized patients. In addition, nurse practitioners provide much of the post-hospital care.

ORGANIZATIONAL ISSUES IN HOSPITAL NEUROLOGY

Deciding how to organize a hospital neurology practice or whether to participate in one is complicated. Some of the major concerns are:

Scope of responsibilities: There is sometimes a disconnect between the scope of practice of the hospital neurologist and the expectations of the facility. Areas of special concern can include pediatrics, trauma, medical coverage of neurosurgical patients, and psychiatric care. The scope of practice should be clear to both the provider and the facility.

Work and call schedule: Most hospitals are accustomed to shift workers. Generally, shifts of longer than 12 hours are uncommon, especially for busier hospitals, and if 24 or more hours are required, contingency plans for overflow need to be defined.

Caseload: Providers need to be rewarded for hard work, but high caseloads correlate with more errors, worse outcomes, and poorer patient satisfaction scores.

A reasonable workload needs to be assured with defined plans regarding how the system will deal with excessive volume.

Quality improvement: Performance on quality measures will be an increasingly important metric on which practice assessment and compensation will be at least partly based.

Compensation: Compensation is most commonly based on a combination of caseload, work hours, quality indicators, and regional norms for comparative practice. Most systems are moving away from purely volume-based compensation.

2 Interface Between Hospital and Outpatient Neurology

Karl E. Misulis, MD, PhD and
Monico Peter Bañez, MD, MBA, FACP, SFHM

CHAPTER CONTENTS

- Continuity of Care
  o Hospital Admission
  o Hospital Discharge
- When Outpatient Neurology Becomes Inpatient
- When a Potential Inpatient Becomes an Outpatient

Progressively fewer neurologists embrace the traditional model of combined outpatient and inpatient care, and this has introduced difficulties with continuity of care. Not only do patients generally want to see the same providers, but many providers may feel that they are left out of the loop if communication is not optimal. Lack of continuity presents greater opportunities for medical errors, such as late-resulting labs being overlooked or planned medication adjustments not being made.

These difficulties are not insurmountable. Most electronic medical record (EMR) systems have the capability of secure messaging to facilitate secure transfer of information and notification of events. Also, Health information Exchanges (HIE) are becoming more robust, aiding communication between enterprises.

However, no technical solution can replace the personal touch. An increasing number of EMRs will notify primary care providers (PCP) if one of their patients has been hospitalized. A brief visit by the PCP can make a major difference for the concerned patient whose life is in the hands of strangers. As hospital neurologists, we should help maintain continuity of care and help PCPs maintain their connections with their patients.

CONTINUITY OF CARE
Hospital Admission

Unless the inpatient and outpatient medical records are in a single database and accessed using a single EMR, the hospital provider does not have easy access to outpatient records. When an admission occurs after normal business hours, manual access of office records is frequently impossible. The best answer for this is an HIE, but these systems are not operational in many markets. One-off connections can be accomplished between EMRs, but this is a huge undertaking for the Information Systems (IS) staff and does not always function smoothly. IS can provide web access in the hospital to select office EMRs. Until a local exchange is functioning, this may be the best solution.

Most PCPs want to know when their patients have been admitted. Communication orders can be built into most EMRs to make this notification automatic.

Hospital Discharge

Post-discharge care: Most patients admitted to the hospital need post-discharge care. One challenge can be finding a provider for this care, both neurologic and medical. Absence of health insurance makes this even more of a challenge. One option is to have community physicians and midlevel providers of both general medicine and specialties aligned with the hospital.

Study follow-up: Studies resulting after discharge have to be reviewed. Almost all systems have the capability of messaging post-discharge results to a provider's inbox. Another technique that is particularly useful is to deliver a message to the provider when the results of all pending studies are complete, thus prompting review of the EMR. However the hospital physician is still responsible for follow-up on these data.

Medication reconciliation assures that specific neurologic meds are considered in the context of other prescribed meds.

Compliance continues to be a problem: One report found that 80% of patients are taking discharge meds after their first stroke, but only 60% after a second stroke. It is hoped that prompt follow-up to address provider and patient lapses will help.[1]

Follow-up appointments for discharged patients depend on the specifics, but, generally, we recommend follow-up at 2 weeks for stroke and transient ischemic attack (TIA), acute and subacute neuromuscular disorders, and seizures. Follow-up at 4 weeks is appropriate for patients seen in the hospital for nonurgent conditions (e.g., dementia, chronic movement disorder).

WHEN OUTPATIENT NEUROLOGY BECOMES INPATIENT

There will be instances when a patient seen in the clinic needs admission either urgently or electively.

Rapid workup needed: Patients with acute or subacute neurological problems may be worked into the clinic when admission is actually necessary. Although same-day diagnostics can sometimes be obtained, action on critical findings or stabilization of the patient can necessitate admission (e.g., mental status change with fever, multiple seizures, recent focal deficit).

Rapid treatment needed: Patients with conditions such a status migraine or myasthenia exacerbation often need admission to facilitate prompt treatment.

Deterioration with chronic disease: Patients with severe dementia or movement disorders are often admitted for aspiration or other complication of their disease.

WHEN A POTENTIAL INPATIENT BECOMES AN OUTPATIENT

The hospital neurologist spends significant time in the ED evaluating patients to be admitted and arranging outpatient care for those who do not need admission. Of the latter, there are those who can receive neurology consultation in the ED and then be discharged to PCP care, and there are those who need further neurologic follow-up after the ED consultation. In addition, there are a few who can have their complete evaluation performed in the office, especially if the system is conducive to urgent workup. Some scenarios that can be so treated include select patients with seizure(s), subacute onset of weakness, TIA, and headache.

All patients who are seen in the ED and discharged to home or clinic should be advised of clinical events that make return to the ED appropriate.

3 Business of Hospital Neurology

Karl E. Misulis, MD, PhD and
Monico Peter Bañez, MD, MBA, FACP, SFHM

CHAPTER CONTENTS

- Stroke Center
  - Acute Stroke-Ready Hospital
  - Primary Stroke Center
  - Comprehensive Stroke Center
- Teleneurology
- Billing and Coding
- Metrics
- Risk Management
- Future Directions

STROKE CENTER

Hospital neurologists are increasingly being asked to treat strokes acutely. Because of this, we are asked to start or participate in Stroke Centers.

There are different levels of stroke center certification, and the key is selecting which is the best fit for each facility. The certifications are designed and granted by The Joint Commission (TJC). Requirements are complex and subject to change, so source documentation from TJC should be consulted (visit https//www.jointcommission.org/facts_about_joint_commission_certification). The criteria presented are active at the time of writing.

The types of stroke centers are:

- Acute stroke-ready hospital (ASRH)
- Primary stroke center (PSC)
- Comprehensive stroke center (CSC)

Many hospitals have the personnel and resources to be a PSC. CSC certification is usually the province of academic hospitals and regional referral medical centers. Smaller hospitals may seek certification as ASRHs.

ACUTE STROKE-READY HOSPITAL

ASRH certification is best suited to hospitals with 24/7 ED service typically without in-house neurology. Basic requirements include:

- 24/7 provider coverage
- Initial evaluation by physician, nurse practitioner, or physician assistant
- Neurologic consultation in person or by telemedicine
- Imaging including computed tomography (CT) and magnetic resonance imaging (MRI) available 24/7
- Ability to administer IV tissue plasminogen (tPA) with subsequent transfer to a stroke center
- Transfer agreement with a PSC or CSC

There are other requirements regarding education, timing of response, record-keeping, and requirement of TJC site visit.

PRIMARY STROKE CENTER

PSC certification is best suited for hospitals with 24/7 neurology coverage, although the criteria do allow for telemedicine to fulfill this requirement. In comparison to the ASRH designation, the PSC must have more extensive access to advanced imaging and neurovascular interventions. Some of the requirements are:

- 24/7 provider coverage, but initial evaluation can be by ED physician
- Neurologic input in person or by telemedicine also 24/7
- Imaging access 24/7 not only including CT and MRI but also computed tomography angiography (CTA), magnetic resonance angiography (MRA), and cardiac imaging
- Ability to provide neurovascular procedures including acute endovascular therapy, carotid stenting, carotid endarterectomy, and intervention for aneurysms
- Access to neurosurgical coverage or a transfer agreement for neurosurgery

COMPREHENSIVE STROKE CENTER

CSC certification is usually for established academic medical centers or regional referral centers. Full-service neurological, neurosurgical, and neuroradiological service is needed. Requirements that distinguish CSC from ASRH and PSC include:

- Neurology expertise available on-site 24/7
- Neurosurgeon and neuroradiologist/neurointerventionalist available 24/7
- Imaging availability including transesophageal echocardiogram (TEE) and catheter angiography in addition to carotid duplex sonography (CDS), transthoracic echocardiogram (TTE), and the other imaging modalities required for PSC
- Participation in patient-centered research requiring institutional review board (IRB) approval
- Sponsor for public educational opportunities

CSCs usually partner with regional PSCs and ASRHs to form a network. Ideally, the CSC should guide the local stroke network on best practices, standards of care, and metrics.

TELENEUROLOGY

Teleneurology has been a logical subset for telemedicine since many busy hospitals either do not have neurologists or do not have sufficient numbers of neurologists to cover calls 24/7. Teleneurology can accomplish at least some of the following:

- Reduce the number of transfers
- Improve urgent evaluation of patients especially with suspected stroke and seizures
- Reduce length of stay and unnecessary tests
- Improve cooperation of local providers and remote specialists

Barriers to more extensive use of teleneurology include:

- Unavailability of participating neurologists
- Concerns over reimbursement
- Concerns over liability
- Concerns that the mechanics of teleneurology can sometimes delay acute care

To address the concerns over reimbursement and staffing, carefully negotiated agreements between facilities have to be established. Preferably, the teleneurology service should be provided by the regional referral hospital that can accept the patient in transfer if needed.

BILLING AND CODING

Billing and coding are complex, and a complete discussion is outside of the scope of this text. However, there are some common issues for consideration.

Timely billing: Providers are better about timely delivery of medical care than timely billing. Most modern electronic medical record (EMR) systems provide the ability to designate a level of service at the time of the encounter, providing the documentation has been completed. Hospital documentation should be completed on the day of service.

Accurate coding: Neurologic coding is complicated, and many capable coders are not facile at the fine points of neurologic coding. Specialty coding expertise is helpful especially for neurology and neurosurgery.

Records and audits: Audits are performed routinely by larger clinics and hospitals to determine quality and completeness of documentation and charge management. Feedback to the providers to correct persistent deficiencies in documentation is essential. In addition, the providers should have the ability to see the performance data regarding the billing performed on their behalf.

METRICS

Quality measures and other metrics for hospital neurology practice present a moving target. The American Academy of Neurology has a series of quality measures for various neurologic disorders. These are available online.[1]

Most of the guidelines pertain to outpatient neurology. However, there are guidelines for some inpatient neurology practice, especially stroke.

In these days of constant push to improve medical care, uneven quality persists. The source of this unevenness is multifaceted and includes:

- Failure to learn new advances in best practices
- Anchoring in the old practice patterns
- Lack of team involvement in practice
- For some providers, high patient volumes

Improved quality and fewer mistakes will help to reduce the casualties that the Institute of Medicine (IOM) reports we are causing in our medical care.

RISK MANAGEMENT

Neurology generally has a relatively low risk of malpractice liability, but this risk can be enhanced with hospital practice.

Case load: Recent changes in hospital practice, including stroke services, have increased the inpatient and ED case load for neurologists. This needs to be controlled. This is accomplished by considering locums, diversion, and telemedicine, in addition to ongoing recruiting.

Shift duration should be controlled. Most medicine hospitalists limit shifts to 12 hours, and, preferably, this should be standard for hospital neurologists.

Continuity of care reduces risk of litigation. As part of hospital practice, where patients are seen on successive days by different providers robust hand-off procedures are essential.

FUTURE DIRECTIONS

Predicting future trends in hospital neurology practice is complicated by uncertainties in the political landscape, regulatory pressures, business pressures from insurers, and evolution in medical education. We expect the trend will continue to have increasing numbers of hospital physicians of all types, including neurology.

An increasing proportion of hospitals are using co-management agreements or call-pay arrangements rather than the traditional obligatory call schedules. This is partly promoted by the need to incentivize providers to meet mandated metrics.

Hospital-at-home has been studied, and there is no evidence that this model is associated with poorer outcomes.[2] But there is no evidence that hospital-at-home for early discharges reduces costs or improves outcomes.[3]

SECTION II
APPROACH TO NEUROLOGIC PROBLEMS

SECTION CONTENTS

4 Motor and Sensory Disturbance
5 Mental Status Change
6 Visual Change
7 Language and Hearing Deficits
8 Cranial Neuropathies
9 Dizziness, Vertigo, and Imbalance
10 Pain and Headache

4 Motor and Sensory Disturbance

E. Lee Murray, MD and
Veda V. Vedanarayanan, MD, FRCPC

CHAPTER CONTENTS

- Overview
- Motor Disturbance
  - Types
  - Physiologic Localization
  - Anatomic Localization
- Sensory Disturbance
  - Types
  - Localization
  - Disorders with Specific Sensory Disturbances
- Localization of Motor and Sensory Disturbance
- Clinical Scenarios in Hospital Neurology
  - Stroke Syndromes
  - Movement Disorders
  - Seizures
  - Demyelinating Diseases
  - Neuromuscular Disorders
  - Psychiatric Disorders
- Approach to Diagnosis of Motor and Sensory Disturbance
  - Evaluation in the Emergency Department
  - Evaluation in the Intensive Care Units
  - Anesthetic Complications from Neuromuscular Disorders
  - Patients with Tumors and Organ Transplantation
  - Patients with Rheumatologic disorders
  - Patients with Diabetes Mellitus
  - Patients with Infectious Diseases

OVERVIEW

This section discusses approach to localization and diagnoses, and this chapter focuses on motor and sensory disturbances.

MOTOR DISTURBANCE

The differential diagnosis for weakness can by quite broad. Narrowing the differential diagnosis starts with a complete history and determining the onset, distribution, and course of the weakness. The examination then determines the type of motor disorder.

Types

Motor disorders can be broadly divided into the following categories:

- Weakness
- Incoordination
- Stiffness
- Abnormal movements

Weakness has the broadest potential localization. Corticospinal tract involvement is most common. Other localizations include basal ganglia, motor nerve, neuromuscular junction, and muscle.

Incoordination also has a broad potential localization. Corticospinal tract, basal ganglia, and cerebellar lesions are most common, although incoordination can occasionally be manifest by other lesions: for example, neuropathy can produce poorly coordinated movements especially if fairly acute or subacute (e.g., acute inflammatory demyelinating polyneuropathy [AIDP]).

Stiffness can be pyramidal or extrapyramidal. Corticospinal tract dysfunction produces flaccidity acutely but ultimately spasticity. Extrapyramidal conditions such as parkinsonism produces stiffness that is clinically distinct from corticospinal dysfunction.

Abnormal movements run the gamut from tremor to seizure. Determining the type of abnormal movement further localizes the lesion.

Physiologic Localization

Corticospinal lesions produce flaccid weakness initially but ultimately produce spasticity. Reflexes are eventually enhanced, although they will not be acutely. Plantar responses are often extensor immediately on clinical presentation in the ED.

Extrapyramidal lesions can produce increased tone with Parkinsonism and a host of related disorders.

Cerebellar lesions produce incoordination rather than weakness although tone may be reduced.

Motor nerve lesions produce weakness with features dependent on localization:

- *Upper motoneuron* lesions produce brisk reflexes, clonus, extensor plantar responses, bowel/bladder compromise, and spasticity.
- *Lower motoneuron* lesions can produce flaccid weakness, depressed or absent reflexes, and prominent muscle atrophy.

Neuromuscular junction lesions produce weakness and fatigue with no sensory symptoms. Reflexes are normal or reduced, depending on the severity of the weakness.

Muscle lesions produce weakness with reduced tone. Reflexes are normal or reduced depending on severity.

Anatomic Localization

Generalized motor disturbance has a broad differential diagnosis. In this case, differentiation between corticospinal, motor nerve, extrapyramidal, muscle, or neuromuscular junction narrows the diagnosis substantially. Few focal lesions produce generalized motor disturbance, although multifocal lesions commonly do.

Focal motor disturbance has a narrower differential diagnosis, although some disorders that produce generalized deficits can initially present with focal findings (e.g., parkinsonism or amyotrophic lateral sclerosis [ALS]).

SENSORY DISTURBANCE

Sensory disturbances can be more vague and subjective than motor disturbance.

Types

Sensory loss is sometimes referred to as *numbness,* although there are varying lay meanings for this term; some patients use numbness to mean abnormal sensation, pain, or even weakness.

Abnormal sensation is distortion of sensory input. Among these are *paresthesias* (abnormal spontaneous sensation) and *dysesthesias* (unpleasant sensation to a non-painful stimulus). These are most commonly due to damage to the peripheral nerves. However, they can be due to lesions in the spinal cord or brain.

Neuropathic pain is produced by abnormal discharge in nociceptive and non-nociceptive afferents that is interpreted as painful. These manifestations can include *hyperesthesia* (enhanced sensory experience that can be perceived as discomfort) and *hyperpathia* (enhanced pain experience). Almost any cause of peripheral nerve damage can produce neuropathic pain.

Sensory ataxia is produced by abnormal sensory input. It can resemble cerebellar ataxia but without other cerebellar signs and with marked exacerbation with eyes closed (i.e., positive Romberg).

Localization

Generalized sensory disturbance is most commonly due to lesions in the peripheral nerves. Polyneuropathy is most common.

Focal sensory disturbance can be due to a lesion at any level. Specifics of the deficits and correlation with motor and reflexes abnormalities narrows the localization (see Table 4.1).[1]

Table 4.1 Localization of sensory deficits

Abnormality	Features	Lesion	Potential cause
Distal sensory deficit	Sensory loss with or without pain distal on the legs; arms may be affected	Peripheral nerve	Peripheral neuropathy
Proximal sensory deficit	Sensory loss on trunk, without limb symptoms	Neuropathy with predominantly proximal involvement	Porphyria, diabetes, plexopathies
Dermatomal distribution of pain and/or sensory loss	Pain and/or sensory loss in the distribution of a single nerve root	Nerve root	Radiculopathy due to disc, osteophyte, tumor, herpes zoster
Single-limb sensory deficit	Loss of sensation on one limb that spans neural and dermatomal distributions	Plexus or multiple single nerves	Autoimmune plexitis, hematoma, tumor
Hemisensory deficit	Loss of sensation on one side of body. May be associated with pain.	Thalamus, cerebral cortex, or projections. Brainstem lesion, spinal cord lesion. Lower lesions do not involve face	Infarction, hemorrhage, demyelinating disease, tumor, infection
Crossed sensory deficit: ipsilateral facial and contralateral body	Pain and temperature disturbance of the ipsilateral face and contralateral body.	Lesions of uncrossed trigeminal fibers and crossed spinothalamic fibers	Lateral medullary syndrome
Pain/temperature vs vibration/proprioception deficits on opposite sides	Unilateral loss of pain and temperature sensation and contralateral loss of vibration and proprioception sensation.	Spinal cord lesion ipsilateral to vibration and proprioception deficit and contralateral to pain and temperature deficit	Disc protrusion, spinal stenosis, intra-spinal tumor, transverse myelitis; intraparenchymal lesions are more likely to produce dissociated sensory loss.
Dissociated suspended sensory deficit	Loss of pain and temperature sensation on one or both sides, with normal sensation above and below	Intramedullary lesion of cervical or thoracic spinal cord	Syrinx, chiari malformation, hydromyelia, central spinal cord tumor, or hemorrhage
Sacral sparing	Preservation of perianal sensation, with impaired sensation in legs and trunk	Lesion of the cord, with mainly central involvement sparing peripherally located sacral ascending fibers	Cord trauma, intrinsic tumors of the cord

Modified From Misulis KE and Murray EL Table 30.4 from Chapter 30 Sensory Abnormalities of the Limbs, Trunk, and Face, from Bradley's Neurology in Clinical Practice, Daroff RB, Jankovic J, Mazziotta JC, Pomeroy SL. Eds. Elsevier 2015

Select disorders with sensory manifestations are described here, and the details of these diagnoses are also found in multiple subsequent chapters. Most of these disorders have motor deficits not discussed here, but some of the disorders are discussed in detail in Chapter 21.

- *AIDP* produces dysesthesias and paresthesias with areflexia early in the course.
- *Sensory neuropathy* is often *sensorimotor neuropathy* with burning pain and superimposed dysesthesias and paresthesias. Reflexes are suppressed.
- *Carpal tunnel syndrome* produces numbness on the thumb, index, and middle fingers without involvement of ulnar and radial distributions.
- *Ulnar neuropathy* produces loss of sensation on the 4th and 5th digits.
- *Syringomyelia* produces a cape-like distribution of loss of pain and temperature with suspended sensory loss.
- *Thalamic infarction* produces an acute onset of unilateral sensory loss and sensory ataxia.
- *Thalamic pain syndrome* produces unilateral burning dysesthetic pain, especially distally on the limbs.
- *Trigeminal neuralgia* produces paroxysms of lancinating, electric shock-like pain in the face.

LOCALIZATION OF MOTOR AND SENSORY DISTURBANCE

Lesions at different levels of the neuraxis can be localized through correlation with the disturbances. Details of localization and diagnosis are addressed well in the recent release of Brazis, Masdeu, and Biller; *Localization in Clinical Neurology*. Comprehensive discussion of stroke syndromes is in the book by Caplan and van Gijn; *Stroke Syndromes*. Both of these are available as Kindle and iBook ebooks.

Cortical lesions produce motor and sensory loss in the portion of the homunculus encompassing the defect. Most common are hand and face, especially with middle cerebral artery (MCA) infarctions. Anterior cerebral artery (ACA) infarctions produce foot and leg deficits.

Internal capsule lesions can produce contralateral motor and/or sensory deficits. Head-to-toe deficit suggest an internal capsule lesion rather than a cortical lesion.

Basal ganglia lesions can produce a wide variety of symptoms but among these can be contralateral weakness and incoordination.

Thalamic lesions produce contralateral sensory loss. Hemisensory loss without weakness suggests a thalamic lesion.

Brainstem lesions produce bilateral weakness that is often asymmetric. In addition, cranial nerve deficits are common. Crossed findings suggest brainstem lesions, with motor involvement on one side and sensory on the other, sensory involvement of the face on one side and body on the other, or cranial nerve deficits on one side and hemiparesis on the other.

Spinal cord lesions (complete) produce loss of sensation and motor function below the level of the lesion, although the level may be somewhat different on the two sides.

Spinal cord lesions (partial but bilateral) produce loss of motor and sensory function below the lesion, which is often incomplete and asymmetric. The levels of clinical involvement may be quite different between the two sides.

Spinal hemisection (Brown-Sequard) produces loss of vibration and proprioception ipsilateral to the lesion and loss of pain and temperature contralateral to the lesion.

Motoneuron lesions produce weakness without sensory findings. Lesions predominately of the upper motoneuron (e.g., primary lateral sclerosis) produce weakness with spasticity, increased reflexes, and upgoing plantar responses in the post-acute phase. Lesions of the lower motoneuron (e.g., progressive muscular atrophy) produce weakness without sensory loss and without hyperreflexia or upgoing toes. Lesion of both the upper and lower motoneuron (e.g., ALS) produces both profiles of deficits.

Nerve root lesions produce motor and sensory deficits that follow a dermatomal distribution. Generally, motor localization is easier than sensory localization.

Plexus lesions produce motor and sensory deficits in more than one nerve root distribution, but they are generally contiguous, suggesting the plexus localization.

Peripheral nerve lesions produce motor and sensory deficits in individual nerve distributions. Motor and sensory deficits with peripheral nerve lesions are more congruent than with lesions of the plexus or spinal cord.

CLINICAL SCENARIOS IN HOSPITAL NEUROLOGY

Some of the most common and most important clinical scenarios encountered in hospital neurology practice with their motor, sensory, and associated findings are presented here.

Stroke Syndromes

Left MCA infarction: Right hemiparesis affecting face and arm more than leg. Sensory loss in the same distribution. If the left hemisphere is dominant, aphasia develops to a variable extent. Infarction of the MCA anterior division produces expressive aphasia and usually preservation of visual fields. Isolated infarction of the MCA posterior division produces mainly receptive aphasia, and right hemianopia may be present. Combined anterior and posterior ischemia produces combined deficits.

Right MCA infarction: Left hemiparesis affecting face and arm more than leg. Sensory loss in the same distribution. If the right hemisphere is nondominant, there is often neglect of the left side. Left hemianopia may be present with involvement of the MCA posterior division.

Thalamic infarction: Contralateral sensory deficit encompassing the entire side with face, arm, and leg involvement. Motor systems are typically not affected.

Basal ganglia infarction: Contralateral weakness and incoordination. No cortical signs such as aphasia or neglect.

Internal capsule infarction: Contralateral motor and/or sensory deficits involving the entire side. Cortical signs are absent.

PCA infarction: Contralateral hemianopia is typical. Confusion and memory deficit is common.

Brainstem infarction: Broad spectrum of disorders related to ischemia in the distribution of the vertebrobasilar system including branches. Some of the most important are:

- LATERAL MEDULLARY SYNDROME: Usually posterior inferior cerebellar artery or vertebral occlusion. Ipsilateral limb ataxia, sensory loss of the face. Contralateral loss of pain and temperature sensation. Associated with nausea, dysphagia, and hoarse voice.

- LOCKED-IN SYNDROME: Usually basilar artery or branch occlusion. Quadriplegia with corticospinal tract signs, impaired horizontal eye movements – relative preservation of vertical eye movements which may be the only way to communicate with the patient. These patients are often initially considered to be in coma until careful neuro exam is performed.
- BASILAR THROMBOSIS: Basilar artery occlusion. Coma with corticospinal tract signs. Usually preceeded by symptoms and signs of brainstem ischemia including dysarthria, dysphagia, and especially varying combinations of extremity and bulbar motor deficits. Visual changes and ultimately congnitive decline are seen.

Movement Disorders

Parkinsonism: Rigidity, bradykinesia, and resting tremor. Associated with shuffling gait, stopped posture, and propensity to forward falls.

Hemiballismus: Flinging movements on one side are usually due to infarction of the subthalamic nucleus. Nonketotic hyperglycemia and some medications can also cause this.

Essential tremor: Tremor of hands evoked by action or posture.

Enhanced physiologic tremor: Exaggeration of normal fine tremor seen with arms and fingers extended.

Seizures

Seizures: Shaking; most commonly focal or generalized depending on the type of seizure. Motor deficit can follow the seizure and produce temporary paresis or paralysis (Todd's paralysis).

Ictal paralysis: Rare paralysis without positive motor activity preceding the weakness.

Demyelinating Diseases

Multiple sclerosis (MS): Weakness that can be monoparesis, hemiparesis, or paraparesis, or cranial nerve deficit of subacute onset. Often has findings of more than one lesion.

Neuromyelitis optica (NMO): Myelopathy that can resemble spinal cord involvement of MS but is associated with visual involvement.

Neuromuscular Disorders

AIDP, critical illness neuromyopathy (CIN), and myasthenia gravis (MG) are the most common neuromuscular disorders encountered in hospital neurology practice. Chronic inflammatory demyelinating polyneuropathy (CIDP) is less common but encountered in hospital practice. Rare neuromuscular conditions are not discussed.

- *AIDP* produces a rapid progression of weakness and sensory change often with neuropathic pain. Areflexia.

- *CIDP* presents with progressive weakness and sensory deficit over months.
- *MG* presents with progressive weakness and fatigue that is worse with activity and improves with rest. Ocular muscles are commonly affected, producing diplopia and ptosis.
- *ALS* presents with progressive weakness with upper and lower motoneuron signs. No sensory findings.
- *CIN* produces weakness in patients in the ICU especially with sepsis or other prolonged illness. Hypotonia and hyporeflexia are common.
- *Inflammatory myopathies* such as polymyositis and dermatomyositis, produce progressive weakness that affects predominately proximal muscles.
- *Toxic myopathies* can present with generalized weakness that is typically symmetrical. Alcoholic myopathy is often accompanied by muscle cramps and muscle tenderness and can lead to rhabdomyolysis and hypokalemia.
- *Periodic paralysis* is a rare group of muscle diseases that can lead to significant situational weakness without respiratory compromise.
- *Botulism* produces descending paralysis with cranial nerve involvement.
- *Tick paralysis* produces progressive paralysis that can resemble AIDP, but there are minimal or no sensory symptoms.
- *Organophosphate poisoning* usually presents with symptoms of cholinergic excess including miosis, bradycardia, lacrimation, urination, emesis, salivation, bronchorrhea, bronchospasm, and generalized weakness.
- *West Nile virus (WNV)* can produce a rapid onset of flaccid paralysis in conjunction with encephalopathy.
- *Multifocal motor neuropathy (MMN)* produces progressive weakness without sensory symptoms.

Psychiatric Disorders

Psychogenic weakness is suspected with motor and often sensory deficit associated with no demonstrable lesion in the motor and sensory systems. Clues to diagnosis can be inconsistency and improbability of localization.

APPROACH TO DIAGNOSIS OF MOTOR AND SENSORY DISORDERS
Evaluation in the Emergency Department

Rapidly progressing muscle weakness suggests consideration of AIDP, MG, and, less often, ALS. Airway, breathing, and circulation are quickly evaluated and addressed. Respiratory and bulbar muscle weakness may require intubation and mechanical ventilation.

Measurement of bedside pulmonary function, forced vital capacity (FVC), and negative inspiratory force (NIF) is helpful in assessing the severity of respiratory compromise.

AIDP is the most common presentation in the ED of severe and generalized weakness with paresthesias of hands, feet, and face, accompanied by areflexia.

Tick paralysis presents similarly to AIDP but tends to occur most commonly in children and has no sensory symptoms.

MG may present in respiratory and bulbar crisis with severe weakness. Ptosis, oculomotor muscle weakness, fatigable weakness, and preserved sensation and tendon reflexes suggest the diagnosis.

Myopathies including inflammatory myopathies and *muscular dystrophies* usually do not present to the ED for first diagnosis. However, the hospital neurologist will see patients with advanced disease who decompensate, thus precipitating ED visit.

Metabolic disorders causing severe weakness in the ED include hypokalemia or hypophosphatemia. These patients may have absent tendon reflexes.

Infectious diseases may present with muscle weakness including especially WNV. Clinical features of encephalitis may be present.

Evaluation in the Intensive Care Unit

Muscle weakness is an important cause for prolonged stay in ICU, long after the primary cause for ICU admission has resolved. Important causes are iatrogenic or from development of an independent neuromuscular disease. In addition, a previously stable neuromuscular disease can be made worse by illness or concurrent medications.

Undiagnosed neuromuscular diseases that can be uncovered by critical illness include:

- Myasthenia gravis
- Myotonic muscular dystrophy
- Mitochondrial disorder
- Acid maltase deficiency (adult form)
- Amyotropic lateral sclerosis

CIN is generalized muscle weakness that can develop in patients with serious illness. Development of weakness is more likely with sepsis, treatment with multiple medications including corticosteroids, and/or neuromuscular blocking agents, and in those with multiorgan failure. Diagnosis can be hampered by coexistent encephalopathy, which makes examination difficult. This is discussed in Chapter 21.

Polyneuropathy may occur in critically ill patients and usually is mild and seldom a cause for weakness in the muscles of respiration The polyneuropathy is due to axonal injury and probably related to nutritional deficiency, toxicities from medications used, organ failures, and effects of cytokines and inflammatory mediators.

Neuromuscular blockade due to pharmacologic agents may be prolonged, especially with renal and/or hepatic failure. Even metabolites of some of these agents have neuromuscular junction (NMJ)-blocking properties.

Anesthetic Complications from Neuromuscular Disorders

Malignant hyperthermia: This is a pharmacologic adverse effect characterized by hyperpyrexia, rigidity, rhabdomyolysis, and myoglobinuria. Mortality risk is 10–30%. The following patients have increased risk:

- Central core myopathy
- HyperCKemia and cramps

- Dystrophin disorder (Becker muscular dystrophy, Duchenne muscular dystrophy, symptomatic female carriers)

Patients with *myotonia congenita* and other myotonic disorders may experience severe trismus and muscle rigidity on exposure to short-acting neuromuscular blocking agents, such as succinylcholine.

Myotonic dystrophy patients are at higher risk for respiratory failure and difficult extubation after exposure to sedating and anesthetic agents.

MG patients should be treated with neuromuscular blocking agents only with caution. They are more likely to experience prolonged weakness.

Mitochondrial disorder patients need careful monitoring of oxygenation during procedures. Lactated Ringer's solution should be avoided and blood glucose monitored.

Patients with Tumors and Organ Transplantation

Lambert Eaton myasthenic syndrome, cholinergic neuropathy, and *sensory ganglionopathy* can be seen with small-cell lung carcinoma.

Necrotizing myopathy causing rapid severe proximal weakness is a rare paraneoplastic presentation seen most often with small-cell lung carcinoma.

Demyelinating polyneuropathy is an uncommon complication seen in patients with lymphoid malignancy and in patients who have had bone marrow transplantation.

Inflammatory myopathy is a rare complication in patients who have undergone bone marrow transplantation.

Progressive polyneuropathy from axonal damage occurs as a side effect of several chemotherapeutic agents, especially vincristine and paclitaxel.

Patients with Rheumatological Disorders

Muscle weakness from myositis occurs in systemic lupus erythematosus, mixed connective tissue disorders, and dermatomyositis.

Mononeuritis multiplex comprises multiple mononeuropathies. This can occur with vasculitis, as in polyarteritis nodosa, Wegener's granulomatosis, sarcoidosis, or isolated peripheral nerve vasculitis.

Small-fiber polyneuropathy is seen most commonly with diabetes but also with vasculitis and Sjögren syndrome.

Dermatomyositis is an autoimmune myopathy. In 20–30% of patients, it is a paraneoplastic syndrome.

Demyelinating neuropathy can occur from biological agents used for a variety of rheumatologic disorders.[2]

Patients with Diabetes Mellitus

Multiple causes of motor and sensory deficit can occur from diabetes mellitus (DM):

- *Predominantly sensory polyneuropathy* is the most frequent neuropathic complication.
- *Sensorimotor polyneuropathy* is the next most frequent presentation.

- *Small-fiber neuropathy* with prominent pain occurs in DM and can precede the clinical diagnosis of DM. This is often associated with autonomic symptoms, orthostatic hypotension, and can be associated with arrhythmia.
- *Focal neuropathies* in upper and lower limbs are common. Susceptibility to compressive neuropathies is increased in patients with DM.
- *Cranial neuropathies* affecting CN 3, 4, 6, and 7 can occur as complication of DM.
- *Diabetic amyotrophy* is a proximal plexopathy seen in patients with DM, especially those with poor diabetic control.

Patients with Infectious Diseases

Human immunodeficiency virus (HIV) infection is associated with a variety of neuromuscular disorders:

- Acute demyelinating polyneuropathy is seen in some patients and usually occurs when seroconversion is taking place. Features are similar to AIDP and is treated with intravenous immunoglobulin (IVIg).
- Small-fiber neuropathy is sometimes seen in patients with HIV.

Herpes viruses (cytomegalovirus [CMV], Epstein-Barr virus [EBV], and varicella zoster virus [VZV]) can cause lumbosacral radiculoplexitis; this is a rapidly developing disorder with progressive asymmetric lower limb weakness with pain and sensory loss. Bladder and bowel incontinence are common.

Arboviruses including WNV and Zika virus can be associated with AIDP as well as with acute disseminated encephalomyelitis (ADEM) or MS.

5 Mental Status Change

Karl E. Misulis, MD, PhD and
E. Lee Murray, MD

CHAPTER CONTENTS

- Overview
- Dementia
  - Degenerative Dementias
  - Nondegenerative Dementias
  - Infectious Dementias
  - Differential Diagnosis
- Confusional State
  - Differential Diagnosis
- Coma
  - Differential Diagnosis
  - Etiology of Coma
- Transient Loss of Consciousness
  - Differential Diagnosis of TLOC
  - Diagnostic Studies
  - Role of the Neurologist

OVERVIEW

Disorders of mental status are among the most common reasons for neurologic consultation, second only to stroke in most institutions. Mental status change may be the reason for admission, or it may develop during hospitalization. The terminology used to describe these states varies, and there is some overlap in terms:

- *Confusional state* is a disturbance of memory and other cognitive functions. Whereas *dementia* is characterized by confusion, the term *confusional state* generally refers to a more acute or subacute state.
- *Dementia* is progressive disturbance of cognitive function that can include memory, reasoning, language, and/or personality.
- *Delirium* is acute to subacute cognitive disturbance with neuropsychiatric manifestations, which may be hyperactive or hypoactive. This can be predisposed by advanced age, dementia, or sensory deprivation.
- *Encephalopathy* is cognitive disturbance that is usually acute to subacute. This term presumes an organic cause. Delirium can be a manifestation.

- *Amnesia* is loss of memory, which can be isolated or a component of a broader cognitive disturbance.
- *Lethargy* is decrease in response, drowsiness, and apathy.
- *Persistent vegetative state* is unawareness of self or the environment with relative preservation of brainstem function.
- *Coma* is unresponsiveness with no voluntary movement or behavior.
- *Brain death* is irreversible cessation of all brain functions. There are established clinical criteria for diagnosis (see Chapter 15).

Concerning hospitalized patients, studies have shown:

- Patients who develop altered mental status in the hospital have an increased likelihood of poor outcome and post-discharge dependence.[1]
- Patients who have cognitive deficits prior to hospitalization have a higher likelihood of complications.
- Patients with advanced age have a high incidence of cognitive impairment not recognized by providers.[2]
- Patients with cognitive deterioration are much more likely to die or be placed in a nursing home.

The distinction between *delirium* and *encephalopathy* is blurred. Many of us consider delirium to be a state of confusion with hyperactivity and perceptual difficulty, whereas encephalopathy refers to the disordered cognitive state with an organic basis, although it has broader range of semantic use.

DEMENTIA

Dementia is progressive cognitive decline that affects up to 10% of patients over the age of 65. Dementia is discussed in more depth in Chapter 18.

Most patients with dementia have a degenerative cause, with the largest proportion having Alzheimer's disease (AD). Other important degenerative dementias include Parkinson disease with dementia (PDD), dementia with Lewy bodies (DLB), and frontotemporal dementia (FTD). Nondegenerative dementias include vascular dementia (VaD), normal pressure hydrocephalus (NPH), and chronic infections.

DLB and PDD are sometimes considered as a single entity since there are similarities in presentation, evaluation, and management.

Degenerative Dementias

Alzheimer's disease (AD): This presents as progressive dementia with relative sparing of other functions early in the course. Diagnosis is suspected by absence of focal signs, behavior, language, or movement deficits. Neuropsych testing can show a specific pattern of deficit. Genetic testing and brain positron emission tomography (PET) are not very useful for nonresearch practice.

Frontotemporal dementia (FTD): This is a group of disorders with dementia associated with behavioral and/or language deficits early in the course. Magnetic resonance imaging (MRI) and computed tomography (CT) may show atrophy, particularly in frontal and temporal regions. Neuropsych testing is supportive. Genetic analysis may be helpful in cases with suspected family history.

Pick disease: This is essentially frontotemporal dementia with pathological findings of Pick bodies. FTD is the preferred term.

Corticobasal degeneration: This presents with Parkinson-like symptoms associated with corticospinal signs. Unilateral arm clumsiness; apraxia, often with rigidity; and bradykinesia are common. Alien-hand syndrome suggests this disorder. Dementia can occur but does not in all patients.

Parkinson's disease with dementia: This is defined as Parkinsonism with dementia developing late in the course. Classically, for this diagnosis, the movement disorder precedes the dementia by at least a year.

Lewy body dementia: This is dementia and behavioral abnormalities with Parkinsonism, where the dementia develops either before or within 1 year of onset of motor symptoms.

Progressive supranuclear palsy (PSP): This is a combination of supranuclear ophthalmoplegia, pseudobulbar palsy, and axial dystonia. Stiffness and slowness can suggest parkinsonism initially. Dementia develops in many but is overshadowed by the motor symptoms.

Huntington disease: This presents with psychiatric symptoms, chorea, and ultimately dementia. Inheritance is autosomal dominant. Diagnosis is suspected by family history and early psychiatric symptoms before motor symptoms develop

Nondegenerative Dementias

Vascular dementia: Presents with dementia with history or signs of stroke or significant vascular risk factors. Cognitive disturbance has an onset which is often abrupt or stepwise. May develop with one or more multiple vascular events, ischemic or hemorrhagic (e.g., amyloid angiopathy).

Normal pressure hydrocephalus (NPH): The triad of dementia, ataxia, and urinary incontinence is often incomplete. Diagnosis is suspected when CT or MRI shows ventricles larger than expected from cortical atrophy.

B$_{12}$ deficiency: Dementia may develop with associated signs of neuropathy or myelopathy.

Hypothyroidism: Confusion is common but usually subacute in onset and seldom confused with degenerative dementia.

Korsakoff psychosis: This presents with marked memory deficit with behavioral change. Occurrence is usually in the setting of previous Wernicke encephalopathy from ethanol.

Infectious Dementias

Creutzfeldt-Jakob disease (CJD): Diagnosis is suspected with dementia that progresses rapidly, often with psychotic features, and especially with motor manifestations of myoclonus, rigidity, and/or cerebellar ataxia. Familial or sporadic.

Neurosyphilis: Presents with dementia, myoclonus, psychiatric disturbance, and often Argyll-Robertson pupils.

HIV–AIDS dementia: Presentation is with subacute or chronic progression of dementia with motor manifestations including ataxia, tremor, corticospinal tract signs, and/or signs of myelopathy.

Differential Diagnosis

The most common causes of dementia, in order, are: *Alzheimer's disease, vascular dementia*, and *frontotemporal dementia*. The other most common causes seen in practice are *Parkinson disease with dementia* and *Lewy body dementia. Corticobasal degeneration* is difficult to diagnose early in the course. The diagnosis is suspected when the patient presents later with parkinsonism and corticospinal signs (see Figure 5.1).

Frontotemporal dementia has subtypes, summarized as follows:

- *Behavioral form of frontotemporal dementia*: Early behavioral issues are often evident before a dementia, including disinhibition, apathy, and difficulty with interpersonal skills.
- *Primary progressive aphasia*: Language defect with expression affected out of proportion to reception. Dementia is evident later.
- *Semantic dementia*: Fluent aphasia, but the semantic defect gives prominent anomia. Reception is preserved initially.

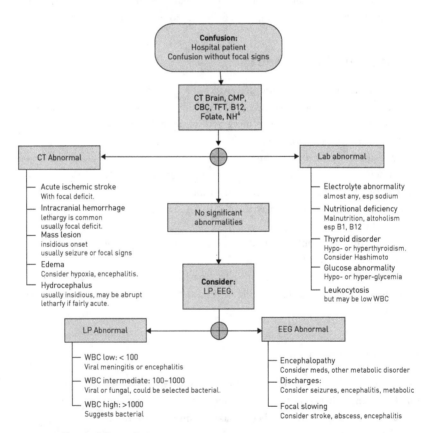

FIGURE 5.1 Flowchart for confusion

CONFUSIONAL STATE

Confusional state often presents with a clinical picture of delirium and often with a history of pre-existing cognitive disturbance. Some of these patients have dementia, either diagnosed or undiagnosed. Delirium is distinct from dementia but is frequently coexistent. Delirium is associated with a disturbance of cognition and perception. Delirium can be hyperactive or hypoactive.[3] Most cases are multifactorial.

Risk factors for hospital delirium include:

- Advanced age
- Pre-existing dementia
- Visual and/or hearing deficits
- Malnutrition
- Alcoholism
- Reduced functional status prior to the hospitalization[4,5]

Hospital delirium is predisposed by situational factors including:

- ICU care
- Fever and/or known infection
- Electrolyte/metabolic disturbance
- Sedative or analgesic medications
- Length of hospital stay
- Severity of illness
- Urinary catheterization

Differential Diagnosis

Differential diagnosis of the confusional state is broad, but among the most common disorders in hospitalized patients are:

Medications: Sedation or agitation can be caused by medications, from especially analgesics, sedative/hypnotics, anticholinergics, some antibiotics (e.g., cefepime).

Hospital encephalopathy: Combination of illness, medications, sleep deprivation, unfamiliarity can result in confusion, agitation, and psychosis. Patients at greatest risk are those with advanced age, multiple medical problems, and pre-hospital cognitive difficulty.

Renal insufficiency: Acute renal failure or exacerbation of chronic renal insufficiency can cause confusion, lethargy, myoclonus, and seizures. Renal failure also predisposes to central nervous system (CNS) vascular disease and infection.

Hepatic insufficiency: Patients present with encephalopathy often with asterixis or myoclonus, and may have seizures. Patients at risk for hepatic encephalopathy are also at risk for Wernicke encephalopathy.

Hypothyroidism: This condition may become evident during concurrent illness. Hashimoto encephalopathy should be considered in hospitalized patients with unexplained confusion; these patients may be euthyroid.

Sleep deprivation: This can produce hospital encephalopathy or psychosis and also can be responsible for pre-hospital cognitive changes. Among the causes considered should be sleep apnea.

Transient global amnesia: This presents as transient short-term memory loss without other deficit; the isolated memory deficit is the clue to diagnosis.

COMA

Coma is a state of unconsciousness where there are no cognitive responses. Stimuli evoke only reflex or primitive responses and not purposeful movements signifying comprehension.

Coma has a broad list of potential etiologies but, in this chapter, the differential diagnosis is the focus.

Differential Diagnosis

Locked-in syndrome: Devastating damage to the caudal brainstem can produce virtual unresponsiveness. Preserved consciousness may only be detected by testing for voluntary eye movements; there are many causes but vascular is most common.

Vegetative state including persistent vegetative state: Severe cerebral damage from a variety of causes (usually trauma or hypoxia) presents with no conscious response, but with responses that signify preserved brainstem function. Eyes are often open and move, but not in response to verbal commands. *Persistent* signifies sustained duration, usually of at least 1–3 months.

Neuromuscular blockade: Unresponsiveness is due to neuromuscular blockade usually from paralytics given in surgery or in the ICU setting. Botulism produces weakness and loss of pupillary response but not usually to the point of appearing to be in coma.

Psychogenic unresponsiveness: This presents with absence of response associated with typical signs of preserved consciousness on detailed exam and electroencephalogram (EEG). No organic pathology is identified.

Etiology of Coma

The etiology of coma is obvious in most cases, but there are some important diagnoses to consider when the cause is not certain.

Trauma: Injuries can produce coma by direct effects of the mechanical injury, resultant edema, contusions, and/or hemorrhage.

Cerebral ischemia: Multifocal ischemia with proximal emboli or single large infarcts with edema, shift, and contralateral compression can cause coma.

Brainstem ischemia: Massive brainstem stroke can produce coma with brain activity not detectable on physical exam.

Cerebral hemorrhage: Single large hemorrhage or multiple smaller hemorrhages can produce unresponsiveness without evident focal signs.

Delayed clearance of sedatives: Patients who are post-op or have had prolonged ICU stay on sedatives can have reduced clearance, especially with renal or hepatic insufficiency. Patients with high body mass index (BMI) may have long-term storage of selected meds, thereby increasing the duration of a medication-induced encephalopathy. Baclofen overdose can mimic brain death.[6]

CNS infection: Encephalitis with direct neuronal damage and/or edema giving secondary damage can cause coma, as can meningitis with secondary vasculopathy.

Hypertensive encephalopathy: This condition can occasionally present as coma.

Intracranial catastrophes may be missed because of the presentation of coma without visible focal signs. We have seen more than a few patients with unresponsiveness presumed to be due to delayed clearance of anesthesia or metabolic encephalopathy who had intracranial catastrophes, especially in these days of avid use of antithrombotics, thrombolytics, and vascular interventions. Large focal brain lesions may not show focal neurological signs because of the global reduction in response.

TRANSIENT LOSS OF CONSCIOUSNESS

Transient loss of consciousness (TLOC) has numerous causes. Syncope is TLOC due to a fall in the perfusion pressure of the brain. Therefore, the focus of this chapter is beyond the usual discussion of syncope and includes other causes of TLOC. When a patient is identified as having true syncope, the most common causes of the cerebral hypoperfusion are orthostatic hypotension, neurocardiogenic syncope, and arrhythmia.

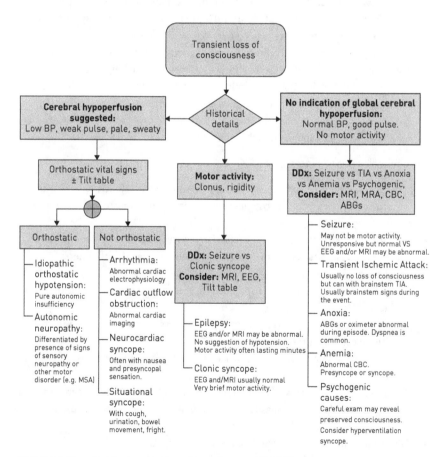

FIGURE 5.2 Flowchart for transient loss of consciousness (TLOC)

TLOC not related to cerebral hypoperfusion can be psychogenic, but this is likely overdiagnosed because long-term cardiac monitoring may document significant arrhythmias in some of these patients.[7]

The role of the hospital neurologist is to assist in determining the cause. While we might occasionally be inundated with consultations for syncope, a neurological consultation is far cheaper than most of our diagnostic tests.

Differential Diagnosis of TLOC

Some of the most important syndromes and causes of TLOC are presented in the following list. Identification of associated features is essential to accurate diagnosis.[8–14]

Common causes of syncope:

- *Orthostatic hypotension*: Presyncope or syncope usually when standing, but not always; can be sitting
- *Neurocardiogenic syncope*: Presyncope from hypotension with a nonpositional trigger such as fright, pain, bowel movement
- *Cough syncope*: Syncope produced by coughing fits, often with COPD
- *Hyperventilation syncope*: Usually reported as shortness of breath.
- *Micturition syncope*: Syncope with urination, especially when standing
- *Arrhythmia*: A wide variety of rhythm disturbances can produce syncope; long-term ambulatory monitoring may be required for diagnosis.
- *Carotid sinus hypersensitivity*: Presyncope or syncope due to bradycardia and vasodilatation; precipitation by carotid stimulation may be noted historically.
- *Convulsive syncope*: Jerking or stiffening as part of the syncope; loss of consciousness occurs first, and motor activity is usually briefer than with seizure.
- *Psychogenic unresponsiveness*: Loss of response with appearance and posture suggesting wakefulness; inconsistencies on exam

Uncommon causes of syncope:

- *Seizure*: Episode of unconsciousness usually with motor activity, which could be misdiagnosed as convulsive syncope; seizure is usually longer and with greater postictal confusion.
- *Transient ischemic attack (TIA), particularly vertebrobasilar*: Episode of marked weakness and fall or unconsciousness; it is usually associated with other brainstem symptoms and signs.
- *Subarachnoid hemorrhage*: Syncope is often preceded and/or followed by severe headache.
- *Nonconvulsive seizure*: Episode of unresponsiveness without motor abnormality; repetitive electrocerebral discharge on EEG
- *Pulmonary embolism*: Rare cause of syncope, usually presents with dyspnea prior to the event.
- *Basilar invagination*: This and other craniocervical abnormalities can result in compromise of the vertebrobasilar circulation and produce syncope, usually with brainstem symptoms and signs.
- *Subclavian steal*: Syncope precipitated by arm exertion.
- *Catecholaminergic polymorphic ventricular tachycardia (CPVT)*: Genetic mutation affecting young patients; it produces syncope often provoked by exercise or emotional stress.

- *Cervical spondylosis*: Vertebral compression can produce brainstem ischemic changes including stroke or TIA but also syncope.

Orthostatic hypotension is the most common cause of syncope in the hospital setting, but not all hypotensive syncope occurs on standing; it can occur when sitting.[15]

TIA is a rare cause of TLOC, although a history of TIA is a risk factor for development of syncope from cardiac causes.[16] Limb-shaking TIAs can be associated with syncope, but this is very rare.[17] Carotid circulation ischemia as a cause for TLOC is rare and occurs only when there is significant carotid disease.[18]

Carotid sinus hypersensitivity (CSH) is often associated with historical clues such as provocation by turning of the head or with tight collars. Carotid sinus massage is strongly supportive of the diagnosis.

Convulsive syncope or *clonic syncope* is easy to confuse with seizure. Cerebral hypoperfusion can produce stiffening and/or shaking, myoclonus, and even automatisms or vocalizations.[19] EEG monitoring may be required to make the differentiation, but generally tongue-biting and postictal confusion favor seizure whereas urinary incontinence and head injury do not help with differentiation.

TLOC that is not syncope may be seizure or TIA. History and observation are usually the keys to this diagnosis. EEG between events is usually unremarkable even if the cause was seizure. MRI of the brain usually shows no acute abnormalities with TLOC of any cause. However, magnetic resonance angiography (MRA) or CT angiography (CTA) might show critical basilar stenosis.

Psychogenic TLOC is in the differential diagnosis of patients with unexplained TLOC. Diagnosis relies on examination during an episode, if at all possible. Elements of the events that suggest a psychogenic component include posture of someone in relaxed sleep (e.g., hands folded, legs crossed, mouth closed), resistance for manual eye opening, resistance to passive limb movement (e.g., forcing the arms by the side).

Diagnostic Studies

Laboratory studies for syncope are commonly overdone. Table 5.1 and accompanying flowchart show the approach to diagnosis of syncope based on clinical suspicion. Of course, all evaluations are individualized. The indicated evaluation depends on the clinical features of the episodes.

Carotid sinus massage is performed specifically to look for CSH. This should not be performed on patients with myocardial infarction, stroke, or TIA in the past 3 months, in patients with a history of known carotid stenosis or occlusion, in patients with ventricular arrhythmia, or in patients with previous adverse effects with the procedure. Carotid sinus massage can be performed by the following steps:

- Patient is supine with neck slightly extended for 5 minutes.
- Massage or pressure in the region of maximal carotid pulsation for 5–10 seconds, with 1 minute between massaging the two sides, starting on the right.
- Monitor BP and HR.
- Watch for any of the following:
  - Asystole for at least 3 seconds
  - Reduction in systolic BP of at least 50 mm Hg with or without reduction in HR

Table 5.1 Diagnostic studies for transient loss of consciousness (TLOC)

Study	Diagnostic value	Indications
Cardiovascular studies		
EKG	Cardiac arrhythmia	Almost all patients
Orthostatic vital signs	Orthostatic hypotension	Most patients, not just ones with a history of positional syncope.
Carotid sinus massage	Carotid sinus hypersensitivity	Suspicion from history—syncope with head turning or tight collars. Usually over age 40.
Transthoracic echocardiogram (TTE or Echo)	Structural heart disease or reduced cardiac function.	Cardiac cause suspected from history, exam, or EKG.
Transesophageal echocardiogram (TEE)	Structural heart disease, especially anatomic lesion, thrombus or cardiac defect.	Seldom indicated for TLOC.
Holter monitor	Arrhythmia	Suspected hypotension due to bradycardia or other arrhythmia not seen on EKG and acute monitoring.
Tilt table	Orthostatic hypotension	Positional hypotension especially if routine orthostatic vital signs are unrevealing.
Implanted loop recorder (ILR)	Arrhythmia	Unexplained TLOC despite aggressive cardiovascular evaluation.
Neurologic studies		
Carotid duplex sonography	Carotid occlusive disease. Often can identify antegrade flow in vertebrals.	Almost never indicated for TLOC. Perhaps if CTA or MRA cannot be done and vertebral flow needs to be assessed.
CT brain	Structural brain lesion—mass, infarct, hemorrhage.	If has unexplained TLOC or focal symptoms/signs. Headache after episode.
CT Angiogram head and neck	Arterial occlusive disease.	If focal neurologic symptoms/signs, or suspected vertebrobasilar ischemia.
MRI brain	Structural brain lesion, ischemia.	If TLOC is associated with focal symptoms or signs, seizure activity, or other suggestion of structural etiology.

Table 5.1 Continued

39

Chapter 5 Mental Status Change

Study	Diagnostic value	Indications
MR angiography (MRA)	Arterial occlusive disease	If cerebrovascular occlusive disease is suspected, especially basilar or bilateral carotid.
Electroencephalography (EEG)	Seizure.	Routine EEG is performed when clinical seizure activity is suspected. Extended-duration EEG is performed when seizure is suspected yet no ictal or interictal activity was observed on routine EEG.
EMG and NCS	Neuropathy	Especially when autonomic neuropathy is suspected. Autonomic testing is performed if possible.

Electrocardiogram (EKG) is performed almost always in patients seen in the ED with syncope, and most of these patients are on telemetry. However, this is no substitute for long-term cardiac monitoring.

Holter monitor provides for one or more days of continuous EKG recording during which the patient can go about most normal activities. Longer term recordings are usually made using an implanted loop recorder (ILR). Holter monitor diagnostic yield is low, reportedly less than 5%.[20]

Transthoracic echocardiogram (TTE) is performed when there is suspicion of cardiac cause on the basis of history, exam, or EKG. Transesophageal echocardiogram (TEE) is seldom needed for evaluation of syncope. Elderly patients with a variety of echocardiogram abnormalities are increased risk of falls.[21] Pulmonary hypertension and a variety of valve abnormalities especially predispose to falls.

ILR is performed in many patients with unexplained syncope especially if there is not a history of positional provocation that would produce orthostatic hypotension. Diagnostic yield may be as high as 46%.[22] Patients older than 65 have a higher incidence of arrhythmia demanding intervention.[23]

Mobile cardiac telemetry (MCT) is a newer technology that provides real-time monitoring using cellular networks. This provides the advantage of being able to record from a patient going about normal daily activities, yet not having to wait for a download of data for analysis.

Tests for neurologic causes are performed only when specifically indicated by history or exam. Carotid duplex sonography (CDS) is almost never indicated for syncope.[24]

Role of the Neurologist

Neurologic consultation is not typically necessary for all patients with syncope. Patients with clear reasons for autonomic insufficiency, such as diabetes, can be managed by our medical colleagues, but, as hospital neurologists, we are often asked to assist with the diagnosis of syncope. We should restrain ourselves from performing an extensive neurodiagnostic evaluation if this is not indicated.

The main role of the neurologic consultation is to obtain the clinical evaluation data needed to narrow the differential and focus the evaluation. The return on investment for the consultation is to avoid performing studies that are more expensive than physician care yet offer little to patient evaluation and management. The neurologist should also discuss safety issues, although there are conflicting opinions regarding when driving and other activities should be restricted. A common-sense approach with attention to applicable laws is best, with documentation of the discussion including rationale.[25]

6 Approach to Visual Deficits

Karl E. Misulis, MD, PhD and
E. Lee Murray, MD

CHAPTER CONTENTS

- Overview
- Visual Loss
  - Monocular Versus Binocular
  - Partial-Field Versus Full-Field
  - Timing of the Visual Loss
  - Localization and Diagnosis
  - Syndromes of Visual Loss
- Eye Pain
- Diplopia
  - Ocular Motor Testing
  - Localization of Lesions Producing Diplopia
- Nystagmus
- Papilledema and Optic Disc Edema
- Anisocoria
- Ptosis
- Other Pupil Abnormalities

OVERVIEW

The most common visual complaints seen by the hospital neurologist are:

- Visual loss
- Diplopia
- Nystagmus
- Ptosis
- Anisocoria
- Eye or periorbital pain

This chapter discusses the presentations of some common visual complaints, localization of the lesions, and possible diagnoses. Specific diagnoses are discussed in their respective chapters. For interested readers, Lemos and Eggenberger recently published an excellent review which is available for free download from PMC.[1]

VISUAL LOSS

Visual loss is organized into diagnoses depending on whether the loss is monocular or binocular, partial field or full-field. Of the partial field defects, a further distinction is made depending on the geometry of the visual loss.

Monocular versus Binocular

Monocular visual loss suggests a lesion affecting the eye or optic nerve. Important causes are optic neuritis (ON), ischemic optic neuropathy, or intraocular pathology (e.g., hemorrhage).

Binocular visual loss indicates a lesion at or behind the optic chiasm or lesions of both optic nerves. If the visual loss is congruent, then a lesion behind the chiasm is indicated. If the lesion is incongruent (e.g., bitemporal hemianopia), a lesion in the region of the chiasm is suggested. Note that patients might report visual deficit in one eye when they actually mean to one hemifield—for example, a right homonymous hemianopia can present with a patient complaining of visual loss in the "right eye."

Partial-Field versus Full-Field

Full-field monocular visual loss suggests catastrophic damage affecting the eye or optic nerve. The spectrum of potential diagnoses is broad, but includes ON, ischemic optic neuropathy, and intraocular hemorrhage.

Full-field binocular visual loss suggests either bilateral occipital ischemia or bilateral ON; speed and mode of onset of the deficit help to distinguish between these two possibilities. Psychogenic visual loss can also present as total visual loss.

Partial-field visual loss also has a broad differential diagnosis partly depending on the geometry of the visual loss:

- *Homonymous hemianopia* indicates a lesion of the contralateral optic radiations or occipital cortex.
- *Bitemporal hemianopia* indicates a lesion of the optic chiasm.
- *Binasal hemianopia* also suggests a lesion in the region of the chiasm, but of a geometry that compresses uncrossed axons laterally in the chiasm. Binasal hemianopia is rare but has been reported to be due to a wide variety of causes and may even be idiopathic or possibly congenital.[2]

Timing of the Visual Loss

Timing of the visual loss narrows the differential diagnosis. Acute visual loss is usually vascular, although ON and acute glaucoma can seem acute. Note that visual difficulty is usually *noticed* acutely, often with a sense of alarm, so an insidious visual loss may be reported as acute because a threshold for symptomatology was reached.

Localization and Diagnosis

Localization and a brief differential diagnosis for specific types of visual loss are presented in Table 6.1. Specific entities are discussed in their respective chapters.

Visual field defect class	Type	Differential diagnoses
Monocular visual loss	Acute monocular visual loss	Ischemic optic neuropathy
		Intraocular hemorrhage
	Subacute monocular visual loss	Optic neuritis
		Optic nerve tumor or compression
		Glaucoma
Binocular homonymous visual loss	Homonymous hemianopia	Infarction of unilateral optic radiation
	Inferior quadrantanopsia	Any lesion of the contralateral parietal region affecting the optic radiations.
		Any lesion of the superior aspect of the contralateral calcarine cortex
	Superior quadrantanopsia	Any lesion of the contralateral temporal lobe.
Binocular incongruent visual loss	Bitemporal hemianopia	Compression of the optic chiasm, usually by tumor.
	Binasal hemianopia	Optic chiasm lesion, esp. tumor. May be idiopathic.
	Asymmetric incongruent field defect	Lesions of the optic tracts with asymmetric involvement
		Lesions of lateral geniculate region.
Bilateral total visual loss	Acute	Bilateral occipital ischemia
		PRES
		Pituitary apoplexy
	Subacute to chronic	Optic neuritis
		Tumor in the region of the optic chiasm
		Glaucoma

Syndromes of Visual Loss

Syndromes of visual loss presenting to the neurologist are described here. Specific entities are discussed in more detail in their respective chapters.

- *Transient monocular blindness*: Acute visual loss in one eye, lasting 5–10 minutes then resolving. Exam is typically normal by the time of presentation.
- *Ischemic optic neuropathy*: Acute visual loss in one eye, which may improve but does not resolve. Exam shows visual loss and often signs of retinal vascular changes.
- *Optic neuritis*: Subacute onset of blurry vision or visual loss over hours to a day. Often with eye pain. May be unilateral or bilateral; exam often shows papilledema, but not invariably.

- *Glaucoma*: Unilateral or bilateral visual loss, often painful with acute exacerbation of glaucoma. Exam may be normal except for tonometry showing increased ocular pressure.
- *Pseudotumor cerebri*: Usually bilateral subacute visual loss is present, often with headache. Exam shows papilledema.
- *Stroke*: Acute onset of visual loss that can be hemianopia, quadrantanopia, or incongruous. Usually associated with signs of other neurologic deficits.
- *Temporal arteritis*: Temporal pain in middle to late age that can lead to blindness from ischemic optic neuropathy. Suspected by temporal artery thickening and/or tenderness.
- *Intraocular hemorrhage*: Acute or subacute onset of monocular visual loss. Ocular exam shows characteristic appearance, whether subretinal, vitreous, or anterior chamber hemorrhage. May produce ocular pain.
- *Retinal detachment*: Acute or subacute onset of visual obscuration as a shadow or curtain over vision. May produce ocular discomfort.

EYE PAIN

Many causes of eye pain do not present with visual loss or other neurologic symptoms and are not considered here, including conjunctivitis, keratitis, or blepharitis. Isolated eye pain usually does not present to the neurologist, but visual disturbance with eye pain may include a number of structural and inflammatory disorders. Differential diagnoses of eye pain include:

- *Glaucoma*: Subacute to acute onset of eye pain with visual disturbance and, ultimately, vision loss with closed-angle glaucoma. Patients may have nausea, vomiting. Conjunctiva may be red.
- *Optic neuritis*: Subacute onset of visual loss, often with eye pain that is exacerbated by eye movement. Exam may show papilledema, but typically not with retrobulbar ON.
- *Temporal arteritis*: Pain in the temporal region more than the eyes, often leading to visual loss if untreated. Temporal artery tenderness and thickening is suggestive of the diagnosis. Associated often with malaise, fever, and other systemic symptoms
- *Uveitis/iritis*: Subacute onset of eye pain, redness, and often blurred vision. Patient may also complain of floaters, flashing lights.
- *Orbital pseudotumor (idiopathic orbital inflammatory syndrome)*: Orbital inflammatory change may produce proptosis, visual loss, and extraocular motor deficits.
- *Orbital cellulitis*: Subacute inflammation of the orbit with bulging of the affected eye(s), limitation of eye movement, and visual loss. Exam shows the obvious orbital inflammatory change.
- *Migraine headache*: Migraine may begin with or be accompanied by eye pain. Ocular migraine is a related transient (1 hour or less) visual disturbance; common manifestations can be visual loss, dark spots, or bright lights.
- *Cluster headache*: Episodes of brief (less than 1 hour) pain around the eye typically with nasal stuffiness, excess ocular tears, and sometimes peri-orbital swelling. Ocular exam is normal.

DIPLOPIA

The differential diagnosis of diplopia is extensive but is narrowed significantly by identification of the anatomy of the deficit.

Ocular Motor Testing

Cranial Nerve Testing

- Abducens (CN 6): Lateral gaze
- Trochlear (CN 4): Depression with medial gaze
- Oculomotor (CN 3): Other movements plus lid elevation, pupil control.

Ocular Muscle Testing

- Superior rectus: Elevation with lateral gaze
- Inferior rectus: Depression with lateral gaze
- Medial rectus: Medial gaze (adduction)
- Lateral rectus: Lateral gaze (abduction)
- Superior oblique: Depression with medial gaze
- Inferior oblique: Elevation with medial gaze

Localization of Lesions Producing Diplopia

Important causes of diplopia include:

- *CN 6 palsy*: Diplopia with affected eye unable to abduct
- *CN 3 palsy*: Affected eye is 'down-and-out', i.e. abducted and depressed. Often associated with ptosis and may have pupil dilation.
- *CN 4 palsy*: Often oblique diplopia, worse with gaze down and medial for the affected eye; failure of internal rotation with medial gaze; often results in compensatory head tilt to opposite side
- *Gaze palsy*: Inability to look in a specific direction, left, right, up, down
- *Gaze preference*: Gaze is spontaneously in one direction (e.g., left or right). Usually with lesions of the hemisphere ipsilateral to the gaze preference.
- *Skew deviation*: One eye is deviated higher than the other. Usually due to brainstem or cerebellar pathology, especially stroke.
- *Muscular ocular palsy*: Individual ocular muscles can be affected, producing gaze defects commensurate with the action of the affected muscle(s). Myasthenia is the most common cause and is usually accompanied by ptosis.

NYSTAGMUS

Nystagmus and other rapid involuntary ocular motor movements are seen occasionally in hospital practice, and there is a broad differential diagnosis that is narrowed substantially by careful characterization of the movements. Nystagmus typically has a slow phase and a fast phase, although not invariably. *Jerk nystagmus* has a fast phase that defines the direction of nystagmus, whereas *pendular nystagmus* has movements in both directions of equal tempo.

Nystagmus is not always pathologic; it is seen in some patients at extremes of lateral gaze. Causes can range from vestibulopathy to medications to primary brainstem pathology. Many presentations of nystagmus are gaze-evoked nystagmus in that the movements develop or are worsened on gaze away from the primary position. Types of nystagmus and their clinical implications are presented in the following list:

- *Vestibular nystagmus*: Vestibular nystagmus is divided into central and peripheral forms.
  - *Central vestibular nystagmus* is usually due to a defect of the brainstem or cerebellum. Nystagmus tends to be worse in the direction of gaze.
  - *Peripheral vestibular nystagmus* is usually due to a defect in the semicircular canals. Nystagmus tends to be worse with gaze in the direction of the fast phase.
- *Gaze-evoked nystagmus*: This is produced by attempted gaze in a particular direction. The fast phase is in the direction of gaze. This can be from toxic or central causes.
  - *End-gaze nystagmus* is a form of gaze-evoked nystagmus especially with far lateral gaze. The eye drifts toward the primary position, and there is a fast phase laterally. This is seen in patients with otherwise normal neurologic function.
- *Nystagmus from medications*: Nystagmus may be present in the primary position but is often exacerbated by lateral gaze. Phenytoin is a classic cause but nystagmus can also be due to alcohol, barbiturates, benzodiazepines, and others.
- *Nystagmus from brainstem lesions*: Nystagmus can be part of a variety of brainstem syndromes, including from infarction, hemorrhage, tumors, and obstructive hydrocephalus, among others. In all of these, there are other clinical findings in addition to the nystagmus.
- *Wernicke encephalopathy*: Nystagmus in either or both the horizontal and vertical planes is associated with other signs such as confusion and/or ataxia; nystagmus would not be expected to be an isolated finding. Due to thiamine deficiency.
- *Nystagmus from ocular muscle weakness*: Weakness of one or more ocular muscles can produce a compensatory nystagmus. Myasthenia is a classic cause.
- *Upbeat nystagmus*: Fast phase is upward with a slow downward drift. Common causes include a variety of intoxications, and brainstem lesions including infarction or hemorrhage.
- *Downbeat nystagmus*: Fast phase is down with a slow upward deviation. Causes are multiple, classically described with Chiari; can be seen with spinocerebellar degenerations, brainstem infarction or hemorrhage, drug toxicity, Wernicke encephalopathy, brainstem encephalitis, and anoxic encephalopathy, among others. Occasional cases are of unknown cause.

PAPILLEDEMA AND OPTIC DISC EDEMA

Optic disc edema is swelling due to a host causes with the common causes being optic neuritis (ON), pseudotumor cerebri and ischemic optic neuritis. *Papilledema* is optic nerve swelling due to increased intracranial pressure. Specific features of each of the disorders are discussed in the section on *Disorders*. Common causes of papilledema and disc edema include:

- *Optic neuritis*: ON can produce unilateral or bilateral disc edema, often associated with pain with eye movements. Optic disc is often normal with retrobulbar optic neuritis.

- *Ischemic optic neuropathy (ION)*: ION can be arteritic (AION; associated with giant cell arteritis) or nonarteritic (NAION). Both can produce disc edema, disc pallor, and ultimately atrophy.
- *Orbital tumor*: Presentation may include proptosis, visual loss, diplopia, and/or orbital pain. Papilledema is commonly seen, although optic disc pallor may be seen.
- *Idiopathic intracranial hypertension (IIH, pseudotumor cerebri)*: Increased intracranial pressure presents usually with headache and papilledema.
- *Intracranial tumor;* Mass effect or obstructive hydrocephalus from intracranial tumor can produce increased intracranial pressure and papilledema.
- *Malignant hypertension*: Malignant hypertension can produce papilledema with associated visual disturbance in addition to other signs of hypertensive encephalopathy.
- *Cavernous sinus thrombosis*: Presentation is usually orbital swelling, pain, and proptosis. Exam can show disc edema and retinal hemorrhages.
- *Central retinal vein occlusion*: Presentation includes visual loss associated with retinal hemorrhages, macular edema, and disc edema.
- *Meningitis;* Causes of subacute and chronic meningitis can cause papilledema, usually bilateral (e.g., *Cryptococcus*, Lyme, neoplastic meningitides).
- *Cerebral edema*: Separately from tumors and hydrocephalus, any cause of intracranial pressure from cerebral edema can cause papilledema (e.g., mountain sickness).
- *Medications*: A wide variety of meds have been associated with increased intracranial pressure and papilledema, including corticosteroid administration and withdrawal, amiodarone, tetracycline, lithium, and naladixic acid.
- *Intoxications*: Heavy metals including lead and arsenic. Hypervitaminosis A.

ANISOCORIA

Unequal pupil size is common, often nonpathologic. Clinical importance depends on specific features and chronicity of the lesion. We ask to see historical pictures of patients with anisocoria, if available, to determine chronicity. Even driver license photos may show previously unappreciated anisocoria. The most common etiologies we seen in hospital practice are physiologic, pharmacologic, and increased intracranial pressure from any cause. Important causes of anisocoria include:

- *Pharmacologic*: Anticholinergics, recent mydriatic agents
- *Horner's syndrome*: Any cause of sympathetic nerve damage
- *Oculomotor palsy*: Trauma and compressive lesions of CN 3 often produce pupil involvement. Ischemic causes are usually pupil-sparing. Increased intracranial pressure.
- *Tonic pupil (Adie)*: Damage to the ciliary ganglion, which may be infectious or idiopathic.
- *Compressive lesion*: Cerebral aneurysm particularly of the posterior cerebral artery.
- *Physiologic anisocoria*: Minimal anisocoria is common, idiopathic anisocoria is present in up to 20% of patients.
- *Cavernous sinus lesions*: Tumors, aneurysms, fistula, thrombosis
- *Migraine and cluster headache*: Migraine can be associated with unilateral mydriasis and/or other ocular motor deficits. Cluster headache can produce ipsilateral miosis.
- *Brainstem stroke*: Brainstem ischemia and hemorrhage can produce anisocoria, but this would not be an isolated finding.

- *Brainstem tumors*: Brainstem tumors, whether intrinsic or extrinsic, can produce anisocoria, but this is typically associated with other signs of brainstem and/or cranial nerve dysfunction.

An occasional cause for neurologic consultation especially in the ICU is unilateral or bilateral pupil dilation, which is sometimes identified as secondary to respiratory therapy treatments (e.g. ipratropium).

Ptosis

The hospital neurologist usually is asked to evaluate ptosis when it occurs in the setting of suspected Horner syndrome or myasthenia. However, senile ptosis is more common. Important causes of ptosis include:

- *Horner syndrome*: Ptosis and miosis is from ipsilateral sympathetic dysfunction.
- *Myasthenia (ocular or gravis)*: Ptosis is usually accompanied by other ocular motor deficits, often not conforming to CN 3.
- *Oculomotor palsy*: Any cause of CN 3 palsy can cause ptosis.
- *Senile ptosis*: Levator stretch or dehiscence; this appears later in life.
- *Bell palsy*: Usually produces inability to close the eye, but mild drooping of the upper lid can occur. Associated with unilateral face weakness.
- *Apraxia of lid opening*: Difficulty in opening eye after closure; it can be idiopathic or associated with a wide variety of conditions.

OTHER PUPIL ABNORMALITIES

Afferent pupillary defect: This presents as decreased response of the pupils due to lesion of the eye or optic nerve. If unilateral, pupil on the affected side shows dilation during the swinging flashlight test—illumination of the side with reduced optic nerve input from primary optic nerve dysfunction or orbital abnormality. Marcus Gunn pupil is a relative afferent defect as described for the swinging flashlight test.

Adie's tonic pupil: The affected eye has a relatively dilated pupil that responds slowly to light but responds more briskly to accommodation i.e. light-near dissociation. Can be seen as a syndrome mainly in females and associated with reduced tendon reflexes and impaired sweating. Can also be seen in patients without these findings, but with no one dominant identified etiology.

Argyll Robertson pupils: This presents as decreased response of the pupils to light but constriction to accommodation, i.e. light-near dissociation. Pupils are usually small and often irregular even prior to accommodation-induced constriction. Once thought to be specific for neurosyphilis, this is seen in other disorders including diabetes.

7 Language and Hearing Deficits

Howard S. Kirshner, MD and
Karl E. Misulis, MD, PhD

CHAPTER CONTENTS

- Aphasia
- Dysarthria
- Hearing Loss

The most common speech and language difficulties to come to the attention of hospital neurologists are *aphasia* and *dysarthria*. Important elements of language and hearing are presented here in overview, with subsequent more detailed discussion in later sections. Additional information on specific diagnostic entities is presented in chapters in Section III, Neurologic Diagnoses.

This chapter discusses the differential diagnoses of the following presentations:

- *Aphasia*: Deficit in language reception and/or expression of a variety of types
- *Dysarthria*: Impaired motor control of speech without an actual language deficit
- *Hearing loss*: Impairment in hearing due to neural degeneration (sensorineural) or mechanical (conductive) defects

Hearing loss can sometimes mimic receptive aphasia or even dementia, especially if the patient is not aware of the deficit or is not willing to report it.

APHASIA

Hospital neurologists will most likely see patients with three subtypes of aphasia: *Global aphasia*, *Broca's aphasia*, and *Wernicke's aphasia*, especially if in a stroke center. The aphasia is characterized by impairment of specific components of receptive and expressive language function. The following list presents some of the subtypes of aphasia and most likely responsible localizations.

- *Broca's (expressive) aphasia*
  FEATURES: Expression is impaired, but comprehension is relatively preserved except for impairment of small, grammatical word relationships.
  LOCATION: Broca's area, inferior frontal gyrus; most commonly middle cerebral artery (MCA) anterior division infarct

- *Wernicke's (receptive) aphasia*

  FEATURES: Speech is fluent but abnormal, with both sound (phonemic or literal) and meaning (verbal or semantic) errors ("paraphasias"), such that the language expression has deficient content. Comprehension of questions and commands is affected.

  LOCATION: Temporal lobe, superior and middle region; most commonly MCA posterior division infarct

- *Global aphasia*

  FEATURES: Deficits of comprehension and expression

  LOCATION: Damage to both Broca's and Wernicke's area; usually MCA infarct, but also seen with inferior cerebral artery (ICA) occlusion, large left basal ganglia hemorrhages

- *Conduction aphasia*

  FEATURES: Chief deficit is in repetition. Reception is relatively preserved although imperfect. Expression is paraphasic, in the literal or phonemic form.

  LOCATION: Parietal lobe, supramarginal gyrus, occasionally temporal lobe

- *Anomic aphasia*

  FEATURES: Prominent deficit in naming, beyond other language difficulties

  LOCATION: Temporal lobe, not one specific region; can be seen with neurodegenerative diseases

- *Transcortical motor aphasia*

  FEATURES: Deficit in initiating speech but repetition and comprehension are preserved.

  LOCATION: Anterior frontal region, either medial or lateral; anterior cerebral artery (ACA) territory strokes

- *Transcortical sensory aphasia*

  FEATURES: Deficit in comprehension, similar to Wernicke's aphasia, but with preserved repetition; speech is paraphasic.

  LOCATION: Temporal-parietal or temporal-occipital junction; can be seen in stroke, occasionally in watershed strokes, mass lesions, neurodegenerative disorders

- *Transcortical mixed aphasia*

  FEATURES: Deficit in both comprehension and expression but preserved repetition

  LOCATION: Watershed region between Broca's and Wernicke's areas, not affecting either directly; can be seen in watershed strokes and also in advanced dementia

- *Pure-word mutism (also called aphemia)*

  FEATURES: Inability to speak, with preserved ability to write; repetition can be preserved, and comprehension is also preserved. Overlaps with transcortical motor aphasia.

  LOCATION: Frontal lobe, often directly in Broca's area, sometimes seen in larger frontal lobe lesions, including tumor, trauma

- *Pure-word deafness*

  FEATURES: Deficit in auditory comprehension but preservation of written comprehension; expression may be paraphasic.

  LOCATION: Superior temporal gyrus, often bilaterally. Disconnection theory: disconnects the primary auditory cortices from Wernicke's area

- *Subcortical aphasia*
  FEATURES: May have elements of receptive, expressive, or global aphasia depending on the location. Expressive aphasia with dysarthria is most common with basal ganglia lesions; fluent aphasia resembling Wernicke's aphasia is most common with thalamic lesions.
  LOCATION: Thalamus and/or basal ganglia

DIAGNOSIS of aphasia in the ED usually begins with emergent evaluation of suspected stroke. Detailed evaluation of stroke is discussed in Chapter 16. A computed tomography (CT) brain scan is often performed emergently, but a magnetic resonance imaging (MRI) scan is more likely to reveal the responsible lesion.

Etiologies of aphasia are multiple:

- *Acute ischemic stroke (AIS):* Infarction in the distribution of the MCA is most common, but the lesion may be proximal in the ICA. The cause can be thrombotic, embolic, dissection, or occasionally watershed from hypoperfusion. ACA ischemia can occasionally produce language difficulty, usually as mutism, aphemia, or transcortical motor aphasia.[1]
- *Cerebral venous thrombosis (CVT):* Usually presents with headache but focal signs can develop, including aphasia. The direct cause can be either a hemorrhage or an infarction, which frequently is noted to cross arterial boundaries on MRI.
- *Tumor:* Lesions of the dominant hemisphere that are suspected tumor are usually associated with a region of edema. Gliomas and metastatic lesions are most common.
- *Intracranial hemorrhage (ICH):* Aphasia can develop with almost any type of intracranial bleeding, including intraparenchymal, subdural, epidural, and subarachnoid hemorrhages. Language function can be worsened by increased intracranial pressure (ICP).
- *Alzheimer's disease (AD):* Patients usually have language difficulty with word finding and comprehension difficulty.
- *Frontotemporal dementia (FTD):* This is a family of disorders, but the common presentations are either prominent behavioral changes or prominent aphasia, the latter referred to as *primary progressive aphasia.*
- *Primary progressive aphasia (PPA):* In the family of FTDs, language difficulty is an early and prominent part of the clinical picture. It has been divided into three forms: progressive nonfluent aphasia, semantic dementia, and logopenic PPA. The logopenic form is usually caused by Alzheimer's disease.
- *Traumatic brain injury (TBI):* Trauma can produce aphasia by contusion, hemorrhage, shear injury, or secondary infarction, but the inciting event is usually known. Occasional patients present to the ED with language deficits or other focal signs without a known history of trauma. Exam can often reveal signs of injury, but they have to be specifically looked for.
- *Seizure:* Patients may develop disordered speech or speech arrest from a focal seizure. Reception is usually markedly impaired and expression is either totally absent or a nonsensical series of phonemes. Absence-type seizures can present with speech arrest, but this is seldom confused with aphasia.

DYSARTHRIA

Dysarthria in a hospital practice is usually due to stroke, which is likely not in the dominant language cortex. A host of other disorders encompass the remaining patients we see urgently. Timing of onset helps to narrow the differential diagnosis.

- *Acute onset*
  - o Stroke, usually subcortical, brainstem/cerebellar
- *Subacute onset*
  - o Myasthenia gravis
  - o Brainstem tumor
- *Chronic*
  - o Hereditary ataxias
  - o Parkinson disease and other degenerative movement disorders

Dysarthrias come in several types, each of which has implications for localization.

- *Spastic dysarthria*
  FEATURES: Slow, dysarthric, and somewhat harsh speech; may have bursts of loud speech
  LOCATION: Corticobulbar tracts
- *Flaccid dysarthria*
  FEATURES: Soft, breathy, nasal, and monotone, often lacking dynamic range
  LOCATION: Lower motoneuron dysfunction
- *Rigid dysarthria*
  FEATURES: Rapid speech that is mumbling and in a monotone
  LOCATION: Extrapyramidal dysfunction (e.g., parkinsonism)
- *Hyperkinetic dysarthria*
  FEATURES: Harsh and generally loud voice, often with involuntary respiratory movements or bulbar movements
  LOCATION: Extrapyramidal lesions
- *Hypokinetic dysarthria*
  FEATURES: Soft voice with rapid speech
  LOCATION: Basal ganglia, especially parkinsonism
- *Unilateral upper motor neuron dysarthria*
  FEATURES: Deficit especially in articulation, prosody; often with dysarthria. This is a subtype of the "spastic" type, usually seen in unilateral strokes.
  LOCATION: Unilateral corticospinal tract lesion
- *Ataxic dysarthria*
  FEATURES: Slow and slurred speech; defect in prosody with irregular timing of phonemes and syllables
  LOCATION: Cerebellar lesions mainly (e.g., multiple sclerosis)

DIAGNOSIS of dysarthrias begins with imaging, preferably MRI but CT is performed if needed urgently or if MRI cannot be performed. If the cause is felt to be vascular, CT angiography (CTA) or MR angiography (MRA) is recommended. If studies are negative, then nonstructural causes need to be considered; however, small infarctions in the brainstem may be missed on MRI. Electromyogram and labs may be done to evaluate for myasthenia gravis and paraneoplastic disorders.

HEARING LOSS

Hearing loss is not typically within the province of a neurology text, but there are some neurologic concerns that the hospital physician might face because hearing difficulty or a language barrier can be misinterpreted as aphasia or even dementia.

PRESENTATION helps to determine the etiology:

- *Sudden unilateral hearing loss* suggests perilymph fistula or Ménière disease. Acute changes are usually associated with vertigo and nausea.
- *Progressive unilateral hearing loss with tinnitus* and/or vertigo suggests Ménière disease or acoustic neuroma.

Disorders affecting hearing are discussed in more detail in Chapter 32, but, briefly, some of the neurologic disorders that are associated with hearing loss are:

- *Ménière disease*: Episodic vertigo, tinnitus, hearing loss, and often ear fullness.
- *Acoustic neuroma*: Hearing loss, tinnitus, and vertigo are typical. Symptoms are usually unilateral, but acoustic neuromas can be bilateral although seldom simultaneous in symptoms onset.
- *Meningitis*: Hearing loss is usually not appreciated initially—the acute manifestations dominate the clinical picture. Several days into the meningitis, hearing difficulty may be appreciated.
- *Cortical deafness*: Bilateral lesions of the superior temporal gyrus can develop from sequential infarction or hemorrhage producing apparent impaired hearing but with preserved functions of the brainstem pathways.
- *Pure word deafness*: Inability to understand spoken words with preserved perception and identification of sounds; Pure word deafness is usually secondary to bilateral lesions involving the temporal lobes, theoretically disconnecting the auditory input to Wernicke's area. This is considered more a form of aphasia than a hearing deficit.

8 Cranial Neuropathies

Karl E. Misulis, MD, PhD and
E. Lee Murray, MD

CHAPTER CONTENTS

- Single Cranial Neuropathies
- Multiple Cranial Neuropathies
- Cranial Nerve Deficits in Hospital Practice

SINGLE CRANIAL NEUROPATHIES

Single cranial neuropathies are much more common than multiple cranial neuropathies but both are discussed here. The most common single cranial neuropathies are facial, abducens, oculomotor, and optic. Chapter 33 discuss ocular motor and other cranial nerve deficits in detail.

- CN 1: Olfactory
  FEATURES: Loss of smell
  ETIOLOGY: Trauma, degenerative disease, chemicals, aging, some brain tumors (e.g., meningioma), malnutrition
- CN 2: Ocular
  FEATURES: Disturbance of vision due to prechiasmatic lesion
  ETIOLOGY: Trauma; demyelination; orbital tumors; pituitary tumors; papilledema from any cause; ischemia including temporal arteritis, retinal artery ischemia; retinal vein thrombosis; infectious optic neuropathy (e.g., cat-scratch disease); optic glioma; toxic optic neuropathy (e.g., methanol, INH, and many others)
- CN 3: Oculomotor
  FEATURES: Diplopia, ptosis, mydriasis
  ETIOLOGY: Oculomotor nerve ischemia from diabetes or other vascular risk factors, aneurysmal compression, brainstem ischemia in multiple locations, cavernous sinus lesions of any type, intraorbital mass or inflammation, increased intracranial pressure from any reason, pineal tumor
- CN 4: Trochlear
  FEATURES: Vertical diplopia, greatest with downward gaze and gaze to the opposite side
  ETIOLOGY: Congenital, brainstem tumors, hydrocephalus, demyelinating disease, aneurysm especially superior cerebellar artery, intracranial hypertension from any cause, orbital tumor or inflammatory lesions

- CN 5: Trigeminal
  FEATURES: Sensory loss in one or more of the trigeminal distributions: V1, V2, or V3
  ETIOLOGY: Trigeminal neuralgia, tumor, trauma
- CN 6: Abducens
  FEATURES: Diplopia, lateral rectus paresis
  ETIOLOGY: Nerve infarction, especially with diabetes; increased intracranial pressure
- CN 7: Facial
  FEATURES: Lower motoneuron facial weakness
  ETIOLOGY: Bell palsy, sarcoidosis, Lyme disease; often idiopathic
- CN 8: Vestibulocochlear
  FEATURES: Hearing loss, tinnitus, and/or vertigo
  ETIOLOGY: Acoustic neuroma, cerebellopontine angle tumors, chronic meningitis either infectious or neoplastic, infarction,
- CN 9: Glossopharyngeal
  FEATURES: Dysphagia, dysarthria, loss of taste from the posterior tongue (likely unnoticed)
  ETIOLOGY: Stroke, tumor, skull-based lesions
- CN 10: Vagus
  FEATURES: Dysphagia, dysarthria
  ETIOLOGY: Stroke, tumors, meningitis
- CN 11: Accessory
  FEATURES: Trapezius weakness, scapular winging
  ETIOLOGY: Trauma, intraoperative damage
- CN 12: Hypoglossal
  FEATURES: Paralysis of the tongue, deviation to the side of the lesion with protrusion
  ETIOLOGY: Infarction, tumor

Although we consider cranial neuropathies as isolated entities, there are many disorders that affect multiple cranial nerves.

MULTIPLE CRANIAL NEUROPATHIES

Multiple cranial neuropathies can develop for a variety of reasons, but among the most common are neoplastic meningitis, vasculitis, and diabetes. Intrinsic lesions of the brainstem can present with multiple cranial neuropathies, but there are usually other signs of parenchymal brainstem dysfunction, including gait ataxia, unilateral or bilateral limb weakness and/or incoordination, or mental status change. Cavernous sinus lesions can result in CN 3, 4, 6, and CN 5 V1 lesions, and, sometimes, Horner syndrome.

Mononeuropathy multiplex from any cause can produce multiple cranial neuropathies although peripheral nerves are commonly affected. Causes can be neoplastic, autoimmune, vasculitis, amyloid, infectious, multifocal tumor infiltration (e.g., lymphoma), or paraneoplastic.

Disorders with multiple cranial neuropathies include:

- *Neoplastic meningitis*: Multiple cranial neuropathies, often with multiple radiculopathies
- *Infectious meningitis*: Usually presents with headache, fever, mental status changes, but can have especially Abducens palsy with increased ICP. Hearing loss is common later in the course; other cranial neuropathies can occur also.
- *Vasculitis*: Multifocal cranial nerve deficits, often associated with peripheral nerve deficits
- *Brainstem lesions*: Gliomas and other infiltrating tumors; ischemia; hemorrhage, including subarachnoid hemorrhage

CRANIAL NERVE DEFICITS IN HOSPITAL PRACTICE

Facial palsy presenting to the hospital is more likely Bell palsy than vascular. Less likely is early acute inflammatory demyelinating polyneuropathy (AIDP).

Ocular motor palsy of a single nerve is most likely to be microvascular in patients with hypertension or diabetes.

Multiple ocular motor deficits such as ptosis with dysfunction of ocular muscles innervated by more than one nerve can be from cavernous sinus lesion, chronic meningeal disease, or brainstem lesion. A non–cranial nerve disorder, such as myasthenia gravis, is also possible.

Cranial nerve palsies without parenchymal brainstem involvement suggests infectious or neoplastic meningitis. Vasculitis is considered.

Cranial nerve palsies with brainstem deficits, such as descending motor or ascending sensory tract involvement, suggest a focal brainstem lesion such as ischemia, hemorrhage, tumor, or demyelination.

Some vascular brainstem syndromes with cranial nerve involvement include:

- *PCA stroke* produces hemianopia and, if bilateral, produces cortical blindness.
- *Basilar thrombosis* can produce deficit in lateral gaze with CN 6 palsies, relative preservation of vertical movements, and miosis, along with quadriplegia or coma.
- *Posterior inferior cerebellar artery (PICA)* occlusion can present with ipsilateral facial sensory loss, Horner syndrome, ataxia, dysphagia, and dysarthria. Contralateral sensory deficit below the brainstem is common.
- *Anterior inferior cerebellar artery syndrome (AICA)* occlusion can vertigo, nausea, vomiting, ipsilateral facial sensory deficit and contralaterai pain and temperature loss of the body and limbs. Horner syndrome, hearing loss, tinnitus, dysphagia, and dysarthria can be seen.
- *Paramedian branch occlusion from the basilar* can produce contralateral hemiparesis and cranial nerve deficits depending on the level of the lesion. Pons involvement affects especially CN 6 and CN 7 with ipsilateral lateral gaze and facial palsies. Midbrain involvement can produce CN 3 palsy with diplopia. Medullary involvement can produce a CN 12 deficit.

9 Dizziness, Vertigo, and Imbalance

Karl E. Misulis, MD, PhD and
E. Lee Murray, MD

CHAPTER CONTENTS

- Terminology
- Syndromes of Dizziness and Vertigo
- Imbalance and Falls
  - Gait Ataxia
  - Falls
- Disorders

Dizziness and vertigo can have central or peripheral generators. The most common etiologies seen by hospital neurologists are complaints due to:

- Benign paroxysmal positional vertigo
- Ménière disease
- Stroke, especially brainstem
- Toxic/metabolic, especially ethanol and medications.

Specific disorders are discussed in detail in Chapter 32 unless otherwise indicated.

TERMINOLOGY

Patients may report "dizziness" or "vertigo," but the specific meaning may be uncertain. Most of these patients are referring to one of the following symptoms:

- *Vertigo*: Sense of spinning.
- *Gait ataxia*: Unsteadiness of stance and/or gait
- *Limb ataxia*: Appendicular ataxia affecting any or all extremities
- *Pre-syncope*: Lightheadedness
- *Syncope*: Loss of consciousness due to cerebral hypoperfusion.
- *Confusion*: Cognitive dysfunction.

Vertigo

Vertigo is a sensation of movement of either the patient or the environment when none has occurred. Vertigo is *central* or *peripheral*. Peripheral vertigo is most common, but the central causes must not missed on clinical evaluation.

Peripheral vertigo includes the follow disorders:

- Benign paroxysmal positional vertigo (BPPV)
- Ménière disease
- Post-traumatic vertigo

Central vertigo includes the following disorders:

- Acoustic neuroma
- Other cerebellopontine tumors
- Migraine
- Stroke
- Multiple sclerosis

Differentiating causes of vertigo depends on character and associated symptoms. Post-traumatic vertigo is considered by many to be a form of BPPV; it is not always paroxysmal, although it is usually positional.

Gait Ataxia

Gait ataxia presents with a propensity to stumble or fall and is sometimes described as "dizziness" even in the absence of true vertigo.

Differential diagnosis of gait ataxia is broad and is narrowed depending on acuity and associated features. Some of the possibilities include:

- *Toxicity*: Common examples are ethanol and phenytoin, but a host of medications and toxins can produce gait ataxia.
- *Stroke*: Ischemic and hemorrhagic stroke especially in the posterior circulation distribution can produce ataxia, but this is almost always associated with other neurologic deficits which localize the lesion.
- *Multiple sclerosis (MS)*: Can present with ataxia and sometimes vertigo, but with MS, the ataxia is more severe than can be explained by vertigo alone.
- *Tumor*: Rarely, tumor in the brainstem or cerebellum can present as predominant gait ataxia. There are usually other findings related to cranial nerve involvement, mass effect, or hydrocephalus.
- *Parkinson disease and related conditions*: Certain diseases result in ataxia plus other motor symptoms depending on the precise disorder.
- *Paraneoplastic syndrome*: Paraneoplastic cerebellar degeneration presents with ataxia often with other brainstem signs.
- *Sensory ataxia*: Neuropathy with a prominent sensory component; Romberg is positive.

Limb Ataxia

Limb ataxia is only rarely referred to as *dizziness* by the patient. Limb ataxia is never due to peripheral vestibulopathy. Limb ataxia in the absence of weakness is usually due to a cerebellar lesion. Weakness with ataxia can be a lesion anywhere from brainstem to cerebral cortex.

Important etiologies of limb ataxia are:

- Stroke
- Tumor
- Multiple sclerosis and other immune-mediated conditions
- Parkinsonism and related movement disorders

One of the most unusual disorders with abnormal limb movements is corticobasal syndrome, discussed in Chapter 23.

Presyncope

Regional terminology sometimes reports presyncope or syncope as "dizziness". Patients report that they feel as if they are going to faint. The common physiological effect is reduction in cerebral blood flow. Possible causes include:

- *Hypotension*
  - Orthostasis
  - Arrhythmia
  - Aortic stenosis
  - Neurocardiogenic (i.e., vasovagal)
  - Blood loss
  - Infection, including sepsis
  - Addison disease
- *Cerebrovascular disease*
  - Bilateral carotid disease
  - Vertebrobasilar insufficiency
- *Anemia*
  - From blood loss or hematologic disorder.
- *Pregnancy*

For some of these etiologies, presyncope may be the presenting complaint. We have seen this especially for anemia, GI bleed, pregnancy, and cardiac outflow impairment. Isolated presyncope due to cerebrovascular disease is rare.

Syncope

Syncope is sometimes used as a generic term for *transient loss of consciousness* (TLOC) but, strictly speaking, loss of consciousness develops because of cerebral hypoperfusion. The complaint of "dizziness" may sometimes precede TLOC or falls. Evaluation of TLOC and syncope is discussed in detail in Chapter 5.

Clonic syncope is shaking of the body in association with syncope. This is due to neuronal hypoxia. Clonic syncope is often mistaken for seizure. Presentation is with TLOC associated with jerking, which can be single or repetitive for a few seconds. Jerking lasting longer than this is unlikely to be clonic syncope.

Confusion

Confusion due to developing dementia usually is not described as "dizziness", but the term is sometimes used for transient cognitive disturbance (e.g., transient disorientation).

Differential diagnosis of this would include:

- *Transient global amnesia*: Memory deficit that is transient but over hours or a day and not momentary.
- *Incipient delirium*: Before more severe symptoms develop, transient confusion can occur.
- *Transient hypotension*: This can present with presyncope or cognitive difficulty. Almost any of the causes of presyncope discussed earlier can cause confusion due to cerebral hypoperfusion.
- *Migraine*: Can occasionally present with confusion.
- *Seizure*: Can rarely cause cognitive dysfunction without prominent motor activity.

A complaint of dizziness associated with a cognitive component indicates that the disorder is central and not peripheral.

SYNDROMES OF DIZZINESS AND VERTIGO

Episodic vertigo without other neurologic symptoms: Peripheral causes are most likely. The possibility of stroke or MS is very low. Diagnoses to consider are:

- BPPV
- Ménière disease

Vertigo with hearing loss:

- Acoustic neuroma
- Ménière disease

Vertigo with appendicular ataxia: Indicates a central lesion.

- Cerebellar stroke
- Cerebellar tumor
- Multiple sclerosis

Presyncope that is positional: Suggests autonomic neuropathy with orthostatic hypotension

- Diabetes
- Parkinsonism and related disorders including MSA

Presyncope that is nonpositional:

- Aortic stenosis
- Anemia
- Sepsis/Systemic inflammatory response syndrome

IMBALANCE AND FALLS

Imbalance and *falls* are common reasons for hospital neurology consultation. Details of the symptoms help to determine etiology. Some of the clinical scenarios are:

- Gait ataxia that is intermittent or constant
- Presyncope or syncope that is or is not positional
- Falls with warning of presyncope, dizziness, or vertigo, or without warning

Some of the associated diagnoses are:

- Orthostatic hypotension
- Drop attack
- Syncope
- Clonic syncope
- Seizure
- Cerebellar ataxia
- Sensory ataxia
- TIA
- Parkinsonism
- Chiari malformation

Gait Ataxia

Gait ataxia can have a broad range of neurologic localizations. Some of the most common clinical scenarios are discussed.

Cerebellar ataxia produces a broad-based gait. Limb ataxia often accompanies gait ataxia, but midline cerebellar lesions, such as ethanol abuse, often do not.

- *Cerebellar infarction* can produce acute onset of gait and appendicular ataxia, depending on location (midline vs. cerebellar hemisphere). Usually presents with associated signs of brainstem dysfunction.
- *Cerebellar hemorrhage* can result in acute onset of ataxia, but there are usually other findings such as headache, nausea, vomiting, ocular motor abnormalities,

or corticospinal deficits. Cognitive dysfunction can rapidly develop. This diagnosis is considered with acute onset of ataxia with progressive deficits, especially in the presence of hypertension.

- *Cerebellar tumor* produces ataxia often with other symptoms such as headache, ocular motor abnormalities, and corticospinal tract abnormalities.
- *Ethanol abuse* produces predominantly gait ataxia without limb ataxia because of the midline vermian involvement.
- *Spinocerebellar degeneration* is suggested by progressive ataxia that may be isolated or associated with other neurologic deficits. Autosomal dominant inheritance supports the diagnosis.
- *Multiple sclerosis* is suspected with cerebellar ataxia in combination with nystagmus, dysarthria, or other neurologic findings.

Corticospinal tract dysfunction usually produces weakness, but can produce ataxia of limb or gait that can eclipse weakness.

- Diagnosis is suspected with ataxia of gait and limbs with corticospinal tract signs. Pure gait ataxia would not be expected from a corticospinal lesion.

Sensory ataxia is due to impaired input for movement feedback circuits. The most common lesions are in peripheral nerves or dorsal columns. Important causes include diabetic neuropathy and B_{12} deficiency. Presentation is with gait ataxia that is worse with eyes closed, when the patient loses visual cues. Position sense and vibration sense are impaired. Specifically absent are nystagmus, speech change, and appendicular ataxia.

Normal pressure hydrocephalus (NPH) is characterized by the triad of ataxia, dementia, and incontinence. The entire triad is often not present. Diagnosis is suspected with gait ataxia along with dementia and supported by increased ventricular size on brain imaging. NPH is discussed in detail in Chapter 26.

Falls

Falls have multiple root causes, some of which include:

- Hypotension
- Ataxia
- Movement disorder
- Weakness
- Vestibulopathy

Hypotension predisposes to fall, especially if the patient is orthostatic. This is suggested by vague dizziness or presyncopal sensations prior to the fall. Observers note pale appearance. Nausea is common.

Ataxia is suggested by imbalance on gait testing even without a fall. Presyncopal sensation, paleness, and nausea are absent. Some patients have evident limb ataxia, but this may be absent with midline cerebellar lesions, such as with chronic ethanol use.

Movement disorders such as Parkinson disease produce impaired leg placement and truncal instability that results in fall. This is suggested by all of the typical findings of the disease as discussed in Chapter 23.

Weakness from almost any cause can predispose to falls. While the list is endless, some of the scenarios presenting to the hospital neurologist are:

- *Focal CNS disorder:*
  - o Stroke, either acute or chronic.
  - o Subdural hematoma or other intracranial hemorrhage.
  - o Tumor
- *Neuromuscular disorder:*
  - o Neuropathy with motor involvement. Fall can be the presenting symptom of acute inflammatory demyelinating polyneuropathy (AIDP) because patients may tolerate weakness until they fall or cannot rise to a stand, thus precipitating ED visit.
  - o Neuromuscular transmission abnormality (e.g., myasthenia gravis).
  - o Myopathy can produce weakness predisposing to falls.
- *Spinal cord lesion:* Any cause of progressive myelopathy can present with falls.
  - o Transverse myelitis (e.g., MS, transverse myelitis)
  - o Compression from tumor or disc
  - o Cord infarction

Vestibulopathy can produce falls usually associated with vertigo and, depending on the disorder, tinnitus or hearing loss. Paroxysmal benign positional vertigo and Ménière disease are most common. These are discussed in Chapter 32.

DISORDERS

Details of these disorders are discussed in their respective chapters, but as an aid to diagnosis, we present here a snapshot of many of the disorders discussed in this chapter.

Benign paroxysmal positional vertigo (BPPV): Brief episodes of vertigo provoked by movement or a specific head position. Duration is usually about a minute. Nausea and vomiting are common. May be off balance because of the vestibular deficit but no other neurologic deficits.

Ménière disease: Episodes of vertigo with nausea, tinnitus, and ultimately hearing loss. No other neurologic deficit. Episodes are longer in duration than BPPV, usually at least an hour and may last days.

Acoustic neuroma: Usually presents with progressive hearing loss, most commonly unilateral. Can present with dizziness, vertigo, imbalance, and a pressure sensation around the ear. Ultimately facial numbness (CN 5) and weakness (CN 7) can occur.

Multiple sclerosis: Attacks of varied neurologic deficit of which ataxia and vertigo can be a component. Unlikely to be isolated vertigo without a detectable deficit.

Cerebellar stroke: Both ischemic and hemorrhagic stroke can present with ataxia and occasional vertigo.

Brainstem stroke: Ischemic and hemorrhagic brainstem stroke produces usually marked motor, cranial nerve, and cognitive deficits.

Orthostatic hypotension: Presyncope or weakness on standing is typical. Some patients will also have orthostatic tremor—a high-frequency tremor in the legs on standing that is not related to hypotension; some patients who are predisposed to orthostatic hypotension also are predisposed to orthostatic tremor.

Sepsis/SIRS: Sepsis produces malaise, weakness, and fever; dizziness might be a part of this, usually manifest as lightheadedness, confusion, difficulty with concentration, and ataxia.

Hypoglycemia: Low glucose can occur in patients with or without diabetes and often produces an inward tremulousness that becomes more of an outwardly visible tremor as the condition evolves.

Anemia: Blood loss or defects in red blood cell manufacture can cause anemia that can present with dizziness, often described as a fogginess of the head. It sometimes has a presyncopal component but can also cause confusion.

Vertebrobasilar insufficiency: Ischemia in a vertebrobasilar distribution can produce vertigo but usually has other signs including cranial nerve deficits, appendicular ataxia, or deficits with speech or swallowing.

Pregnancy: Pregnancy can present with fatigue or nausea as the first sign. Alternatively, patients with known pregnancy can present with dizziness due to anemia, any cause of hypotension, or neurologic conditions such as cerebral venous thrombosis, arterial infarction, or intracranial hemorrhage.

10 Pain and Headache

E. Lee Murray, MD and
Karl E. Misulis, MD, PhD

CHAPTER CONTENTS

- Overview
  - Localization and Diagnosis of Pain Syndromes
  - Psychology of Pain
- Headache
  - Overview
  - Evaluation
    - Headache Scenarios
    - When to Obtain Neuroimaging
    - Laboratory Testing
    - Lumbar Puncture
  - Differential Diagnosis
- Neuropathic Pain
  - Clinical Scenarios
  - Management of Neuropathic Pain
  - Compressive Neuropathies
  - Surgical Injuries
  - Needle and Catheter Injuries
- Spine Pain
  - General Principles of Spine Pain
  - Spine Pain Syndromes
- Chronic Pain Syndromes
- Nonorganic Pain
- Role of the Hospital Neurologist

OVERVIEW

Pain can be classified into different types that have anatomic, physiologic, and symptomatic distinctions:

- *Neuropathic*
  FEATURES: Shooting, stabbing, or burning; abnormal perception of temperature
  CAUSE: Neuropathy from any cause, tumor infiltration, ischemia

- *Visceral*
  FEATURES: Deep steady pain especially abdominal or pelvic, often with intermittent paroxysms
  CAUSE: Distortion or distension, ischemia, infiltration
- *Muscular*
  FEATURES: Deep muscular-area pain that may be crampy and movement-related
  CAUSE: Trauma, inflammation, ischemia
- *Skeletal*
  FEATURES: Bone-area pain, often deep and with activity-dependent exacerbations
  CAUSE: Trauma, arthritis, ischemia, tumor
- *Vascular*
  FEATURES: Aching pain with tenderness
  CAUSE: Ischemia from occlusive disease, inflammation

Neuropathic pain has a character that depends on the involved nerves but also on the nerve types:

- *Large-fiber neuropathic pain* is typically shooting or stabbing. Large-fiber pain may be associated with cutaneous sensory loss, but may be less noticeable than the sensory deficit of small-fiber neuropathy.
- *Small-fiber pain* is more steady, dull, aching or burning. Small-fiber neuropathic pain is often accompanied by impaired sensation of pain and temperature.

Neuropathic pain syndromes encountered in hospital practice can include:

- *Peripheral neuropathy*: Diabetic peripheral neuropathy is the most common cause and is usually characterized by distal burning pain and sensory loss.
- *Mononeuropathy*: Compression or infarction of single nerves can cause both small- and large-fiber pain in the distribution of the nerve.
- *Plexopathy*: Compression, section, infiltration, or inflammation of either the lumbosacral or brachial plexus can cause prominent pain and often weakness.
- *Cranial nerve pain*: Trigeminal neuralgia is the most common cranial nerve pain. Glossopharyngeal neuralgia is occasionally seen.

Muscular pain can be generated in the muscle fibers, associated nerves, or surrounding tissues. Some of the most common syndromes of muscle pain are:

- *Muscle cramp*: Often this is precipitated by a specific movement. There is often palpable muscle contraction with the cramp. Causes are many, from local muscle and innervating nerve damage to inflammation. Generalized or multifocal cramps often have a metabolic cause.
- *Muscle pain with exertion*: Muscle pain and cramp is common after exertion, even in athletes. This can be exacerbated by coexistent fluid or electrolyte disturbance.

Pain may bridge some of the subdivisions; for example, limb injury may result in a combination of muscular, skeletal, and neuropathic pain.

Localization and Diagnosis of Pain Syndromes

Localization and characterization of the pain are essential to diagnosis; for example, headache can have vascular or inflammatory features, but within those categories there are multiple etiologies. Some important classifications are presented in Table 10.1.

Psychology of Pain

Acute and chronic pain have distinct effects on the psychological makeup of patients.

Table 10.1 Localization of pain syndromes

Disorder	Type	Features	Etiologies
Headache	Vascular	Migrainous headache with throbbing of steady headache, often associated with nausea and/or photophobia	Migraine Temporal arteritics Dissection
	Inflammatory	Steady pain, often severe, with pain with motion of the neck	Infectious meningitis, encephalitis, neoplastic meningitis
	Increased intracranial pressure	Holocephalic pain sometimes with visual disturbance	Tumor, infection, pseudotumor cerebri
Limb pain	Bone origin	Aching pain centered in bony elements often worse with weight-bearing or change in position	Trauma, tumor
	Muscle origin	Aching and/or cramping pain in muscular area often worse with activation of affected muscle(s)	Trauma, inflammation,
	Nerve origin	Lancinating and/or steady pain, usually over a defined cutaneous distribution	Neuropathy from any cause, trauma
Spine pain	Bone origin	Aching or crushing pain worse with weight-bearing and torsion	Arthritis, trauma, tumor
	Nerve origin	Local pain with radiation in the segmental distribution	Cord or cauda equina compression Nerve root compression
	Muscle origin	Steady paraspinal pain worse with standing and movement	Strain, trauma

Chronic pain: Chronic pain often produces affective disturbance, anxiety, and/or depression. Psychological response to chronic pain can be an impediment to effective pain management.

Pain without identified pathology: Limitations in diagnostic capabilities may result in misattribution of pain as being of nonorganic origin, but pain in the absence of detectable disease or pain exceeding expected symptoms raises the possibility of a psychological component to the pain.

HEADACHE
Overview

While most headache patients will present in an outpatient setting, headache remains a frequent reason for ED visits. Many times, ED physicians will manage the work-up and treatment of headache, but the neurologist may be consulted for patients with refractory headache, sudden severe headache, atypical features of headache, or those associated with abnormal neuroimaging, focal signs, or seizure.

Evaluation

Primary versus secondary headache: Primary headaches, such as migraine, cluster, and tension headache, are not related to underlying pathology. Secondary headaches are a manifestation of an underlying pathology, such as a tumor, stroke, infection, or other etiology. Features suggestive of secondary headaches should be red flags:

- Change in headache type
- Sudden onset of new headache
- Sudden severe headache
- Headache associated with positional changes
- Headache after trauma
- New headache over the age of 50
- Abnormal neurological examination
- Fever
- Nuchal rigidity
- Seizure
- Mental status change

Headache Scenarios

Select scenarios seen in the ED or hospital setting include:

First severe headache without deficit: Usually migraine in younger patients. With severe headache, imaging with computed tomography (CT) is often needed and if subarachnoid hemorrhage (SAH) or meningitis is suspected then lumbar puncture (LP) is often needed.

Recurrent severe headache without deficit: If the patient has a history of migraine, cluster, or other recurrent headache and has a typical headache, then management is the focus. Not every headache needs imaging.

Headache with cognitive change: Stroke, SAH, hydrocephalus, encephalitis, or meningitis can be causes. Evaluation starts with brain imaging. LP should be considered even in the absence of fever.

Headache with focal deficit: Stroke is of principal concern, although migraine can also produce focal deficits. Imaging must be performed.

Headache with fever: Headache can be a component of many systemic illnesses, particularly viral syndromes. LP usually has to be done to look for meningitis.

Headache with rhinorrhea: A history of head trauma associated with rhinorrhea might point toward intracranial hypotension due to a CSF leak.

New-onset headache over the age of 50: Mass lesions or temporal arteritis (giant cell arteritis) should be considered.

Headache with cough or exertion: Often a sign of primary exertional headache; however, magnetic resonance imaging (MRI) of the brain along with imaging of the vascular structures is often needed.

When to Obtain Neuroimaging

Not all patients with headache need neuroimaging. Those with episodic headache without any atypical features and with a normal neurological examination usually do not need neuroimaging.

Neuroimaging is usually indicated when the diagnosis is not known, and especially if the features suggest a serious etiology. Some of these features include:

- Sudden onset of severe headache (thunderclap)
- Headache associated with fever and/or systemic illness
- Change in personality
- Headache associated with seizure
- Headache associated with a focal neurological examination finding
- Headache exacerbated with positional changes
- Papilledema
- New onset headache over the age of 50
- Changes in headache pattern

Neuroimaging modality depends on the overall clinical presentation. Those with acute neurological change should usually start with an urgent noncontrast CT of the head. Those with more subacute/chronic presentation or nondiagnostic CT will likely need MRI.

Laboratory Testing

Complete blood count (CBC) should be done in those patients with fever or possible immunocompromised state looking for any leukocytosis or anemia. Thrombocytosis can cause a hypercoagulable state, which can lead to venous occlusions and thus headache.

Erythrocyte sedimentation rate (ESR) and *C-reactive protein (CRP)* should be obtained on every patient over the age of 50 presenting with headache. While these tests are not specific, significant elevations can point to possible temporal arteritis.

Arterial blood gases (ABG) can be obtained in those patients with respiratory issues. Hypoxia and/or hypercapnia can cause headache.

Lumbar Puncture

LP should be considered in patients who present these headache scenarios:

- Fever with the headache
- Mental status changes with headache
- Signs of a systemic process, such as inflammation
- Thunderclap headache if CT is negative for SAH or other structural etiology

LP should usually be performed after neuroimaging has been performed and no mass lesions have been identified.

Differential Diagnosis

Specific conditions are discussed in Chapter 20 unless otherwise indicated.

Migraine with or without aura produces pain that can be unilateral or bilateral, regional or global. Character is often throbbing with scalp tenderness. Associated symptoms are often nausea, vomiting, photophobia, or phonophobia. Visual changes such as flashing lights, kaleidoscope effects, or heat wave sensations are often described in migraine. Migraine often has a crescendo worsening of pain over the 20- to 30-minute period. Patients usually prefer a quiet dark environment during the headache.

Cluster headache is often seen in middle-aged males. Headaches are often unilateral and associated with severe stabbing-type pain in conjunction with conjunctival injection, unilateral tearing, or rhinorrhea. In contrast to migraine patients, cluster patients are often very anxious and seek activity as an ameliorating intervention. Alcohol can often exacerbate cluster-type headaches.

Primary stabbing headache is a rare form of headache that is characterized by sudden sharp (stabbing) pain often in a consistent location, typically in the distribution of the first division of the trigeminal nerve. Although the pain is intense, the duration is often just a few seconds.

Primary exertional/sexual headache is a rare headache that will often present to the ED due to the circumstances surrounding the headache and the severe/intense nature of the headache. Exertional headache occurs most often with strenuous activity and seems to be more common in hot and/or high-altitude environments. Sexual headache often becomes most intense near or at the time of orgasm. Both headaches are described as intense throbbing headache that is often the worst the patient has ever experienced. Patients warrant neuroimaging of the brain and cerebrovasculature. Indomethacin can be effective in these headaches.

Other presentations include:

Short-lasting unilateral neuralgiform headache with conjunctival injection and tearing (SUNCT): Unilateral headache is characterized by severe, short-lasting (seconds) headache that is associated with tearing and conjunctival injection. Lidocaine or phenytoin have been helpful for some patients. Select anticonvulsants are helpful. Indomethacin does not help.

Paroxysmal hemicrania: Similar presentation as SUNCT; however, headaches are longer lasting and often occur consistently on the same side of the head. Tearing, conjunctival injection, and rhinorrhea are often associated. Headaches are typically responsive to indomethacin.

Occipital neuralgia: Pain originating from the posterior portion of the head with radiation over the convexity. Typically exacerbated by palpitation of the greater and/or lesser occipital grooves. Pain is often improved with occipital nerve blocks.

Temporal arteritis: This should be considered and ruled out in any patient over 50 presenting with a headache. Headache is often unilateral, temporal, or periorbital but may be more extensive. Associated symptoms can include jaw claudication, visual changes, weight loss, malaise, ischemic optic neuropathy, and joint pains/polymyalgia rheumatica.

Pseudotumor cerebri: Most commonly seen in obese female of childbearing age. Diagnosis is made based on findings of optic nerve swelling on funduscopic examination, normal neuroimaging, and evidence of increased intracranial pressure over 25 cm H_2O during LP. Symptoms include severe headaches, blurred vision, and possibly CN 6 nerve palsy.

Cerebral venous thrombosis (CVT): This should be considered in patients presenting with a possible hypercoagulable state with new-onset headache, seizure, focal weakness, or other signs of increased intracranial pressure. Pregnancy and the postpartum state predispose to CVT. (Chapter 16)

Intracranial hemorrhage: Any patient with an acute headache with mental status changes, focal weakness, and/or seizure activity should undergo immediate CT imaging of the head to rule out any intracranial hemorrhagic process. Those patients with a posterior fossa hemorrhage will often present with nausea, vomiting, and ataxia. (Chapter 16)

Cerebral ischemia/Transient ischemic attack (TIA): A small percentage of ischemic stroke patients experience headache along with a focal neurological deficit. Headache along with neck or facial pain should also raise a concern for a possible cervicocephalic arterial dissection. (Chapter 16)

Meningitis: Central nervous system infections should be considered in patients with headaches associated with mental status changes, fever, neck stiffness, cranial neuropathy, or seizure activity. (Chapter 17)

Intracranial hypotension: Patients presenting with marked positional nature to the headache and resolution in a supine position, should be evaluated for low-pressure headache, often from a CSF leak. (Chapter 26)

Acute glaucoma: Can present acutely as orbital headache, often exacerbated by eye movement, blurred vision, pupil changes. Glaucoma should be considered in patients with acute headache who are taking topiramate.[1]

Cerebral mass lesion: Headache from a mass lesion, either tumor or abscess, will likely present in a subacute manner. However, patients are often seen in the ED due to associated focal weakness, cranial nerve abnormality, severe worsening of the headache due to hemorrhage, and/or seizure activity. (Chapter 25)

NEUROPATHIC PAIN

Neuropathic pain rarely necessitates hospitalization, but patients may have symptoms while in the hospital for unrelated issues. Some of the painful scenarios of neuropathic pain that we are asked to consult include:

- Diabetic neuropathy
- Peripheral nerve or plexus injury
- Radicular pain
- Trigeminal neuralgia (Chapter 20)
- Glossopharyngeal neuralgia (Chapter 33)
- Herpes zoster and postherpetic neuralgia (Chapter 17)

Clinical Scenarios

Acute neural injury: Neuropathic pain from injury can be from trauma precipitating admission or hospital-related injury. Inpatients are particularly susceptible to compressive neuropathies, needle-stick injuries, plexus injuries from direct exploration, or bleeding into the region of the plexus. Bleeding into the region of the nerves or plexus can occur from extravasation of blood around the site of an arterial stick, such as for angiography.

Cancer-related neuropathic pain: Cancer patients can develop multifocal radicular pain from neoplastic meningitis. Tumors can also directly infiltrate peripheral nerves or plexus, often causing severe neuropathic pain. Bone metastases can result in collapse, indirectly producing neuropathic pain. These are discussed in Chapter 25.

Spine disease: Painful radiculopathy from spinal degenerative disease can precipitate admission to facilitate rapid diagnosis and for pain control. Radiculopathy is most likely in the lumbar region, followed by the cervical region and, more rarely, by the thoracic region.

Idiopathic: Neuropathic pain in the absence of injury can be one of the painful idiopathic cranial nerve syndromes. These are discussed in Chapter 33.

Diabetic neuropathy: The distal burning pain of diabetic neuropathy is seldom a reason for inpatient consultation, but it is important to differentiate chronic neuropathy from a superimposed developing syndrome such as acute inflammatory demyelinating polyneuropathy (AIDP) or toxic neuropathy (e.g., chemotherapy- or antibiotic-related).

Trigeminal neuralgia: Lancinating pain in the distribution of the trigeminal nerve; this condition is discussed in Chapter 20.

Postherpetic neuralgia: This neuropathic pain in the distribution of a nerve root previously affected by herpes zoster is discussed in Chapter 17.

Management of Neuropathic Pain

MANAGEMENT of neuropathic pain usually consists of medications plus physical therapy.[2] Agents usually used for neuropathic pain include:

- Antiepileptic drugs (AEDs): especially gabapentin, pregabalin, carbamazepine, oxcarbazepine

- Antidepressants: especially tricyclic antidepressants (TCAs) and serotonin norepi-nephrine reuptake inhibitors (SNRIs)
- Muscle relaxants: especially baclofen and tizanidine
- Analgesics: wide range of opiates and nonopiates

Muscle relaxants are used for neuropathic pain even in the absence of muscle spasm or rigidity.

Analgesics used should be nonopiate if possible. If opiates are used, transition to sustained-release preparations may be appropriate.

Antidepressants are used because some have a specific effect on neuropathic pain in addition to a benefit for patients who have depression along with their pain. TCAs are often effective at doses that are subtherapeutic for depression.

Compressive Neuropathies

Compressive neuropathies in the hospital can be of almost any type, but there is a particular propensity to peroneal (fibular) and ulnar compression when patients are bed-bound. In addition, nutritional deficiencies in hospitalized patients exacerbate a number of conditions including neuropathies.

PRESENTATION is usually with decreased sensation and often pain in the affected distribution. Weakness may occur with more severe compression but might not be noted initially.

Surgical Injuries

Direct surgical injuries to peripheral nerves are uncommon. Neuropathic pain can be an associated problem, although the duration is usually limited. Medical and possibly surgical therapy may be needed, but these conditions often improve spontaneously. These are discussed in more detail in Chapter 12.

Needle and Catheter Injuries

Needle stick can directly impale a nerve or cause bleeding in the region of the nerve. Unless the patient is sedated, direct needle stick injuries of nerves are exquisitely painful from the onset. If pain begins some hours or days later, then direct stick was not the cause. Hematoma or blood extravasation produces pain that develops some minutes or hours after the event. Some of the more common needle stick neural injuries are:

- *Gluteal IM injection*: Sciatic nerve injury; this should be largely avoidable with attention to technique.
- *Arterial line placement in the wrist*: Medial or radial nerve injury
- *Phlebotomy in the antecubital fossa*: Medial or lateral antebrachial cutaneous nerves
- *Phlebotomy at the wrist*: Superficial radial nerve
- *Phlebotomy at the hand*: Dorsal sensory branches
- *Catheterization of the femoral artery*: Femoral nerve

SPINE PAIN

Spine pain is usually in the cervical or lumbar region, occasionally in the thoracic region. Differential diagnosis is discussed here, and specific disorders are discussed predominately in Chapter 24.

General Principles of Spine Pain

Generators of pain in the spine region are bone, paraspinal muscles, and nerves. Neural elements include spinal cord, nerve roots, and surrounding nerves. Relative contributions to the pain depend on the localization, and localization can depend on the character of pain:

- *Bone pain*: Poorly localized steady pain
- *Muscular pain*: Regional, steady, often cramping pain
- *Neural pain*: Usually well-localized burning, shooting, or stabbing pain

Spine Pain Syndromes

Musculoskeletal spine pain: Pathology in the vertebral body elements can be associated with tightness and cramping pain of the paraspinal muscles. Radicular symptoms and signs are absent unless accompanied by neural compression or destruction. Causes can include degenerative, traumatic, neoplastic, or inflammatory etiologies.

Cervical radiculopathy: Pain from the neck radiating into the arm, sometimes with weakness. Pain and deficit often do not have a simultaneous onset.

Lumbar radiculopathy: Pain from the low back radiating into the leg, sometimes with weakness. Pain and deficit often do not have a simultaneous onset.

Thoracic radiculopathy: Pain and sensory disturbance in a thoracic dermatome; common etiologies include herpes zoster (shingles), diabetes, thoracic disc, bony compression, and tumor. Degenerative causes are less likely than in the cervical and lumbar spine.

Conus medullaris syndrome: Compression or infiltration of the conus medullaris usually presents with back pain, leg weakness, and incontinence.

Cauda equina syndrome: Compression of the nerve roots below the conus medullaris commonly produces back and leg pain, ultimately progressing to weakness of the legs and incontinence.

Infectious meningitis: Inflammatory involvement affects the meninges and nerve roots. Chronic meningitis is especially likely to produce cranial nerve and nerve root symptoms and signs.

Neoplastic meningitis: Tumor involvement of the CSF with involvement of the meninges can cause nerve root pain and motor and/or sensory deficits.

CHRONIC PAIN SYNDROMES

Chronic pain management is beyond the scope of this book and usually is not the province of the hospital neurologist. The care given during hospitalization should be sufficient to control pain enough to make discharge possible, and the patient should be set up with a comprehensive pain management program.

MANAGEMENT of chronic pain is usually multimodal, using a combination of medications, therapy, and psychological counseling. Patients must have realistic expectations.

Sources of information on comprehensive pain management can be found in the notes to this chapter.[3,4] Some brief guidelines include:

- *Antidepressants* are often used for their effect especially on neuropathic pain but also to treat the depression that accompanies chronic pain in many patients.[5] Patients with depression tend to have poorer outcomes and higher disability scores. For patients with neuropathic pain, TCAs are particularly helpful for pain from small-fiber neuropathy (e.g., diabetic neuropathy).
- *Analgesics* are almost always used. In general, these are used in a controlled fashion, and, if narcotics are used, a contract should be established with close monitoring of use. Sustained-release formulations should be considered where appropriate.
- *Antiepileptic drugs (AEDs)* are often used for neuropathic pain. Large-fiber neuropathic pain is often treated with AEDs, including carbamazepine, oxcarbazepine, gabapentin, or pregabalin.
- *Smoking cessation* is recommended for almost all patients with nonmalignant pain. There is evidence that smoking makes pain more likely to be chronic, and smoking cessation may reduce the chronicity of pain.[6,7]

Cancer pain is treated differently than nonmalignant pain. Since many of these patients are expected to have progressive disease and have a limited life expectancy, we are more liberal about our use of analgesics. However, the non-narcotic options should be considered also since they may allow the patient to be more alert and thereby enjoy a better quality of life.

NONORGANIC PAIN

Pain is a subjective sensation, so proving that a report of pain is unreal is almost impossible. With nonorganic pain, neurologic workup usually reveals no likely source of pain that would be expected to produce the reported symptoms. Neuropsychological testing is performed on many patients with chronic pain and can help identify individuals who have psychological factors at least as a component of their pain.

ROLE OF THE HOSPITAL NEUROLOGIST

The role of the hospital neurologist in pain management depends on the capabilities and interests of the neurologist. Many pain specialists do not keep an active hospital practice, so pain management falls on the hospital attending, with assistance from neurology and anesthesiology. Our role is usually twofold: to identify the source of the pain and to advise on effective treatment.

SECTION III
NEUROLOGIC DIAGNOSES

SECTION CONTENTS

11 Neurologic Complications in Medical Patients
12 Neurologic Complications in Surgical Patients
13 Neurologic Manifestations of Systemic Disease
14 Hypoxic-Ischemic Encephalopathy
15 Brain Death and Persistent Vegetative State
16 Vascular Disease
17 Infectious Diseases
18 Cognitive Disorders
19 Seizures and Epilepsy
20 Headache
21 Neuromuscular Disorders
22 Demyelinating Diseases
23 Movement Disorders
24 Spinal Cord Disorders
25 Neuro-Oncology
26 CSF Circulation Disorders
27 Pregnancy and Neurology
28 Endocrine Disorders
29 Nutritional Deficiencies and Toxicities
30 Neurotoxicology
31 Neuro-Ophthalmology
32 Neuro-Otology
33 Cranial Nerve Disorders
34 Autonomic Disorders
35 Traumatic Brain Injury
36 Sleep Disorders
37 Developmental and Genetic Disorders
38 Psychiatric Disorders

11 Neurologic Complications in Medical Patients

Karl E. Misulis, MD, PhD and
E. Lee Murray, MD

CHAPTER CONTENTS

- Overview
- Infections
  - Sepsis and SIRS
  - Encephalopathy
  - Seizures
  - Focal Deficit
- Cancers
  - Local Tumor Invasion
  - Metastases
  - Paraneoplastic Disorders
  - Metabolic Effects
  - Cerebrovascular Disease
  - Neurologic Complications of Cancer Treatment
- Diabetes Mellitus
  - Stroke and Transient Ischemic Attack
  - Neuropathy
  - Hypoglycemia and Hyperglycemia
- Cardiac Disease
  - Stroke in Patients Admitted for Cardiac Disease
  - Confusion After Cardiac Catheterization
- Renal Disease
- Hepatic Disease
- Rheumatologic Disease
- Hypertension
  - Hypertensive Emergency
  - Posterior Reversible Encephalopathy Syndrome
- Neuromuscular Disorders
  - Critical Illness Neuromyopathy
  - Mononeuropathies
  - Botulism

OVERVIEW

This chapter presents a review of some of the most important neurologic complications seen in hospitalized patients. An issue of *Continuum* was devoted to this topic.[1]

INFECTIONS

Systemic infections predispose to neurologic complications by metabolic, ischemic, and direct inflammatory effects. Most patients with neurologic complications have *sepsis* or *systemic inflammatory response syndrome* (SIRS).

Sepsis and SIRS

SIRS is usually but not invariably due to infection, other causes being ischemia, trauma, burns, and inflammation due to autoimmune and other reasons. SIRS is defined as having at least two of the following[2]:

- Temperature of at least 38°C or less than 36°C
- Heart rate of greater than 90 beats per minute.
- Respiratory rate of more than 20 breaths per minute or a $PaCO_2$ of less than 32 mm Hg.
- WBC of greater than 12,000/µL or less than 4,000/µL or immature (bands) at greater than 10%.

Sepsis is defined as at least two SIRS criteria, and the cause is known or suspected infection.

Severe sepsis is defined as sepsis with acute organ dysfunction caused by the sepsis, usually from hypotension and hypoperfusion. Organ dysfunctions can include altered mental status.

Septic shock is defined as sepsis with persistent or refractory hypotension or tissue hypoperfusion despite adequate fluid resuscitation.

Multiorgan dysfunction syndrome (MODS) is defined as the presence of organ dysfunction in an acutely ill patient such that homeostasis cannot be maintained without intervention.

Neurologic complications are most prominent with increasing severity of the sepsis.

Encephalopathy

Encephalopathy is the most common neurologic complication of systemic infections and SIRS. Mild confusion from urinary tract infections (UTIs) or other infections is often overlooked initially.

PRESENTATION of the encephalopathy can begin with delirium, with difficulties with attention, disorientation, and confusion. Lethargy may develop, especially with metabolic derangements from the underlying condition. The disorder may progress to coma.

DIAGNOSIS is clinical, but the specific label of *septic encephalopathy* is given when other diagnoses have been eliminated.

Differential Diagnosis

Differential diagnoses to consider include:

- Metabolic encephalopathy
- Meningitis
- Encephalitis
- Brain abscess
- Nonconvulsive seizures
- CNS infarction
- CNS hemorrhage

Studies which should be considered include:

- *Computed tomography (CT) of the brain*: For possible infarction, hemorrhage, or abscess
- *Magnetic resonance imaging (MRI) of the brain*: If MRI is possible, it is more sensitive than CT for structural lesions, but it cannot be done in some ICU patients and in those with a permanent pacemaker (PPM) or many other devices.
- *Electroencephalogram (EEG)*: For encephalopathy and for identification of focal or nonconvulsive seizure activity
- *Lumbar puncture (LP)*: To evaluate cerebrospinal fluid (CSF) for meningitis or encephalitis
- *MRI of spine*: For possibility of epidural abscess
- *Labs*: for a wide range of metabolic, inflammatory, and infectious markers

Nonconvulsive seizure in critically ill patients is underdiagnosed. Patients with nonconvulsive seizures are usually lethargic or minimally responsive.

Meningitis can be missed or diagnosed late. Although hospital-acquired bacterial meningitis is uncommon in a patient who has not had CNS instrumentation, a patient admitted with presumed pneumonia or other systemic infection with mild delirium may ultimately be found to have meningitis.

Encephalitis may present with nonspecific symptoms initially, and, if the patient is found in the ED to have a UTI or other systemic infectious source, diagnosis of encephalitis may be delayed until more dramatic neurologic findings develop, such as marked encephalopathy, seizures, or focal signs.

Lumbar epidural abscess can rarely present with encephalopathy with systemic signs of infection.[3] MRI of the spine may be indicated, especially if there is a history of spine pain or if the patient has limb weakness in a distribution suggesting a cord lesion.

Seizures

Seizures in the ICU can be convulsive or nonconvulsive. Seizures in a patient with SIRS or sepsis can be due to CNS infection or vascular disease. Also, some antibiotics, such as cefepime and meropenem,[4] predispose to seizures. Renal insufficiency increases the risk of medication-induced seizures, as does renal failure itself.

PRESENTATION of seizures in the ICU can be generalized motor, focal motor, multifocal motor, or subtle. Patients with marked unresponsiveness without an obvious cause on labs and imaging should be evaluated by EEG for *nonconvulsive status epilepticus* (NCSE).

DIAGNOSIS of seizure is obvious with marked motor activity, but can be suspected by subtle motor activity, spontaneous nystagmus, or unexplained encephalopathy.

The differential diagnosis of seizures with systemic infection includes:

- Medication-induced seizure
- CNS infarct or hemorrhage
- CNS infection: Abscess, meningitis, encephalitis
- Metabolic: Hepatic or renal failure or electrolyte abnormality
- Cessation or dose reduction of anticonvulsant in a patient with known seizure disorder
- Hypoxia or hypoperfusion due to hypotension or profound anemia

Studies can include:

- MRI brain for structural lesion
- CT brain if MRI cannot be performed
- EEG for focal slowing and/or epileptiform discharges
- Long-term EEG monitoring
- CSF for meningitis or encephalitis.
- Labs for metabolic abnormalities

Long-term EEG monitoring is increasingly available in hospitals with neurology services, either as a mobile EEG device or with at least two channels on bedside monitors. An EEG machine with video capture is preferable; this may obviate transfer to an epilepsy monitoring unit (EMU).

CSF analysis should be obtained for most patients with seizure and sepsis unless there is another definite cause (e.g., cerebral infarction, abscess). Even then, septic emboli or meningitis should be considered.

Focal Deficits

Focal deficits are occasionally seen in patients with sepsis, but they may be missed because of encephalopathy. Focality can be due to a host of etiologies, but principal concern is focal structural lesion or the rare possibility of focal nonconvulsive discharge. Pre-existing (i.e. not acute) neurologic lesion is a common cause of focal findings in this setting.

PRESENTATION is of a patient with sepsis or SIRS noted to have weakness of one or more limbs or the face. Anatomic localization guides diagnostic study:

- *Cerebral lesions*: Hemiparesis or monoparesis
- *Cervical spine lesion*: Unilateral or bilateral arm weakness and often associated leg weakness
- *Cord lesion below the cervical spine*: Bilateral leg weakness

- *Peri-vertebral or plexus lesion* (e.g., abscess): Unilateral arm or leg motor and/or sensory deficit, usually with significant pain

DIAGNOSIS is suspected by any focal deficit in a patient with sepsis or SIRS, and clinical anatomic localization directs the diagnostic studies.

Studies that may be indicated include:

- *MRI or CT brain*: Hemiparesis
- *MRI spine*: Paraparesis or quadriparesis
- *Nerve conduction studies (NCS) and EMG*: Weakness involving all extremities with or without the face.
- *EEG*: Focal weakness without a structural etiology
- *LP*: Focal or multifocal weakness without structural etiology
- *MRI brachial plexus*: Unilateral arm weakness
- *MRI lumbosacral plexus*: Unilateral leg weakness

Plexus lesion[5] is suspected by prominent pain that involves the extremity more than the spine. Spinal lesions producing unilateral limb symptoms usually have significant regional spine pain and also are likely to have a distribution restricted to one or two dermatomal levels, whereas plexus lesions are more likely to span at least two or three dermatomal distributions.

CANCERS

Most neurologic complications related to cancer that we see are from metastases, but remote effects are the most difficult to diagnose.

The role of the hospital neurologist is largely to help with localization and diagnosis in these patients and to help with management of the neurologic complications of cancers: e.g. pain, seizure, altered mental status, cerebral edema. The hospital neurologist can also help to direct and facilitate therapy especially when time is of the essence (e.g., cord compression or malignant cerebral edema). Management of neurologic complications of cancer is discussed in Chapter 25.

Cancers can present to the neurologist through the following basic mechanisms:

- Local tumor invasion
- Metastases
- Remote effects of cancer (e.g., paraneoplastic syndromes)
- Metabolic effects (e.g., hypercalcemia)
- Secondary effects of cancer and treatment (e.g., sepsis, abscess, radiation plexopathy)

Differential diagnosis of a neurologic abnormality can be narrowed by classification of the features:

- Hemiparesis
  - Cerebral metastasis
  - Brain abscess
  - Stroke

- Monoparesis
  - Cerebral metastasis
  - Plexopathy from tumor invasion or radiation
  - Spinal metastasis
- Paraparesis
  - Metastasis to the vertebral column with cord compression
  - Metastasis to the vertebral column with bony collapse
  - Meningeal carcinomatosis
  - Paraneoplastic myelitis
- Quadriparesis
  - Tumor affecting upper cervical spine
  - Acute inflammatory demyelinating polyneuropathy (AIDP)
  - Paraneoplastic encephalomyelitis
- Confusion without focal signs
  - Multifocal metastases
  - Metastasis producing hydrocephalus
  - Metabolic effect (e.g., electrolyte, hepatic, renal encephalopathy)
  - Sepsis
  - Limbic encephalitis
  - Paraneoplastic encephalomyelitis
- Diffuse weakness
  - Paraneoplastic peripheral neuropathy (e.g., AIDP)
  - Lambert-Eaton myasthenic syndrome
  - Chemotherapy-induced peripheral neuropathy
  - Myasthenia gravis (with thymoma)

Stroke is particularly common with lung, pancreatic, and colorectal cancers and occurs generally within the first 3 months from diagnosis, when the patient is in the midst of chemotherapy and/or radiation. Patients with lung cancer have a relative risk of stroke of more than 4.[6]

AIDP has been described in patients with cancer, especially small-cell lung cancer.[7] This is believed to be a paraneoplastic syndrome. *CIDP* may have a paraneoplastic association.[8,9]

Paraneoplastic encephalomyelitis can produce cerebral and/or spinal involvement. There are also other related autoimmune conditions well presented in the paper by McKeon.[10] Some of these are discussed in the Chapters 22 and 25.

Local Tumor Invasion

Neurologic presentation of local tumor invasion is usually from one of the following mechanisms:

- Nerve compression and infiltration
- Spine or skull invasion
- Vascular compromise

Opportunity for local tumor invasion depends on location. Paraspinal tumors can invade the vertebrae and either directly compress nerve roots and spinal cord (e.g., lymphoma) or cause vertebral collapse with resultant neural compression.

Lung cancer of the upper lobes can directly invade the lower brachial plexus, as opposed to radiation plexopathy which tends to affect the upper plexus, since there is less surrounding tissue to attenuate radiation.

Lumbosacral plexus infiltration can occur from a variety of tumors including gastrointestinal, gynecological, and urological cancers.[11] These can, in turn, have intradural extension.

Metastases

Metastases to the brain and spine are much more common than primary tumors of the neuraxis. The most common primary tumor sources for brain metastases are lung, breast, gastrointestinal, renal, and melanoma.[12]

PRESENTATION can include headache, focal neurologic deficit, mental status change, and seizure.

- *Headache* is by far the single most common symptom and, in a patient with known cancer, should trigger evaluation for metastasis before development of other symptoms.
- *Focal deficit* can be progressive or acute in onset and can be of almost any localization. Gradual progression suggests expanding mass effect. Acute change suggests infarction or hemorrhage. Intracranial hemorrhage can occur with many types of cancers but suggests melanoma, lung, renal, or thyroid cancer.
- *Seizures* raise the concern for brain tumor at all ages, although this as a cause is relatively unlikely in the absence of known malignancy.
- *Asymptomatic metastases are common.* Up to a third of brain metastases can be asymptomatic,[13] yet the prognosis for survival is poor after diagnosis.

Diagnosis is best done by MRI of the brain with contrast. If MRI cannot be done, then CT of the brain with contrast is an alternative. Positron emission tomography (PET) is not an optimal study for identification of brain metastases, having a 25% false-negative rate and a 17% false-positive rate.[14]

Spine metastases are the third most common site for metastasis after the lung and liver. Primary cancers include lung, breast, prostate, biliary, hematologic including myeloma, and thyroid.[15] Most of these tumors are adenocarcinomas. Spine metastases commonly produce spine pain and weakness of the extremities appropriate to the level of the lesion.

Diagnosis of spine metastases is best with MRI spine with contrast. CT spine with contrast is performed if MRI is contraindicated; however, although MRI gives superior visualization of the neural elements, CT shows additional details of the bony elements and may need to be done along with the MRI. If MRI cannot be done, CT myelography can show details in the canal that plain CT cannot. For myelopathy, if no lesion is identified at the clinically identified level, then imaging must be done above the level of the lesion, including a brain scan if a midline cerebral lesion might fit the clinical presentation.

Meningeal metastases are most commonly seen in small-cell lung cancer, breast cancer, and melanoma.[16] Patients present with symptoms related to nerve root, spinal cord, cranial nerve, or cerebral involvement. Nerve root symptoms are usually pain and sometimes motor and sensory deficits in the nerve root distribution. Spinal cord involvement can produce pain near the segment of the metastasis, weakness from myelopathy or cauda equina involvement, and sphincter disturbance. Cranial nerve involvement produces diplopia with ocular motor (CN 3, 4, 6) involvement, facial weakness (CN 7), facial sensory change (CN 5), or almost any combination of cranial nerve deficits.

Diagnosis of meningeal metastases is suspected when a patient with cancer presents with cranial nerve or nerve root symptoms, myelopathy, or a cauda equina lesion. Confusion or behavioral disturbance in the absence of visible brain metastasis also raises concern for meningeal metastases.

MRI of the region of neurologic localization is performed with contrast and can visualize the metastases in approximately half of patients.[17] CSF analysis often shows malignant cells on cytology although high-volume analysis or repeated LPs may be needed to show this. Cell count is usually increased, protein is high, and glucose is often low. Very high protein levels suggest cord compression. Note that in patients with encephalopathy, symptoms and signs of myelopathy from cord compression can be subtle enough to be missed. Bone scans are sensitive for bony involvement but not for neurologic involvement.

Paraneoplastic Disorders

There are many paraneoplastic disorders affecting the nervous system. These are discussed in more depth in Chapter 25.

Lambert-Eaton myasthenic syndrome (LEMS) is a defect in neuromuscular transmission that can be a remote effect of cancer. Presentation is with progressive weakness, proximal more than distal. Bulbar muscles can be affected.

Paraneoplastic cerebellar degeneration is due to anti–Purkinje cell antibodies. Presentation is with vertigo and ataxia that affects both gait and appendicular coordination.

Paraneoplastic neuropathies affect sensory and autonomic function. If they present after treatment, they may be misdiagnosed as neuropathy from chemotherapy or nutritional causes.

Metabolic Effects

Patients with cancer are predisposed to neurologic complications due to a host of metabolic abnormalities that can include:

- Hepatic failure
- Renal failure
- Protein-calorie malnutrition
- Electrolyte abnormality
- Hypoxia/hypercarbia

These are discussed in detail in Chapters 13 and 29.

Cerebrovascular Disease

Stroke is more common in patients with cancer. Cancers can affect coagulation, as can chemotherapy and radiation therapy. This discussed further in Chapter 25.

- *Hypercoagulable state* can produce either arterial or venous infarction.
- *Thrombocytopenia* can produce intracerebral hemorrhage.
- *Metastases* of some tumors have a propensity to bleed, and the first sign of the metastasis may be the resultant intercerebral hemorrhage (ICH).
- *Radiation therapy* can produce secondary vascular changes that make stroke more likely.

Neurologic Complications of Cancer Treatment

Cancer treatment can have neurologic complications due to chemotherapy, radiation therapy, or surgery. Surgical complications are discussed in Chapter 12. Detailed discussion of neurologic complications of cancers is found in Chapter 25.

Chemotherapy neuropathy develops in response to a number of treatments including but not limited to vinca alkaloids, platinums, and taxanes. Neuropathy typically begins during chemotherapy and progresses with additional treatment.

Radiation vasculopathy predisposes to stroke, and this has been best described for children who received whole-brain radiation[18] and in patients with head and neck cancers who received radiation to the carotid region.[19]

Radiation plexopathy involves the brachial plexus, especially with lung but also breast cancer, and the lumbosacral plexus, especially with pelvic cancers. Presentation is with motor and/or sensory deficit with little or no pain.

Radiation myelopathy can be early or late. Presentation is with myelopathy with leg weakness and sensory loss. Often there is neuropathic pain.

Radiation cerebral edema can develop during the course of radiation therapy. Presentation is usually increased focal deficit and encephalopathy from increased intracranial pressure.

Neutropenia predisposes to uncontrolled infection and associated encephalopathy and weakness. Inflammatory change from neutropenic sepsis predisposes to vascular occlusion. In addition to bacterial infections, fungal and viral infections can occur.

DIABETES MELLITUS

Neurologic complications of diabetes mellitus (DM) are also discussed in Chapters 13 and 28.

Stroke and Transient Ischemic Attack

Stroke risk is increased at least threefold in patients with diabetes, even more in patients at middle age.[20] Outcome of stroke is substantially worse in patients with diabetes, with an incidence of mortality at least twice that of nondiabetics.

Stroke and transient ischemic attack (TIA) are discussed in Chapter 16. Diabetes risk should be assessed in every patient admitted with stroke who does not already have the diagnosis; a new diagnosis of DM is common during stroke/TIA admission. Of patients who already have diagnosed DM, good glycemic control may improve outcome, and education and encouragement on DM self-care further reduces the risk of recurrent stroke.

Neuropathy

Neuropathies due to DM are discussed in Chapters 21 and 28. DM is associated with:

- Polyneuropathy
- Mononeuropathy
- Mononeuropathy multiplex
- Ocular motor palsy
- Autonomic neuropathy
- Lumbar radiculoplexopathy (diabetic amyotrophy)

Diabetes should be considered in virtually all patients seen in the hospital with neuropathy.

Hypoglycemia and Hyperglycemia

Hypoglycemia usually produces altered mental status, progressing to lethargy and ultimately coma. If the duration of the hypoglycemia is prolonged, the damage can be irreversible (e.g., a patient not waking in the morning is found to be profoundly hypoglycemic). Seizures[21] are much less common. With milder hypoglycemia, exacerbation of migraines can be seen.[22]

Hyperglycemia can present as diabetic ketoacidosis (DKA), usually in type 1 diabetics, and as hyperosmolar hyperglycemic state (HHS), usually in type 2 diabetics.

- *DKA* is a state of hyperglycemia, ketosis, and metabolic acidosis. Medical presentation is usually with polyuria, polydipsia, and rapid weight loss. Neurologic presentation is usually altered mental status from confusion to lethargy and coma. Stroke syndromes, seizures, and posterior reversible encephalopathy syndrome (PRES) can occur with DKA.[23] Patients with these neurologic presentations will occasionally be identified with DKA in the ED.
- *HHS* occurs usually in older patients with known DM or may be the presenting manifestation of DM. Presentation is often neurologic with encephalopathy, which may range from confusion to lethargy to coma. Focal deficits can be seen that can suggest stroke. Seizures can occur and can be focal or generalized and can suggest encephalitis, especially if HHS occurs in the setting of a precipitant illness.

CARDIAC DISEASE

Neurologic complications of primary cardiac disease are common. Some of these include:

- *Focal deficit*: Usually from stroke due to atrial fibrillation, atrial or ventricular thrombus, embolus from a faulty valve, or right-to-left shunt

- *Brain abscess*: From subacute bacterial endocarditis (SBE)
- *Syncope*: From arrhythmia or other cardiac cause of hypotension
- *Hypoxic encephalopathy*: From cardiac arrest
- *Confusion*: From congestive heart failure (CHF), stroke

CHF is associated with cognitive decline that begins often with subtle memory difficulty and may progress to frank dementia.[24] While some of these cases are due to strokes, other mechanisms include reduced cerebral perfusion.[25] Patients with CHF are predisposed to decompensation with hospitalization and concurrent illness.

Stroke in Patients Admitted for Cardiac Disease

Stroke is more common in patients hospitalized with cardiac disease, either as a complication of their cardiac condition or procedure or because of coexistent cerebrovascular disease. Complications of cardiovascular surgery are discussed in Chapter 12. This discussion concerns neurologic complications not related to surgery.

Etiologies of stroke in patients hospitalized for cardiac reasons include:

- Valvular emboli
- Right-to-left shunt
- Cardiac catheterization
- Arrhythmia
- Aortic plaque with embolization.
- Subacute bacterial endocarditis
- Myocardial infarction

Patients with *acute myocardial infarction* (MI) are more likely than the general population to have stroke. Predictors of increased risk include diabetes, hypertension, advanced age, atrial fibrillation, heart failure, anterior location of MI, and history of prior stroke or MI.[26]

Diagnosis and management of stroke is discussed in detail in Chapter 16.

Confusion After Cardiac Catheterization

Confusion is common after cardiac catheterization. Some of the reasons can include:

- Stroke, especially multifocal
- Medications, especially sedatives and analgesics
- Contrast reaction
- Secondary metabolic abnormality (e.g., exacerbation of renal insufficiency after contrast)

At least 16% of patients admitted to the cardiac ICU develop delirium.[27] Onset is most commonly between 1.5 and 2.0 days, with a duration of about 1.5 days. No one etiology had been identified to cause the majority of delirium, but electrolyte abnormalities are most common.

PRESENTATION can be with lethargy or delirium. Focal findings are usually absent and, when present, suggest acute ischemic stroke (AIS) or ICH. Seizures can occur and can be subtle. A rare syndrome of contrast-induced neurotoxicity has been described, with confusion being the principal finding, but some patients have associated ophthalmoplegia, cerebellar ataxia, oocal motor deficits.[28]

DIAGNOSIS begins with basic labs for electrolyte abnormalities, brain imaging urgently with CT, and ultimately MRI if needed. LP is usually not needed unless subarachnoid hemorrhage (SAH) is suspected. EEG is appropriate if no other cause is identified or if the patient exhibits subtle symptoms suggesting seizure, such as nystagmus or facial or limb repetitive movement.

MANAGEMENT depends on the etiology. If no AIS or other acute neurologic event is identified, the goal should be to maintain good vital signs, avoiding hypotension or hypertension; normalize electrolytes and maintain appropriate fluid balance; avoid nonessential meds, including especially unnecessary sedatives and analgesics, and vigilance for concurrent illness.

RENAL DISEASE

Patients with renal insufficiency and failure are predisposed to a host of neurologic complications due to direct effects on metabolism plus the effects of associated conditions.[29] Reduced renal clearance not only produces metabolic changes directly contributing to encephalopathy, myoclonus, and seizure, but also reduces clearance of drugs. Stroke is more common, both ischemic and hemorrhagic, partly because of associated hypertension or diabetes. Complications of renal disease are discussed further in Chapter 13.

Neurologic consultation on hospitalized patients with renal insufficiency is often for one of the following reasons:

- Seizure in the dialysis unit; usually due to electrolyte changes
- Stroke, often precipitated by coexistent hypertension or diabetes
- Encephalopathy, usually from metabolic disorder such as worsening renal failure. Encephalopathy sometimes occurs with seizures, often as a component of *dialysis disequilibrium*, in which electrolyte and fluid changes produce a constellation of symptoms from cerebral edema including headache, nausea and vomiting, encephalopathy, and seizures.[30]

HEPATIC DISEASE

Hepatic failure is associated with neurologic complications which can be related to the accumulation of ammonia, manganese, and lactate; increased permeability of the blood–brain barrier; or a CNS inflammatory response.[31] Complications of hepatic disease are discussed further in Chapter 13. Common neurologic presentations include:

- Encephalopathy
- Asterixis
- Myoclonus
- Seizure

Asterixis is the most specific of these findings—outstretched arms and hands show episodic loss of maintained hand posture.

Encephalopathy with hepatic failure is generally screened for by ammonia level, but since this is not the only mediator, lack of ammonia elevation does not rule out the diagnosis.

Seizure can be treated with many antiepileptic drugs (AEDs) but generally avoided are those agents that have hepatic metabolism, such as valproate.

Less common neurologic complications include intracranial hemorrhage, CNS infection, and demyelination. Causes of hepatic insufficiency may have their own additional features (e.g., alcoholism that produces hepatic insufficiency plus Wernicke encephalopathy).

RHEUMATOLOGIC DISEASE

A host of rheumatologic conditions can be cause for neurologic consultation in the hospital, and a review in *Continuum* was devoted to this topic.[32] Among the most common are:

- Temporal arteritis/giant cell arteritis
- Systemic lupus erythematosus (SLE)
- Rheumatoid arthritis (RA)
- Scleroderma

Temporal arteritis or *giant cell arteritis* is a specific inflammatory change that prominently affects the temporal artery, although it is not confined to it. Neurologic presentation is temporal headache, thickened and tender temporal artery, and, if untreated, blindness from involvement of branches of the ophthalmic artery (see Chapter 20).

SLE predisposes to a host of neurologic complications, including:

- Stroke
- Encephalopathy
- Seizures
- PRES

Antiphospholipid antibody syndrome (APS) is often but not invariably associated with SLE and predisposes to stroke. Testing for APS should be considered in younger patients with stroke, especially in those with SLE but even in those without this diagnosis.

Rheumatoid arthritis (RA) can be associated with neuropathy. Some of this is due more to entrapment from deformation in the extremities than from entrapment in the spine. Vasculopathy associated with RA can also predispose to neuropathy. Stroke is more likely in patients with RA because of systemic inflammation and also because of the effects of corticosteroids used to treat the condition.[33]

Fibromyalgia and *chronic fatigue syndrome* are commonly treated by rheumatologists and are also seen by neurologists although seldom in the hospital setting; these conditions will not be considered further here.

Scleroderma or *systemic sclerosis* is an autoimmune condition with excessive deposition of connective tissue. Neurologic manifestations can include weakness from muscle involvement, facial pain from trigeminal involvement, carpal tunnel syndrome from median nerve involvement, or visual loss from retinal artery involvement.

Sjögren syndrome is an inflammatory condition of autoimmune pathogenesis. Most symptoms are non-neurologic, with xerostomia or xerophthalmia. Neuropathy and autonomic dysfunction can develop. PRES has been reported,[34] and optic neuropathy and other cranial neuropathies also have been rarely reported.[35]

HYPERTENSION

Hypertension predisposes to a variety of neurologic disorders, particularly cerebrovascular. We consider here two common reasons for neurologic consultation: *hypertensive emergency* and *PRES*. Closely related *eclampsia* is discussed in Chapter 27.

Hypertensive Emergency

Hypertensive emergencies occur when marked hypertension is associated with organ damage. The term *malignant hypertension* is sometimes used interchangeably. Blood pressure is at least 180/120 mm Hg and there are signs of organ damage, usually to eyes or kidneys. Ocular damage is manifest as papilledema, which may or may not be symptomatic; blurred vision or frank visual loss can occur. Renal damage is manifest by edema and laboratory findings indicating renal insufficiency. Other findings may be confusion and signs of pulmonary edema. Focal deficits suggest stroke, which can be ischemic or hemorrhagic, especially if mental status is normal. Focal deficit with encephalopathy may be a manifestation of hypertensive emergency without visible cerebrovascular occlusion.

All patients with hypertensive emergency are evaluated for renal and ocular function. CT or MRI brain scan is indicated if there are any neurologic deficits, whether encephalopathy or focal deficit.

Posterior Reversible Encephalopathy Syndrome

PRES can occur from hypertensive emergency, although there are nonhypertensive causes, including immunosuppressive agents, cancers,[36] chemotherapy, and renal insufficiency.[37] The term is a bit of a misnomer since the encephalopathy is not always posterior and not always reversible. This is discussed in detail in Chapter 13.

NEUROMUSCULAR DISORDERS

Neuromuscular disorders, such as myasthenia gravis or amyotrophic lateral sclerosis (ALS), can be exacerbated during hospitalization, but here we discuss disorders that are products of the hospitalization and concurrent illness. Neuromuscular disorders are discussed further in Chapter 21.

Critical Illness Neuromyopathy

An acute neuromyopathy can occur in patients who have had prolonged hospitalizations, especially those who have been critically ill, received high-dose corticosteroids, and/or undergone neuromuscular blockade. Patient will often have generalized weakness along with difficulty weaning from the ventilator. EMG/NCS can show evidence of both neurogenic and myopathic features. Other potential causes need to be ruled out, including structural lesions in the brain and spinal cord, such as infarct. Neuromuscular junction disorders such as myasthenia gravis should also be considered.

Mononeuropathies

Multiple causes for mononeuropathies can manifest in hospitalized patients. Among these are compressive neuropathies, operative injuries, damage from compartment syndromes, perineural bleeding, or inflammation. These are discussed in Chapters 12 and 21.

Botulism

Toxin is usually food-borne or develops in infected wounds. Presentation is with dry mouth, vomiting, and diarrhea along with cranial nerve involvement. Descending paralysis is then seen and continues to progress to involve respiratory muscles. This is discussed in Chapter 21.

12 Neurologic Complications in Surgical Patients

E. Lee Murray, MD and
Karl E. Misulis, MD, PhD

CHAPTER CONTENTS

- Common Events
- Surgery
  - Nerve Injuries
  - Orthopedic Surgery
  - Cardiovascular Surgery
  - Trauma
  - Transplant Patients
  - Bariatric Surgery
- Anesthesia
  - Delirium
  - Seizure
  - Malignant Hyperthermia
  - Prolonged Neuromuscular Paralysis
  - Myelopathy

COMMON EVENTS

Neurologic complications in surgical patients can be directly related to surgery, indirectly related to hospitalization, or related to exacerbation of underlying medical conditions. In addition, trauma patients requiring surgery may have had neural trauma as a component of their injury that may not be recognized at intake.

Some of the neurologic scenarios unrelated to surgical specialty are:

- Encephalopathy and delirium
- Stroke
- Seizure
- Withdrawal syndrome

Encephalopathy and delirium develop commonly especially in elderly patients and patients with pre-existing medical conditions who are hospitalized. This is commonly exacerbated by effects of sedative/hypnotics, sleep deprivation, protein-calorie deficit, and any of a host of other medications including antibiotics. Hospital delirium is further discussed in Chapter 18.

Stroke in the peri-operative period is most commonly ischemic but can be hemorrhagic.

- *Ischemic stroke* can be related to being off antithrombotics for surgery, right-to-left shunt, hypercoagulable state related to a medical condition, or systemic hypotension producing watershed infarction.
- *Hemorrhagic stroke* is more likely in patients who had transient or sustained hypertension and in patients who are or had recently been anticoagulated or had been on antiplatelet agents.

Seizure is a common cause for hospital neurology consultation. In the peri-operative state, conditions predisposing to seizure include metabolic disturbance with electrolyte, renal, or hepatic dysfunction; medications, including select antibiotics; withdrawal state; stroke (ischemic or hemorrhagic); and in patients with known seizure disorder missing meds.

Withdrawal state with encephalopathy or seizures can develop when a patient admitted for surgery is abruptly withdrawn from agents such as ethanol or opiates. If regular use is known, precautions can be taken, but often the history of use or abuse is not revealed. Less common withdrawal events can be from dopaminergic agents such as those used for Parkinson disease.

SURGERY
Nerve Injuries

Direct surgical injuries to peripheral nerves are uncommon but do occur. Decreased sensation after abdominal or chest or breast surgeries is expected. Neuropathic pain can be an associated problem, although the duration is usually limited. Prognosis depends on the type of injury, whether stretch, crush, or cut. Crush injuries can be from hemostats or retractors intraoperatively or from positioning of the limb (e.g., ulnar or peroneal compression).

PRESENTATION can be with any combination of pain, motor, and sensory deficit in the distribution of the affected nerve.

DIAGNOSIS is usually evident immediately with acute intraoperative trauma. Crush injuries may not be appreciated immediately and, because of symptoms related to the postoperative course, might not be noticed for a few days following surgery.

MANAGEMENT depends on the type of injury. Transection of the nerve warrants consideration of epineurial repair. Partial transections might be amenable to fascicular anastomosis depending on size and anatomy. Stretch and crush injuries leave the epineurium intact.

Orthopedic Surgery

Shoulder surgery has been described as producing damage to the suprascapular, axillary, or musculocutaneous nerves. Incidence is usually far less than 5%.[1]

Spine surgery of a variety of types has been associated with a variety of deficits, some due to mechanical damage to the spinal cord. Scoliosis surgery has a small risk of nerve damage.

Hip surgery can be associated with neural injury that is usually transient, just as dislocation can produce neural manifestations. The peroneal division of the sciatic nerve is most commonly affected.[2]

Long bone fracture and surgery may result in fat embolism, which can present neurologically as delirium progressing to coma. Seizures can occur. Associated symptoms are dyspnea and often petechiae.

Cardiovascular Surgery

Cardiovascular surgery has the principal complications of stroke and hypoxic encephalopathy.

Stroke can be ischemic or hemorrhagic. Ischemic stroke is likely from proximal emboli or from hypotension producing watershed infarction. Hemorrhage is usually related to present or recent anticoagulation or an epoch of hypertension.

Hypoxic encephalopathy can occur after an episode of cardiac arrest prior or subsequent to cardiac surgery. A nontrivial episode of hypotension can produce hypoxic encephalopathy or cause watershed infarction.

Seizure in the peri-operative period raises concern over cerebral infarct or hemorrhage. Acquired CNS infection during hospitalization is rare. However, if the patient has cardiac infection, cerebral abscess can develop.

Trauma

Trauma patients have numerous potential reasons for neurologic consultation. Among the most common are:

- Head injury
- Seizure
- Encephalopathy and delirium
- Peripheral nerve injury

Head injury is discussed in Chapter 35. Most facilities have patients with traumatic intracranial hemorrhage evaluated by neurosurgery rather than neurology.

Seizure can develop early or late. The seizures can be focal or generalized. Antiepileptic drugs (AEDs) as part of initial therapy reduce the risk of recurrent early seizure but do not appear to alter the chance of late seizures.[3]

Encephalopathy and delirium can be associated with concussion but also can develop from conditions associated with the hospitalization. Some of these are:

- Withdrawal state (e.g., opiates, ethanol)
- Metabolic encephalopathy (e.g., renal or hepatic insufficiency)
- Toxic encephalopathy (e.g., analgesics, sedative-hypnotics)

Hospitalization encephalopathy is discussed further in Chapter 18.

Peripheral nerve injury can occur at almost any location. This can be from the primary injury or later complication, such as compartment syndrome or compressive neuropathy.

Transplant Patients

Neurologic complications of transplantation are an occasional cause for neurologic consultation. Possible causes of neurologic complications include:

- Direct operative and perioperative effects
- Effects of the failed organ
- Immune suppression
- Opportunistic infection

A detailed discussion of each transplantation and correlated neurologic complications is beyond the scope of this book; see the edited volume by Biller and Ferro for detailed discussion on this topic.[4] Patients with neurologic complications often have shorter life expectancies than those without, so managing and possibly preventing these is a focus of study.

Immune suppression from antirejection therapy predisposes to infection, which may range from mild to life-threatening sepsis. This is mainly an issue in the weeks to months following transplantation, at a time when antirejection therapy cannot be reduced or discontinued without risk to the transplanted organs.

Peri-operative complications of principal concern to the neurologist are local neural injury and peri-operative stroke.

- *Kidney transplant*: Femoral nerve or lumbosacral plexus injury[5]
- *Heart transplant*: Stroke, hypoxic encephalopathy
- *Lung transplant*: Hypoxic encephalopathy, stroke
- *Liver transplant*: Central pontine myelinolysis, stroke, Posterior reversible encephalopathy syndrome (PRES)[6]
- *Bone marrow transplant*: Idiopathic hyperammonemia, neuromuscular complications from graft versus host reaction, immune-mediated encephalomyelitis

Failed organ effects including renal and hepatic dysfunction that cannot be immediately reversed after transplantation. Hence, persistent metabolic encephalopathy may be slow in clearing after successful transplantation.

Underlying disease predisposes to neurologic complications. If the patient is being transplanted because of diabetes, hypertension, or other systemic cause of organ failure, these also increase the risk of metabolic, hemodynamic, and vascular neurologic complications.

Opportunistic infection is possible in transplant patients not only because of the immune suppression from antirejection medications but also often by virtue of the metabolic effects of the organ failure itself.

Bariatric Surgery

Bariatric surgery has a host of potential neurologic problems. Most are related to nutritional deficiency.

Important neurologic presentations following bariatric surgery can be:

- Encephalopathy
- Polyneuropathy
- Mononeuropathy
- Myelopathy
- Optic neuropathy

Among the deficiency states with neurologic manifestations that can be encountered are:

- B_1 deficiency
- B_{12} deficiency
- Copper deficiency

Specific complications are as follows. These are all discussed in Chapter 29.

- *Encephalopathy* is usually due to B_1 deficiency but can be due to B_{12} deficiency.
- *Polyneuropathy and mononeuropathy* can be seen with any of these deficiencies.
- *Myelopathy* is usually from B_{12} or copper deficiency.
- *Optic neuropathy* is usually from B_{12} or B_1 deficiency.

Wernicke encephalopathy from B_1 deficiency presents more acutely than the other disorders.

ANESTHESIA

Potential neurologic complications of anesthesia depend on the route, whether general, regional block, or spinal block. Among some of the most important complications that can be related to anesthesia are:

- Delirium
- Seizure
- Malignant hyperthermia
- Prolonged neuromuscular paralysis
- Myelopathy

Delirium

Delirium is common postoperatively. Issues specifically within the sphere of anesthesiologists that can make delirium more likely include:

- *Medications* including but not limited to benzodiazepines, opiates, antihistamines, anticholinergics, corticosteroids, anesthetic agents such as propofol.
- *Electrolyte abnormalities.* Fluid imbalance predisposes to difficulty with electrolyte abnormalities and the potential for either dehydration or fluid overload. Any of these can predispose to delirium.

- *Withdrawal syndromes* are common, especially with ethanol, opiates, and benzodiazepines.

Clearance of medications can be delayed by renal or hepatic insufficiency or increased storage of the medication in patients with high body mass index (BMI).

Seizure

When seizures occur around the time of surgery, they are often in patients with known epilepsy, but they can be seen with no prior known history. Seizure is most common during induction, although seizure during recovery can occur.

Enflurane can lower seizure threshold and is often avoided in patients with known epilepsy. Nitrous oxide does not have a major consistent effect but may exacerbate seizures. Halothane, on the other hand, can terminate seizures.

Details of seizure presentation and management are discussed in detail in Chapter 19.

Malignant Hyperthermia

Malignant hyperthermia is a disorder affecting a subgroup of calcium channels. These are most commonly activated by inhalation anesthetics such as halothane plus succinylcholine. Marked increase in skeletal muscle calcium produces muscle activation, hyperthermia, acidosis, and, ultimately, rhabdomyolysis. Propensity has autosomal dominant inheritance with variable penetrance.

PRESENTATION is with muscle rigidity and hyperthermia after receiving precipitant agents. This is associated ultimately with tachycardia, tachypnea, and fever. Patients may develop markedly elevated CPK and rhabdomyolysis.

DIAGNOSIS is often suspected when a patient who has received precipitant agents develops muscle rigidity and hyperthermia even before development of rhabdomyolysis and myoglobinuria. The main differential diagnosis is severe sepsis.

MANAGEMENT includes cooling and management of any electrolyte abnormalities. Dantrolene is commonly used.

Prolonged Neuromuscular Paralysis

Prolonged neuromuscular blockade after induction and intubation for anesthesia has become less common with newer agents. However, it can occur especially in patients with delayed clearance.

Myelopathy

Myelopathy following epidural and spinal anesthesia is very rare but has been described. Most commonly, this presents with asymmetric motor and sensory deficits that progress over hours. Magnetic resonance imaging (MRI) of the spine is performed to rule out epidural hematoma or other structural lesion. Occasionally, T2 hyperintensity in the cord may be seen. Most patients improve. Some patients have been treated with corticosteroids.

13 Neurologic Manifestations of Systemic Disease

Karl E. Misulis, MD, PhD and
E. Lee Murray, MD

CHAPTER CONTENTS

- Overview
- Hypertension
  - Hypertension with Acute Ischemic Stroke
  - Hypertension with Acute Intracranial Hemorrhage
  - Hypertensive Crisis
- Posterior Reversible Encephalopathy Syndrome
- Renal Insufficiency
  - Seizure
  - Dialysis Disequilibrium
  - Stroke
  - Altered Clearance of Medications
- Hepatic Failure
  - Hepatic Encephalopathy
  - Seizures
  - Myoclonus
- Diabetes Mellitus
  - Diabetes Ketoacidosis
  - Hyperosmolar Hyperglycemic State
  - Hypoglycemia
- Rheumatologic Disease
  - Systemic Lupus Erythematosus
  - Rheumatoid Arthritis
- Sarcoidosis
- Respiratory Abnormalities
  - Hypoxia
  - Hypercapnia
- Electrolyte and Fluid Disorders
  - Hypernatremia
  - Hyponatremia

- Hypercalcemia
- Hypocalcemia
- Hypomagnesemia
- Water Intoxication
- Central Pontine Myelinolysis
- Role of the Neurologist

OVERVIEW

Presentation and differential diagnosis of acute neurologic complications of medical diseases were discussed in Chapter 11. In this chapter, we discuss selected disorders in greater detail. Other chapters discuss manifestations of systemic diseases in the context of clinically related disorders, as follows:

- Neurologic complications of cancers: Chapter 25
- Infectious diseases: Chapter 17
- Hypoxic-ischemic encephalopathy: Chapter 14
- Stroke: Chapter 16
- Hospitalization encephalopathy: Chapter 18
- Diabetic neuropathy: Chapter 28

HYPERTENSION

Hypertension has a multiplicity of neurologic implications, but in the hospital the following scenarios are of special concern:

- Hypertension with acute ischemic stroke
- Hypertension with acute intracranial hemorrhage
- Malignant hypertension/hypertensive crisis

Hypertension with Acute Ischemic Stroke

Blood pressure (BP) is commonly increased at the time of acute ischemic stroke. Implications of this include increased risk of bleeding with IV tissue plasminogen activator (tPA) if BP remains high, but also a higher baseline blood pressure prior to the stroke worsens outcome. Recent advances in BP management may be responsible for some of the improvement in stroke outcome seen independently of thrombolytic therapy.[1]

Decisions on BP management are governed by many factors. Guidelines from 2013 are freely available.[2]

Some of the most important factors governing BP management in acute stroke are:

- Elevated BP at time of presentation can be either or a combination of baseline hypertension plus reactive BP from the acute ischemia.
- Contraindication to IV tPA presently is severe uncontrolled hypertension, often defined as systolic BP of greater than 185 or diastolic of greater than 110 mm Hg.[3]
- Marked lowering of BP with acute stroke can worsen deficit by reducing perfusion of affected tissue.

MANAGEMENT of BP depends on the clinical scenario:

- *Acute stroke that is a candidate for IV tPA but with BP too high*: The goal is to bring the BP into a range that would allow IV tPA to be given yet not so low as to reduce perfusion pressure. Acute management is often with nicardipine or labetalol intravenously by titration. After administration of tPA, the BP must be continued to be controlled in the same manner.
- *Acute stroke that is a candidate for endovascular therapy*: Most hospital neurologists follow the BP management guidelines for IV tPA when managing the BP of a patient who is undergoing endovascular therapy.
- *Acute stroke that is not a candidate for IV tPA*: There is less consensus for this scenario. However, the Guidelines recommend lowering of BP by 15% during the first 24 hours after the stroke. But the antihypertensive agents should be withheld unless the systolic blood pressure is greater than 220 or the diastolic BP is greater than 120.
- *Acute stroke with cerebral edema*: Patients with cerebral edema following acute ischemic stroke are difficult to manage. Edema peaks at about 4 days following the acute stroke. There are less-defined guidelines, other than that marked hypertension can produce hemorrhage into the infarction, and hypotension reduces perfusion especially with cerebral edema. Antihypertensive therapy is usually minimized unless there is marked elevation. As discussed in Chapter 41, medical and, if needed, surgical management of the edema can help.
- *Acute stroke has been managed, and the patient is preparing for post-hospitalization care*: Details of routine BP management will not be presented here, but, as the patient is being readied for discharge or rehab, a regimen of antihypertensive therapy appropriate for outpatient therapy is established. Algorithms for routine management of BP are beyond the scope of this text, but the JNC-8 guidelines should be part of the hospital neurologist's library.[4]

Hypertension with Acute Intracranial Hemorrhage

Hypertension after acute intracranial hemorrhage is common and presents a management problem since we want to lower the BP to reduce further bleeding yet do not want to reduce perfusion pressure in a patient with increased intracranial pressure (ICP). Medical and surgical management of acute intracranial hemorrhage are discussed in more detail in Chapter 16. Several studies have examined BP management in this scenario without a clear consensus. Generally, traditional management is to aim for a systolic BP of less than 180 within 6 hours from symptom onset.[5] It is likely that more aggressive management will be used and guidelines will be revised.

Hypertensive Crisis

The term *hypertensive crisis* is predominately used, although the term *malignant hypertension* is widely used interchangeably. Strictly speaking, malignant hypertension includes papilledema. Both diagnoses indicate marked hypertension with organ damage involving cerebrovascular, cardiovascular, and/or renal systems.

PRESENTATION is hypertension with a complaint of headache, visual disturbance, or other neurologic or cardiac findings. Neurologic findings can include focal weakness or sensory change, confusion, or seizures.

DIAGNOSIS is suggested to the neurologist by headache or focal deficits associated with severe hypertension. Then it is confirmed by identification of other organ damage and absence of a fixed structural or vascular defect in the brain. Focal deficits due to hypertensive emergency must be distinguished from acute stroke in order to decide whether tPA should be offered. In general, rapidly fluctuating deficits favor hypertensive emergency. Neurologic symptoms that are fixed suggest infarction or hemorrhage.

- A *computed tomography (CT) of the* brain is performed emergently to look for bleeding or early edema.
- A *magnetic resonance imaging (MRI) of the* brain is ultimately performed to look for ischemia not seen on the CT.
- *CT angiography (CTA)* or *magnetic resonance angiography (MRA)* is performed at some point. MRA is generally preferable to CTA in the case of renal insufficiency, but when acute vascular event and intervention is considered, CTA may be performed emergently despite renal status.

MANAGEMENT consists of prompt reduction in blood pressure, and IV meds are generally favored, especially nicardipine or labetalol. Goal is typically a 20–25% reduction in mean arterial pressure (MAP) over 1–2 hours. After resolution of the acute event, long-term aggressive antihypertensive therapy is given.

POSTERIOR REVERSIBLE ENCEPHALOPATHY SYNDROME

Posterior reversible encephalopathy syndrome (PRES) is a constellation of findings due to vasogenic edema usually caused by uncontrolled hypertension. It is also seen in cancer patients receiving immunosuppressant chemotherapy and in eclampsia/pre-eclampsia.[6]

PRESENTATION is typically with headache and confusion, often associated with visual difficulty or seizures. ED presentation may resemble acute stroke, and appropriate protocols are performed.

DIAGNOSIS is suspected when a patient with encephalopathy or stroke-like symptoms has MRI findings suggestive of PRES. Note that, despite the name, the findings are not always posterior and can be watershed, frontal or temporal, or even brainstem in distribution. Depending on the appearance, encephalitis can be in the differential diagnosis.

MANAGEMENT is generally supportive. Seizures are treated by typical meds, especially phenytoin, valproate, or levetiracetam. Uncontrolled seizures can be managed by midazolam. BP is reduced gently if elevated. If the cause is believed to be an immunosuppressive agent, administration should be discontinued.

RENAL INSUFFICIENCY
Seizure

Seizures are common in patients with renal failure, especially around the time of dialysis, but they may also occur independently of the timing of dialysis.

PRESENTATION of is usually with generalized motor seizure activity during dialysis or shortly thereafter. Focal or subtle seizures can occur but are less likely.

DIAGNOSIS begins with imaging, with MRI being preferable. If MRI is not immediately available, emergent CT may be indicated especially if mental status has not returned to baseline. Lumbar puncture (LP) should be considered if there is fever or other signs of potential CNS infection. The differential diagnosis should include dialysis disequilibrium (discussed later), stroke, metabolic derangement, and PRES.

MANAGEMENT of seizures in renal insufficiency requires different medication approaches. Some of the newer antiepileptic drugs (AEDs) have fewer adverse effects and metabolic disturbances and have fewer drug–drug interactions than some of the older drugs.[7] During maintenance treatment for seizures in renal failure, doses of many AEDs have to be adjusted, as well as the timing of doses in relation to dialysis times.

AEDs in which the renal system plays less of a role and therefore may be preferable include[8]:

- Valproate
- Lamotrigine
- Benzodiazepines

AEDs that have a propensity to accumulate in patients with renal insufficiency include topiramate, levetiracetam, gabapentin, and pregabalin.

Dialysis Disequilibrium

Dialysis disequilibrium is a disorder of fluid balance occurring around the time of hemodialysis.[9] Most of these patients have just started hemodialysis, but it can occur later in the course.

PRESENTATION is with headache, restless, nausea, and confusion. Seizures can occur. Onset is usually during dialysis, but can be delayed until several hours after dialysis. Occurrence on a non-dialysis day suggests an alternative diagnosis.

DIAGNOSIS is clinical, with headache being the most common symptom. Development of nausea, confusion, and especially seizures is supportive. CT brain is performed emergently to look for intracranial hemorrhage and edema. MRI is ultimately performed in most circumstances. An electroencephalogram (EEG) is performed to look for nonconvulsive seizures, especially if mental status has not improved. CSF analysis is usually not needed but is considered especially with fever or persistent symptoms.

MANAGEMENT is supportive. If cerebral edema develops, then standard measures are used; however, since these patients are on dialysis, hyperosmolar agents have to be used with care.[10] Patients with dialysis disequilibrium can rarely develop PRES[11] or central pontine myelinolysis (CPM).[12]

Stroke

Patients with renal failure, especially those on dialysis, are predisposed to both hemorrhagic and ischemic strokes.[13] Complicating factors include frequent coexistence of diabetes, hypertension, and coagulation abnormalities. Unfortunately, patients with renal failure have often been excluded from some trials, so we have less robust treatment guidelines for these patients.

PRESENTATION and DIAGNOSIS of patients with stroke and renal failure does not differ from in other patients (Chapter 16). There is some hesitation about the contrast load when performing CTA, but this is a minor issue for most patients and the diagnostic information provided usually more than eclipses the risk.

MANAGEMENT of patients with stroke and renal failure does not differ from other patients. Renal failure and dialysis are not in the exclusion criteria for IV tPA. However, many of these patients are anticoagulated, which could exclude them. Endovascular therapy should be considered if appropriate.[14]

Altered Clearance of Medications

Renal insufficiency affects the elimination of many meds even prior to necessity of dialysis. Also, altered protein binding can affect free fractions of meds. Some examples are:

- *Cefepime*: Encephalopathy can develop with cefepime,[15] and this is usually in patients with renal insufficiency. Patients can present with variable severity of encephalopathy and seizures. Nonconvulsive status epilepticus can occur[16] and can be missed if EEG is not performed.
- *Phenytoin*: Altered protein binding with renal insufficiency increases the free fraction of phenytoin so that a therapeutic free level is achieved with a generally low total level.

Neurologists practicing in the hospital should be particularly attuned to renal insufficiency in prescribing antiepileptic drugs, anti-infectives including many antibiotics and acyclovir, and sedatives.

HEPATIC FAILURE
Hepatic Encephalopathy

Hepatic encephalopathy is a disorder of cognition that is seen in patients with liver failure from a variety of causes. Portal-systemic shunts can also produce hepatic encephalopathy in the absence of hepatic failure.

PRESENTATION is with confusion, memory loss, behavioral change, and deficits in coordination, ultimately progressing to asterixis and then to more marked encephalopathy and to coma.

Stages have been described[17]:

- *Stage 0*: No visible changes in behavior; no asterixis is present.
- *Stage 1*: Impaired attention and concentration; sleep disorder of hypersomnia or insomnia, asterixis may be present.
- *Stage 2*: Disorientation, lethargy, behavioral change; asterixis is prominent.
- *Stage 3*: Disorientation, marked behavior change; asterixis might not be evident.
- *Stage 4*: Coma

Hepatic encephalopathy typically develops in the setting of a precipitating event such as concurrent infection, GI bleeding, or even constipation.

DIAGNOSIS is suspected by increased liver function tests (LFTs) and elevated ammonia. However, the measured ammonia level does not correlate precisely with clinical severity.

- EEG is most helpful diagnostically if it shows triphasic waves, but these are not specific.
- CT or MRI of the brain is needed to look for structural abnormality such as hematoma, infarction, or edema.
- CSF analysis may be needed to look for CNS infection, especially if there is fever or elevated WBC.

MANAGEMENT includes:

- Giving medications to reduce ammonia, such as lactulose.
- Addressing precipitating events (e.g., GI bleed or concurrent infection).
- Adjusting concurrent meds appropriate to the hepatic insufficiency, which might necessitate changing to meds that do not have hepatic metabolism.
- Using antibiotics to reduce ammonia production in the GI tract.
- Reducing protein in the diet, with vegetable protein being predominant.

Seizures

Seizures can be part of the presentation of hepatic encephalopathy, or seizures can occur for another reason in patients with hepatic insufficiency as a comorbid condition (e.g., liver failure developing in a patient with epilepsy). In general, we select meds with less hepatic metabolism. Among these are[18]:

- Levetiracetam
- Pregabalin
- Gabapentin

For patients with seizures who are critically ill, levetiracetam is first line for most patients.

Myoclonus

Myoclonus can occur with hepatic failure and usually does not need treatment other than for management of the underlying hepatic disorder and any precipitating concurrent illness. Also, it is important to review the patient's current medications for responsible agents that may be new or at increased dose. Treatment is usually not needed, but, if so, levetiracetam may be considered.

DIABETES MELLITUS

Patients with diabetes mellitus (DM) have a propensity to more complications and poorer outcomes from medical conditions, so neurologic consultation is common. Among the disorders discussed elsewhere in this text are stroke (Chapter 16) and neuropathy (Chapter 21). Here, we discuss disorders that are not discussed in detail elsewhere: the hyperglycemic states, diabetic keotacidosis (DKA) and hyperosmolar hyperglycemic state (HHS), and hypoglycemia.

Diabetic Ketoacidosis

DKA is hyperglycemia, ketosis, and metabolic acidosis. This is predominant in type 1 diabetics although it can occur with type 2 DM.

PRESENTATION neurologically is with altered mental status, but it can progress to marked encephalopathy, coma, and can develop focal deficits or seizures associated with PRES,[19] but this mainly occurs in children.[20] Stroke can be a precipitant for DKA. Medical presentation is polyuria, polydipsia, and usually a history of rapid unintentional weight loss.

DIAGNOSIS at the time of a neurologic presentation is suspected when initial labs show hyperglycemia. Subsequent follow-up labs show ketosis, acidosis, and prominent anion gap. Urgent CT brain is indicated, but MRI is preferable if it can be done urgently. EEG is ordered if there are overt seizures or marked encephalopathy.

MANAGEMENT of the neurologic complications of DKA depends on the complication. Stroke symptoms and seizures are more often seen in children than adults with DKA. Treatment is described in Chapters 16 and 19, respectively.

Hyperosmolar Hyperglycemic State

HHS is mainly seen in type 2 diabetics and is hyperglycemia, hyperosmolarity, with dehydration, but without ketosis. Onset is over days to weeks.

PRESENTATION neurologically can be varied and includes encephalopathy, focal deficits, and/or seizures. The encephalopathy can range from delirium to coma.

DIAGNOSIS is suspected when a neurologic presentation is accompanied by hyperglycemia but without ketoacidosis. CT or MRI brain is needed urgently to exclude a focal structural lesion.

MANAGEMENT of the medical aspects of HHS is per the internist. Neurologic complications including seizures are treated by standard meds. The main objective is to differentiate between focal deficits from HHS and acute stroke.

Hypoglycemia

Hypoglycemia can present to the hospital neurologist with encephalopathy, focal deficits, or seizures. Cause is usually a diabetic who took excessive insulin or who took regular doses of meds but did not eat. Nondiabetics can develop hypoglycemia although usually not severe enough to prompt emergency neurologic evaluation.

PRESENTATION is usually with tremor, nervousness, palpitations, or diaphoresis. With more severe hypoglycemia, patients can develop mental status change, speech change, or weakness that is usually generalized. With profound hypoglycemia, seizures or coma can develop.

DIAGNOSIS is established by documentation of hypoglycemia when symptomatic. However, documentation of glucose level at the time of the event may not be possible. Brain imaging with CT or MRI is needed for patients with mental status changes or other neurologic deficits or seizures. EEG is indicated for seizures and persistent encephalopathy.

MANAGEMENT includes emergent glucose administration. With insulin overdose in diabetics or nondiabetics, persistent monitoring of serum glucose and retreatment is often needed.

RHEUMATOLOGIC DISEASE

Neurologic complications of rheumatologic disease is usually due to either autoimmune attack of the nervous system by the disorder or by effects of agents used for treatment, often immunosuppressants.[21]

Systemic Lupus Erythematosus

Systemic lupus erythematosus (SLE) is an autoimmune disorder that affects multiple organs. Skin and bone marrow involvement are frequent medical manifestations. Neurologic complications of SLE can be stroke from vasculitis or antiphospholipid antibody syndrome (APS), encephalitis, inflammatory myelopathy, neuromuscular disorder, or psychiatric disorder.[22] The term *neuropsychiatric SLE* is commonly used.

PRESENTATION depends on the specific neurologic complication.

- *Stroke* may present as almost any conventional stroke syndrome. Young patients have a higher relative risk of SLE-related stroke than do older patients.
- *Encephalitis* can manifest as confusion, memory loss, and headache, which can progress to significant cognitive impairment. Seizures can also develop.
- *Psychiatric manifestations* of SLE can present with behavioral or mood disorder and sometimes with psychosis.
- *Inflammatory myelopathy* can present with fairly abrupt onset of clinical myelopathy, which can be severe. Clinical and MRI appearance can resemble transverse myelitis.
- *Neuromuscular complications* of SLE include polyneuropathy, sometimes as acute inflammatory demyelinating polyneuropathy (AIDP), myasthenia gravis, plexopathy, or cranial neuropathy.

DIAGNOSIS of the neurologic complications depends on the specific manifestation—with MRI of brain or spinal cord, EEG, nerve conduction studies (NCS)/electromyography (EMG), or LP as appropriate. Association with SLE is established by rheumatologic evaluation. Note that SLE can present with neurologic manifestations.

MANAGEMENT of the SLE is per rheumatology methodology. Immune treatment of the underlying condition is needed.

Rheumatoid Arthritis

Rheumatoid arthritis (RA) is an autoimmune inflammatory disorder with mainly bony involvement. Cerebral involvement is uncommon, whereas myelopathy and neuropathies are more common. Neuropathic involvement can be vasculitis or compressive.

PRESENTATION *of myelopathy* is with paralysis and segmental pain. The most common cause is atlantoaxial subluxation with cord compression.

PRESENTATION *of neuropathy* is with mononeuropathy, multiple mononeuropathies, or asymmetric polyneuropathy.

DIAGNOSIS of the myelopathy and neuropathy are by standard methods, usually MRI and EMG, respectively. Treatment of myelopathy from atlantoaxial subluxation is surgical.

SARCOIDOSIS

Sarcoidosis is a multisystem inflammatory disorder of unknown etiology. Neurologic complications develop in about 10% of patients.

PRESENTATION depends on area(s) of involvement. Among the most common are:

- *Peripheral neuropathy*: Motor and/or sensory polyneuropathy or mononeuropathy multiplex; marked pain and/or weakness can develop.
- *Cranial neuropathy*: Facial palsy is most common which may be unilateral or bilateral. Optic neuropathy can develop, as can diplopia from involvement of ocular motor nerves.
- *Meningeal inflammation*: Meningitis can develop, which is typically chronic with headache, nausea/vomiting, and possibly mental status changes.
- *Brain inflammatory lesions*: Mass lesions can develop that can present with focal deficits or seizures.

DIAGNOSIS is usually known at the time of neurologic presentation, and a minority of patients present with neurologic findings as the first sign of their disease. Biopsy of an affected site is typically diagnostic, such as pulmonary lesion, lymph node, or skin. MRI brain and spine may show enhancement of nodules in the brain or of the meninges. CSF is usually normal with neuropathy, but with CNS involvement it often shows a mild pleocytosis, increased protein, and normal or low glucose. CSF ACE levels can be increased, although this is less likely with pure peripheral manifestations.

MANAGEMENT usually begins with corticosteroids. IV methylprednisolone can be given for acute symptoms followed by oral corticosteroids. Other immunosuppressants are used, but decisions in this regard should include consultation with our colleagues in rheumatology and/or pulmonology.

RESPIRATORY ABNORMALITIES

Hypoxic ischemic encephalopathy is discussed in depth in Chapter 14. Hypoxia and hypercapnia are discussed here.

Hypoxia

Hypoxia can be acute or chronic. Acute hypoxia is usually associated with respiratory compromise including pulmonary disorder, cardiac disease, or anemia. Other potential causes are near-drowning and altitude sickness. Among the cardiac disorders are low-output states from congestive heart failure (CHF) and aortic stenosis. Chronic hypoxia is usually associated with COPD, but other chronic pulmonary and cardiac conditions can predispose to this.

Acute hypoxia presents with agitation, confusion, and, with increasing severity and duration, lethargy, myoclonus, and coma.

Chronic hypoxia can present with more subtle symptoms such as personality change and mild cognitive dysfunction. Many patients with chronic hypoxia also have hypercapnia.

Hypercapnia

Hypercapnia is most often seen in the hospital setting with patients with COPD. Presentation is commonly with drowsiness, confusion, often with headache. More severe hypercapnia can produce asterixis, lethargy, and coma.

ELECTROLYTE AND FLUID DISORDERS

Fluid and electrolyte disorders are common causes of presentations to the ED but can also often develop during a hospitalization. Neurologic consultation is commonly when encephalopathy or seizures are present.

Hypernatremia

Hypernatremia is commonly caused by dehydration from GI losses, decreased water intake, diabetes insipidus, excessive losses through sweating or tachypnea, or mineralocorticoid excess from adrenal tumor.

PRESENTATION is usually with confusion and lethargy, and can progress to coma. Seizures can occur. Before coma develops, irritability and hyperreflexia are common.

DIAGNOSIS is made by elevated sodium; other electrolyte abnormalities are commonly also present. Brain imaging with CT or MRI is usually needed to look for other causes of the neurologic presentation.

MANAGEMENT is by gentle reversal of the hypernatremia with cautious fluid management, attention to other electrolytes, and close neurologic follow-up. Rapid correction can exacerbate neurologic manifestations.

Hyponatremia

Hyponatremia is commonly asymptomatic when mild but can be profound in the settings of GI losses from vomiting or diarrhea, psychogenic polydipsia, and alcoholism. Some medications predispose to hyponatremia, especially carbamazepine and some diuretics. Heart failure and hepatic failure predispose to hyponatremia, as do rhabdomyolysis and burns.

PRESENTATION with mild to moderate hyponatremia is with altered mental status, confusion, and behavioral change. More marked hyponatremia can cause lethargy and seizures, progressing to coma if not treated.

DIAGNOSIS is made by labs showing significantly low sodium. Brain imaging with CT or MRI is needed for patients with encephalopathy, coma, or seizures to look for other diagnoses. EEG is also often indicated for these patients.

MANAGEMENT is by gentle correction of the electrolyte disorder with attention to fluid balance. Too-rapid correction can predispose to CPM.

Hypercalcemia

Hypercalcemia seen in the hospital is usually due to malignancy or hyperparathyroidism.[23]

PRESENTATION is malaise, nausea, weakness, and confusion, progressing to lethargy and ultimately coma if untreated. Neurologic symptoms are often associated with acute renal insufficiency.

DIAGNOSIS is suspected when routine labs show hypercalcemia. Evaluation for the etiology includes measurement of not only calcium but also phosphorus and parathyroid hormone (PTH); if osteolytic activity is suspected, skeletal studies are performed.

MANAGEMENT often begins with volume replacement since most of these patients are dehydrated. Medical treatments include loop diuretics, bisphosphonates, and reduction of dietary calcium and vitamin D.

Hypocalcemia

Hypocalcemia is defined as a reduction in total calcium with normal plasma protein, or a reduction in ionized calcium. Causes include hypoparathyroidism, vitamin D deficiency, and renal disease.

PRESENTATION is usually subtle, with minimal symptoms for most patients; hypocalcemia is identified on routine labs. Neurologic manifestations can begin with muscle spasms and aching. Paresthesias occur but are often not a prominent complaint in the hospital setting. More severe symptoms can be irritability, seizures, and marked encephalopathy.

DIAGNOSIS is often suspected only when routine labs results show hypocalcemia. A clue should be muscle cramps and spasms. Additional labs to examine calcium balance are warranted when hypocalcemia is diagnosed. Patients with encephalopathy or seizures should have brain imaging and EEG.

MANAGEMENT is with careful calcium replacement with supplemental vitamin D if appropriate.

Hypomagnesemia

Hypomagnesemia is reduction of serum magnesium (Mg). Important causes are reduced intake, intracellular Mg shunting, increased GI loss, and renal loss. Decreased intake is usually seen in alcoholics and other states of starvation. Intracellular movement of Mg is seen with refeeding syndrome, alcohol withdrawal, and pancreatitis. GI loss is from vomiting or diarrhea. Renal loss is from a host of conditions but particularly diuretics. Neurologic symptoms are often exacerbated by coexisting hypocalcemia and hypokalemia.

PRESENTATION begins with weakness, tremor, and paresthesias. Progression can be to muscle spasms, nystagmus, encephalopathy, and seizures. Neurologic symptoms can be accompanied by cardiac arrhythmias.

DIAGNOSIS is made by the low Mg identified on lab studies. Assessment of other electrolytes is important when this diagnosis has been made. Brain imaging with CT or MRI is needed for patients with encephalopathy or seizures. EEG is indicated for seizures or marked encephalopathy.

MANAGEMENT consists of replacement of Mg, with simultaneous monitoring and management of other electrolyte abnormalities, especially hypokalemia and hypocalcemia.

Water Intoxication

Water intoxication is usually by polydipsia, which can be part of a psychologic disorder. Manifestations include those of especially hyponatremia. Cerebral edema can develop if severe.

Central Pontine Myelinolysis

CPM is also known as *osmotic demyelination syndrome (ODS)*. This is a demyelination of especially the central pons, but demyelination can occur elsewhere in the brain. Cause is usually attributed to hyponatremia, specifically with rapid correction. However, there are other causes including liver disease, cancers, and pregnancy.

PRESENTATION is with confusion, weakness with spasticity, and ocular motor abnormalities including nystagmus. Encephalopathy may make motor and cranial nerve exam more difficult. *Locked-in syndrome* is usually due to brainstem infarction, but CPM is in the differential diagnosis.

DIAGNOSIS is suspected by the finding of spasticity and ocular motor abnormalities with encephalopathy. Differential diagnosis includes Wernicke encephalopathy. MRI brain shows characteristic signal changes at the basis pontis.

MANAGEMENT begins with ensuring that, if hyponatremia is being corrected, the rate of correction is slow. Patients at risk for Wernicke encephalopathy (e.g., alcoholism, cancer) should be given vitamin supplementation including thiamine.

ROLE OF THE NEUROLOGIST

The disorders discussed in this chapter are not the primary province of the neurologist. A common theme is encephalopathy, weakness, and seizures.

While we are often focused on infections and structural abnormalities, we must check electrolytes if that has not been very recently done. Particularly check for electrolyte and metabolic derangements that might not have been recently assessed: ammonia, ABGs, calcium, magnesium, and creatinine, as well as thyroid function tests and nutritional assessments.

The role of the consulting neurologist is to make sure that these common disorders have been considered and assist with immediate neurologic management.

14 Hypoxic-Ischemic Encephalopathy

Karl E. Misulis, MD, PhD and
E. Lee Murray, MD

CHAPTER CONTENTS

- Overview
- Evaluation
- Management
- Role of the Neurologist
  - Medical Management
  - Prognosis
  - Discussion with Family

OVERVIEW

Hypoxic-ischemic encephalopathy (HIE) is one of the most common reasons for hospital neurology consultation. The reasons for neurologic consultations are usually:

- Medical management
- Evaluation and management of myoclonus and seizure activity
- Prognosis

EVALUATION

Initial evaluation of a patient with encephalopathy following cardiac arrest includes extensive cardiac evaluation, but neurological evaluation often includes computed tomography (CT) of the brain to look for intracranial catastrophe as a precipitant of the cardiac arrest.

MANAGEMENT

Following the return of spontaneous circulation (ROSC), most institutions recommend therapeutic hypothermia (TH). As employed in routine practice, the target temperature is 33°C; recent evidence suggests that a target temperature of 36°C may be effective, although this is not routine therapy at the time of this writing.

TH has been used predominantly for patients with shockable rhythms, ventricular tachycardia (VT or V-tach), and ventricular fibrillation (CF or V-fib), but it also has been used for nonshockable rhythms, such as pulseless electrical activity (PEA) or asystole. This field is moving quickly, so the reader is advised to consult the most recent guidelines.

ROLE OF THE NEUROLOGIST

The reasons for neurologic consultation are generally for guidance on medical management, opinion on prognosis, and for involuntary motor activity. These are addressed individually.

Medical Management

Patients with V-fib and V-tach are optimal candidates for TH, and presently 33˚C is the most commonly used target temperature. Protocols are in place in most institutions for these interventions. Patients with PEA and asystole are not considered ideal candidates, although TH is used and there are some data on this,[1] although we echo the concerns of Hessel[2] regarding expansion of use of TH in clinical situations such as nonshockable rhythms.

Prognosis

Before the days of TH, there was a fairly extensive literature that helped to determine prognosis. However, with any of the temperature manipulation protocols, there is concern that these data are not necessarily valid, so the implications of the clinical and diagnostic findings are being re-examined. New data are needed.

AAN Practice Parameter[3] 2006, established on data obtained prior to extensive TH use, indicated that poor prognosis for good neurologic recovery was suggested by absent pupil reflexes, or absent or extensor motor responses 3 days after arrest, or myoclonic status epilepticus within the first day.

Although we do not have extensive data on prognosis for patients who have received TH, we generally believe that features on day 1 prior to institution of hypothermia that indicate poorer prognosis are absent pupil response, absent corneal response, and no motor response.

Before routine use of TH, findings suggesting better prognosis included pupil response, eye movements, and any motor response.

Seizures are common and indicate a poorer prognosis, particularly myoclonic status epilepticus. The poor prognosis is not because of the seizures per se, but rather the seizures are indicative of severe neuronal damage.

Discussion with Family

Discussion with the family should always be frank and realistic. Unfortunately, public expectations for outcome after cardiac arrest may not be realistic. In most fictional accounts, approximately 70% of cardiac arrests result in total recovery, whereas in real life the chance of independence is less than 15%, with many of those surviving patients having neurologic deficits.

No single approach to discussion will be appropriate for all families. Anger and projection are common coping mechanisms for some members. Exacerbating this is conflict within some families. Keeping a cool head during the discussions is essential, and usually even the most difficult family members eventually evolve their thought processes. This may take longer ICU time than the clinician feels is appropriate. While utilization is a concern for all healthcare systems, we recommend being a bit generous on maintenance of advanced care when we believe the clinical outlook does not justify the effort. If this is particularly prolonged or if family members do not seem to have confidence in the opinions or actions of the clinician, then a second opinion is warranted. Further discussion on this topic is found in Chapter 42.

15 Brain Death and Persistent Vegetative State

Karl E. Misulis, MD, PhD and
E. Lee Murray, MD

CHAPTER CONTENTS

- Brain Death
- Persistent Vegetative State
- Differential Diagnosis
- Role of the Neurologist

BRAIN DEATH

The Medical Consultants on the Diagnosis of Death to the President's Commission for the Study of Ethical Problems in Medical and Biomedical and Behavioral Research published criteria for determination of brain death in 1981.[1] Subsequent guidelines were published by the American Academy of Neurology in 1995,[2] and further recommendations were published by Wijdicks in 2010.[3] The criteria depend on absence of brain function, known cause, and irreversibility of the condition:

- Absence of all cerebral function
  - Coma with absence of response to any stimuli except spinal reflexes
  - No spontaneous movement
- Absence of brainstem function
  - No signs of cranial nerve function including:
    - Eye movements
    - Pupil responses
    - Negative corneal, cough, gag
    - Negative cold caloric testing
  - No respiratory effort on apnea testing
- Irreversibility of the dysfunction
  - Known cause and not due to reversible etiology (e.g., intoxication)
  - Period of observation between two exams
  - Confirmatory test (e.g., electroencephalogram [EEG]) may be performed and shorten the required period of observation

Armed with criteria, the following list relates the procedures for establishing brain death:

- Steps for determination of brain death:
  o Establish irreversible and proximate cause of coma.
  o Achieve normal core temperature.
  o Achieve normal systolic blood pressure.
  o Perform a neurologic exam for brain death.
- Clinical examination for brain death:
  o *No responsiveness*: Including no eye opening or movement to noxious stimuli
  o *Absence of brainstem reflexes*: Pupil responses, oculocephalics, oculovestibular reflex, corneal reflex, facial movement to noxious stimuli, pharyngeal and tracheal reflexes
  o *Apnea*: Absence of breathing drive using standard procedures
- Ancillary tests:
  o Ancillary tests are performed especially if there is uncertainty about the reliability of parts of the neurologic exam or if apnea testing cannot be safely performed. Depending on protocols used, ancillary testing may reduce the period of observation before diagnosing brain death.
  o Preferred ancillary tests include EEG, radionucleotide flow study, and angiography.

Apnea testing is often performed by ventilating the patient with 100% O_2 then disconnecting ventilatory support for several minutes. No respiratory effort despite a $PaCO_2$ of at least 60 mm Hg is supportive of the diagnosis of brain death.

PERSISTENT VEGETATIVE STATE

Persistent vegetative state (PVS) is condition of unconsciousness while appearing awake. This can follow a variety of CNS insults including trauma, hypoxia, bilateral hemisphere damage from strokes, or encephalitis.[4] PVS is defined as unconsciousness lasting at least 1 month from the onset, whether from a traumatic or nontraumatic cause (AAN 1995).[5] Some investigators recommend longer times of observation, up to 3 months for nontrauma and 12 months for trauma patients.

The vegetative state can have some appearance of responsiveness, with roving eye movements, tearing, and grimacing to stimulation, but true cognitive response does not occur. EEG can show a variety of abnormalities, but typically does not show an alerting response to stimulation.

Families often have a particularly difficult time coping with and understanding the vegetative state. They frequently believe that there is more cognition than is present.

DIFFERENTIAL DIAGNOSIS

Differential diagnosis of brain death and persistent vegetative state is limited. Encephalopathy and other patterns of decreased response are seen commonly, but reversible causes resolve within hours to days, if addressed, and are not prominent in this differential diagnosis.

- Brain death differential diagnosis
  - *Neuromuscular paralysis*: Paralytics can produce total absence of response but with marked decrease in tone. EEG shows preserved activity.
  - *Locked-in syndrome*: Unresponsiveness, but voluntary vertical eye movements are typically preserved. EEG shows preserved activity.
  - *Toxic/metabolic encephalopathy*: Decreased tone and unresponsiveness, but pupil responses are usually preserved.
  - *Hypothermia*: Decreased response is seen, but usually with preserved pupil and other brainstem responses.
- Vegetative state differential diagnosis
  - *Psychogenic unresponsiveness*: Unresponsiveness with preserved tone and usually body and limb positioning rarely seen in organic unresponsiveness; the EEG is normal. Not persistent.
  - *Global aphasia*: Total lack of response to language and expression of language

ROLE OF THE NEUROLOGIST

Neurologists are commonly consulted for determination of brain death and for determining prognosis in patients who are not brain dead. While there are established guidelines for brain death, there is less consensus regarding prognosis for patients with brain damage.

Some of the factors that make prognosis complicated include the following:

- *Assessment of quality-of-life*: Patients, families and even healthcare providers have very disparate views on what is considered a quality of Life (QoL) that would be justify continuing medical supports.
- *Laws*: State laws differ in the determination of who is authorized to make medical decisions. In the absence of advanced directives, making these decisions can be particularly difficult, even more so if there is disagreement between family members on what is considered appropriate for the patient. Involvement of Ethics Committees and/or legal counsel may be needed.
- *Imperfect prognostic indicators*: Prognosis with properly determined brain death is on solid scientific grounds, but prognostic indicators for patients with some preserved neurologic function is complex and sometimes uncertain.

The concepts of brain death and irreversible brain damage are becoming increasingly well-known to the public so, in discussions, these are seldom new concepts. Yet many laypersons harbor misconceptions that are, in part, due to mass media reporting. Reports in the press of patients who were dead yet recovered impair efforts to advise loved ones about realistic prognoses. These news stories are often poorly investigated, and the facts do not live up to the hype. We do not find it helpful to discuss these media events unless asked. Even then, discussing the veracity of the reports can be dicey, damaging the credibility of the clinician. We prefer to discuss the facts of the case at hand, and, if asked about these reports, state that we do not have all the information needed to comment on that particular report but that often important data are not included in mass media. These issues are further discussed in Chapter 42.

16 Vascular Disease

E. Lee Murray, MD and
William C. Barrow, MD

CHAPTER CONTENTS

- Overview
- Ischemic Stroke
  - Emergent Evaluation and Management
    - IV Thrombolytics
    - Special Considerations in IV tPA therapy
    - Endovascular Therapy
    - IV Heparin
    - Antiplatelets
  - Stroke Mimics
  - Post-Acute Evaluation
    - Stroke Risk Factors
    - Cardioembolic Source
    - Carotid Stenosis
    - Cryptogenic Stroke
  - Post-Acute Management
    - Secondary Prevention
    - Therapy
- Intracerebral Hemorrhage
  - Types of Hemorrhage
  - Evaluation and Management
- Vascular Abnormalities
  - Cerebral Aneurysms
  - Arteriovenous Malformations
  - Cavernous Malformations
  - Dural Arteriovenous Fistulas
  - Carotid Cavernous Fistula
  - Developmental Venous Anomaly
  - Arterial Dissections
  - Amyloid Angiopathy
- Central Venous Thrombosis
  - Cavernous Sinus Thrombosis
- Spinal Infarction
- Role of the Hospital Neurologist

OVERVIEW

In 2011, stroke dropped from the third leading cause of death to the fourth in the United States. Much of this is likely related to improvements in treatment options for acute stroke care and better collaboration between emergency medicine, radiology, and neurology.

ISCHEMIC STROKE

Between 80% and 85% of strokes are ischemic, whether due to embolism, large-vessel disease, or small-vessel thrombotic occlusion. We will consider both acute and sub-acute ischemic stroke. (Stroke syndromes were discussed in Chapter 4.)

Emergent Evaluation and Management

The approach to *acute ischemic stroke (AIS)* begins with a rapid and thorough evaluation to determine diagnosis and eligibility for reperfusion therapy. Figure 16.1 presents a flowchart but evaluation of every patient is individualized.

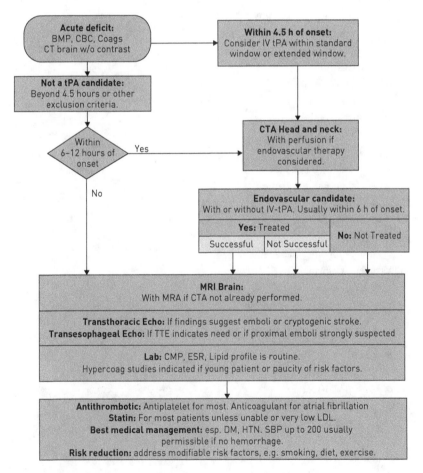

FIGURE 16.1 Flowchart for acute stroke

Key first actions:

- ABCs
- Vital signs
- Brief history
- Brief exam
- CT brain

History will ultimately be complete, but in the ED as part of the urgent evaluation we need the basics:

- *Best history of the event*: With sources as available from patient, EMS, family, friends, and other sources as immediately available
- *Past medical history*: As available from preceding sources and also as evidenced from brief exam (e.g., PPM, sternotomy scar, dialysis shunt)
- *Electronic medical record (EMR) review*: For evidence of prior medical conditions predisposing to stroke as well as for non-stroke conditions that should be considered.

Initial examination is far simpler than the subsequent comprehensive neurologic exam. Details of the exam are governed by present findings, but, in general, we recommend the following basics on presentation:

- *Mental status*: Alertness, orientation
- *Language*: Comprehension, expression
- *Motor*: Strength and tone in all extremities
- *Sensory*: Focused assessment considering results of motor exam
- *Reflex*: Tendon reflexes and plantar responses
- *Ocular*: Pupils, ocular movements, visual fields
- *Medical*: Cardiac, pulmonary, peripheral vascular, skin

Examples of scenarios where the history and exam are specifically tailored to the presentation can include:

- *Hemiparesis with inconsistent findings*: Consideration of atypical stroke, demyelinating disease, migraine, or functional weakness. Query specifically about headache, previous events, stressors. Review EMR for previous related conditions. Perform additional examination for deficits of multiple lesions or inconsistency.
- *Encephalopathy*: Marked encephalopathy raises concern over multifocal acute strokes, brainstem or cerebellar infarct with edema, or intracranial hemorrhage. Nonstroke etiologies are considered including intoxication, electrolyte or metabolic abnormality (e.g., high or low glucose, renal failure, hepatic failure), seizure, head injury.
- *Ataxia*: Ataxia in the absence of other neurologic deficits suggests cerebellar lesion, but alternatives include intoxication, paraneoplastic cerebellar degeneration.
- *Seizure*: Seizure can be subtle and occasionally nonconvulsive. If seizures are considered, then look for nystagmus or even subtle limb movements.

The *National Institutes of Health Stroke Scale (NIHSS)* is performed whenever stroke is suspected, usually by nursing or physician staff who are specifically trained in its performance and interpretation. Details of the NIHSS are presented in Chapter 39.

Computed tomography (CT) of the brain without contrast is performed urgently, within a few minutes of arrival. Some facilities have direct-to-CT protocols for suspected stroke. This requires coordination between EMS and ED staff with urgent notification of the stroke team.

Lab studies on presentation typically include BMP or CMP, CBC, and coagulation studies. Bedside glucose is commonly performed to rule out marked hyper- or hypoglycemia.

This initial evaluation is to determine if the patient is a candidate for immediate reperfusion therapy with intravenous tissue plasminogen activator (tPA) and/or endovascular therapy.

Key points in deciding to proceed with reperfusion therapies:

- Time patient was last known normal
- NIH Stroke Scale (NIHSS)
- Current blood pressure
- Significant past medical history
- Blood glucose level
- Coagulation studies if patient may be on anticoagulation therapies
- Neuroimaging: CT of the head without contrast.
- Risk vs. benefits: 3–6% risk of an intracerebral hemorrhage (ICH) and 2–3% risk of a fatal ICH

IV Thrombolytics

Inclusion criteria for IV tPA (<3 hours from symptom onset): Intravenous tPA is indicated for adult (≥ 18 years of age) patients with acute ischemic stroke if it can be given within 3 hours from onset of symptoms.

Exclusion criteria for IV tPA (<3 hours of symptom onset): Initial exclusion criteria were quite lengthy and limited the number of patients who qualified for IV tPA. Revised guidelines were published in 2013 and 2016, and a new package insert was released in February 2015.[1] These narrowed the contraindications significantly; this, however, opened the door for inconsistent interpretation of some criteria:

- Contraindication for bleeding diathesis
- Warning for recent intracerebral hemorrhage
- Warning for blood pressure 175/110
- Contraindication for subarachnoid hemorrhage
- Warning for pregnancy category C
- Warning for age over 77

The 2016 guidelines further liberalized criteria for administration of IV tPA. These are freely available online and should be in every neurologists files; only a selection of the recommendations is discussed here.[1] Among the changes were:

- *Stroke severity:* Initial guidelines cautioned against using tPA in patients with severe stroke or with mild stroke. 2016 guidelines recommend consideration in patients with severe stroke and in patients with mild stroke which is disabling.

- *Clinical improvement*: Initial guidelines did not encourage tPA administration for patients who were improving. 2016 guidelines recommend considering tPA despite improvement if the deficit is still disabling.
- *Timing of administration*: Initial guidelines recommended treatment only within the 3 hour-from-symptoms-onset time window. 2013 guidelines recommended consideration of tPA in the 3-4.5 hour window but excluding age > 80 years, patients with NIHSS > 25, imaging evidence of MCA stroke involving more than 1/3rd of the distribution, or patients with a history of both previous stroke and diabetes. The 2016 guidelines liberalized consideration of use in the 3-4.5 hour window to include selected patients over 80 years of age and in select patients with a history of prior stroke and diabetes.
- *Pregnancy*: Initial guidelines had pregnancy as a contraindication. New guidelines recommend consideration of tPA for moderate to severe stroke, with urgent involvement the OB physician.
- *Myocardial infarction*: Initial guidelines recommended not giving tPA with MI within 3 months. New guidelines recommend consideration if AIS and MI are concurrent, and also if MI has been within 3 months under certain circumstances.
- *Seizure*: Initial guidelines recommended not giving tPA if there was a seizure at onset. New guidelines recommend considering tPA if residual deficit is not felt to be due to postictal effect.

Administration of thrombolytic: The only Federal Drug Administration (FDA)-approved IV medication for acute stroke is recombinant tPA. Once the decision is made to proceed with IV tPA, 0.9 mg/kg of medication is mixed for a maximum dose of 90 mg. The first 10% of the total amount mixed is given as a bolus. The remaining 90% is infused over 1 hour.

Patients must be monitored closely over the next few hours for signs of bleeding or acute neurological change. Any acute change in neurological status requires stopping the infusion of tPA and obtaining a stat CT of the head to rule out bleeding.

Precautions should be used in patients who are taking concomitant angiotensin-converting enzyme (ACE) inhibitors because angioedema can occur during or immediately after the administration of tPA. If it develops, tPA infusion should be stopped, and medical treatment with corticosteroids, antihistamines, and possibly epinephrine be considered.[2]

Patients who have received either IV thrombolytics and/or endovascular therapies should be monitored in an ICU or stroke unit for at least 24 hours after treatment.

Post IV t-PA care:

- No anticoagulants or antiplatelet agents for 24 hours following tPA infusion
- Blood pressure control of less than 180/100 for the first 24 hours post infusion
- No arterial punctures, invasive procedures, or intramuscular injunctions for 12 hours post infusion
- Repeat CT scan of the head or MRI of the brain before initiating antiplatelet or anticoagulant therapy to rule out asymptomatic hemorrhage
- Frequent evaluation by nursing staff of the patient's neurological status

If all the preceding criteria are not available at the administering facility, transfer to a stroke center should be arranged immediately.

Special Considerations in IV tPA Therapy

Patients with improving deficits are sometimes not given tPA because of initial recommendations that suggested that treatment was not needed for patients showing rapid improvement. However, we now recommend consideration if the patient has significant deficit even if improved.

Patients with aphasia and no other deficit are functionally devastated yet can have a low NIHSS. While strict adherence to original recommendations resulted in these patients not being treated, we now recommend consideration of tPA even if aphasia is the only deficit.

Informed consent may not be obtainable. If no family is available and the patient cannot give informed consent due to aphasia, then administration of IV-tPA within the 3-hour window is appropriate since it is adherent to accepted medical practice. Treatment in the extended 3–4.5 hour window is not FDA approved, so, in our working practice, we do not recommend this without informed consent from patient or family. Likewise, endovascular therapy within 6 hours can be considered without necessitating informed consent, but beyond this time window in our practice we ask that consent be obtained.

Endovascular Therapies

Multiple clinical trials have been published recently showing added benefit of endovascular therapies in patients with amenable occlusions. Most patients in these studies, however, also received IV tPA, which currently remains the "gold standard" for treatment of acute stroke. Endovascular therapy should be considered especially in patients seen within the 6-hour window even if they are receiving tPA, and we extend that consideration beyond 6 hours depending on clinical details.

IV Heparin

Presently, there is no clinical evidence supporting the routine use of IV heparin in acute ischemic stroke. However, IV heparin is frequently used in acute/subacute stroke patients with simultaneous myocardial infarction, pulmonary embolism, or other medical comorbidities that necessitate urgent anticoagulation.

Extra caution and close monitoring of neurological status is needed in patients with large infarcts receiving IV heparin due to the risk of hemorrhagic conversion of the ischemic region.

Antiplatelets

Aspirin is recommended by AHA/ASA guidelines[3] for patients with AIS unless contraindicated (e.g., coagulopathy, significant hemorrhage). In most facilities, aspirin is administered in the ED as soon as the CT demonstrates no hemorrhage if the patient is not a candidate for IV tPA or endovascular treatment. If the patient does receive treatments, then aspirin is withheld for 24 hours.

Clopidogrel does not have the supportive data that aspirin does for AIS and is not recommended if aspirin can be used.

Aggrenox is a combination of aspirin and dipyridamole and is FDA approved for secondary prevention of AIS and transient ischemic attack (TIA).

Stroke Mimics

Several other neurological conditions can present with acute to subacute focal deficits in addition to infarct. A thorough stroke workup should be performed while alternative diagnoses are considered. The suspicion of a *stroke mimic* should not preclude the administration of IV thrombolytics if indications for IV tPA are present and contraindications have been ruled out. Luckily, the risk of hemorrhage from tPA in patients with most stroke mimics is low. Common stroke mimics include:

- Migraine
- Seizure
- Mass lesion (no tPA if responsible mass seen on CT)
- Encephalopathy
- Multiple sclerosis lesion
- Encephalitis
- Hypertensive encephalopathy
- Conversion reaction and malingering

Clues to stroke mimic include:

- *Gradual onset and progression* may suggest migraine, demyelinating lesion, or tumor.
- *Headache* suggests migraine or tumor but can occur in AIS.
- *Fever* suggests encephalitis but can occur with stroke from septic emboli.

Chapter 4 discusses in more detail the differential diagnosis of focal motor and sensory symptoms.

Post-Acute Evaluation

Post-acute evaluation begins as soon as emergent management of AIS is initiated. This includes the following elements:

- Etiologic determination
  - Structural assessment (e.g., thrombus, occlusive disease)
  - Medical assessment (e.g., hyperlipidemia, diabetes, hypertension, vasculitis, other inherited, metabolic, or inflammatory condition)
- Secondary prevention
  - Antithrombotics (e.g., antiplatelets, anticoagulants)
  - Statins (for patients with and without hyperlipidemia)
- Best medical management (especially diabetes and hypertension
  - Risk reduction (address modifiable risk factors)
- Functional improvement
  - Therapy and rehab if needed
  - Assistive devices if needed
  - Feeding tubes if needed

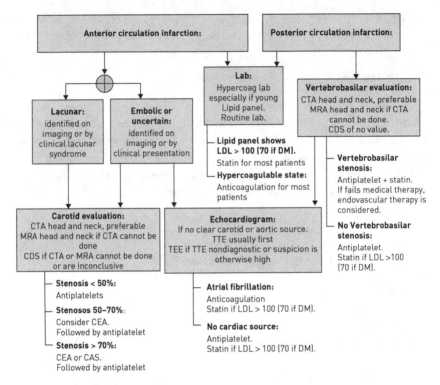

FIGURE 16.2 Flowchart for post-acute care

The flowchart in Figure 16.2 suggests a general approach to post-acute evaluation and management, but all approaches are customized to the specific patient's clinical situation.

Studies that can be performed include:

- MRI brain to identify the infarct
- CT brain if MRI cannot be done, especially if reperfusion therapy is performed, to look for bleeding
- CT angiography (CTA) or MR angiography (MRA) if not already done; for most patients, CTA is preferable.
- Carotid duplex sonography (CDS) if better study cannot be performed, but CTA or MRA are preferable.
- Transthoracic echocardiogram (TTE) if the stroke is possibly embolic (likely not needed for lacunar strokes). Transesophageal echo (TEE) is considered if TTE is negative yet there is still significant concern for proximal emboli or if the TTE shows abnormalities that need further evaluation.
- Lipid profile should be performed on almost all patients.
- Hypercoagulation panel is recommended for young patients or those without significant risk factors for stroke.
- Cardiac evaluation for arrhythmia: EKG and telemetry to start, then consider a Holter or implantable loop recorder (ILR) depending on clinical suspicion.

Stroke Risk Factors

Research has demonstrated multiple risk factors for both ischemic and hemorrhagic strokes. Many of these risk factors are considered *modifiable*.

Hypertension is the most prevalent modifiable risk factor. Atrial fibrillation also carries a significant risk of embolic infarcts.

Modifiable risk factors include:

- Hypertension
- Atrial fibrillation
- Diabetes
- Dyslipidemia
- Carotid stenosis
- Smoking
- Obesity
- Alcohol use

Nonmodifiable risk factors include:

- Family history
- Race/ethnic background
- Age
- Sex
- Previous stroke/TIA
- Cardiac anomaly (e.g., PFO)

Cardioembolic Source

From 20% to 30% of cerebral infarctions are the result of a cardioembolic source. Although there are several sources that can lead to cardioembolic infarcts, some are more prone to causing an infarct. Major cardiac risk factors include:

- Atrial fibrillation
- Left ventricular thrombus
- Dilated cardiomyopathy
- Atrial myxoma
- Recent myocardial infarction
- Mitral valve stenosis
- Prosthetic valve

Minor cardiac risk factors include:

- Mitral valve prolapse
- Patent foramen ovale
- Calcified aortic stenosis
- Atrial septal aneurysm

Patients with atrial fibrillation have a higher risk for thromboembolism with concomitant histories of hypertension, congestive heart failure, advanced age, diabetes, or previous stroke/TIA. Anticoagulation is superior to aspirin for secondary prevention in patients with atrial fibrillation.[4]

Patent foramen ovale (PFO) is an abnormality encountered during routine echocardiograms or as part of a stroke workup. Recent guidelines from the AAN recommend closure of the PFO not be performed in patients with cryptogenic stroke. In rare circumstances, such as recurrent strokes despite adequate medical therapy with no other mechanism identified, The Amplatzer PFO Occluder is an option. Antiplatelet therapies instead of anticoagulation should be used in the absence of other indications for anticoagulant therapies.[5]

Carotid Stenosis

Patients with significant (50–99%) stenosis of the ipsilateral symptomatic lesion should be considered for possible carotid endarterectomy. The North American Symptomatic Carotid Endarterectomy Trial (NASCET) showed the 2-year ipsilateral stroke rate was 26% in medically treated versus 9% in patients treated with carotid endarterectomy (CEA).[6]

Medical management of symptomatic internal carotid artery disease ipsilateral to stroke/TIA in corresponding vascular territory[7]:

- *0% to less than 50%*: Aspirin plus statin
- *50% to less than 69%*: CEA plus aspirin superior to aspirin only in selected patients. CEA only shows a moderate reduction in risk of stroke.[8]
- *70% to less than 99%*: CEA plus aspirin superior to aspirin alone
- *Total occlusion*: Aspirin plus statin

Carotid endarterectomy versus angioplasty and stenting: Studies comparing CEA to angioplasty/stenting have shown similar results in reduction of recurrent stroke. However, current recommendations suggest reserving angioplasty/carotid stenting for patients who are at high risk for complications of CEA. High-risk patients include those with significant cardiac disease, severe pulmonary disease, contralateral internal carotid artery occlusion, recurrent stenosis after endarterectomy, age over 80 years, and previous neck surgery or radiotherapy. After CEA or angioplasty/stenting, antiplatelet plus statin are recommended for most patients.

Cryptogenic Stroke

Cryptogenic stroke is defined by the TOAST criteria as a brain infarction that is not attributable to a definite cardioembolism, large-artery atherosclerosis, or small-artery disease despite extensive vascular, cardiac, and serologic evaluation.[9]

The CRYSTAL AF trial further clarified the workup to include extended cardiac monitoring for at least 24 hours and evaluation of hypercoagulable states along with transesophageal echocardiogram.[10]

Atrial fibrillation is likely the cause for many recurrent strokes; however, this can be difficult to diagnosis due to the asymptomatic and intermittent nature of the disease.

Long-term cardiac monitoring including implantable recorders should be considered in those with recurrent stroke. Those patients with a clear recurrent embolic infarct pattern could be considered anticoagulation candidates even without documentation of atrial fibrillation.

Post-Acute Management

Secondary Prevention

Reducing the risk of recurrent stroke can potentially be medical or surgical. For most patients, secondary prevention consists of:

- *Antithrombotics* usually with antiplatelets
- *Statins*
- *Best medical management* of comorbid conditions such as diabetes and hypertension

Antiplatelet agents include aspirin and clopidogrel, usually used individually, seldom in combination.[11] Combinations are occasionally used for intracranial stenosis. Aggrenox (aspirin + dipyridamole) is an alternative.

Anticoagulation is recommended for patients with stroke secondary to atrial fibrillation.[12] Dabigatran, apixaban, and rivaroxaban are alternatives to warfarin for select patients. If the patient is unable to take anticoagulants, then aspirin is recommended.

Surgery or *stenting* is recommended for select patients with significant occlusive disease.

Statins

Statins are routinely used for lipid management but have benefits in secondary stroke risk even in patients without hyperlipidemia. While many patients are concerned about the risk of adverse effects from statins, for most, the potential benefits outweigh the risks. AHA/ASA guidelines recommend statin for patients with stroke or TIA who have a low-density lipoprotein (LDL) level of 100 mg/dL or greater, 70 if diabetic.

Therapy

Rehabilitation consultation is recommended for all patients with functional deficits after stroke. Any combination of physical therapy, occupational therapy, or speech therapy may be needed. Stay in a rehab facility may be needed.

INTRACEREBRAL HEMORRHAGE

The role of the hospital neurologist in ICH differs depending on facility. In many large hospitals, neurology takes the lead in care of ischemic strokes, whereas neurosurgery cares for hemorrhages even if they are not evidently surgical; this is partly because it is not uncommon for a nonsurgical hemorrhage to ultimately require surgery.

Types of Hemorrhage

The major types of intracranial hemorrhage are:

- Subdural hematoma
- Epidural hematoma
- Subarachnoid hemorrhage
- Lobar hemorrhage
- Cerebellar hemorrhage
- Basal ganglia and thalamus hemorrhage
- Brainstem hemorrhage

Subdural Hematoma

Subdural hematoma (SDH) is blood collection between the dura and brain. Most common cause is head injury.

PRESENTATION can be acute or chronic:

- *Acute SDH* usually has a history of unconsciousness at the time of the injury. Increasing headache, mental status change, focal deficit, or seizures may develop.
- *Chronic SDH* may have no memorable traumatic event. Headache, altered mental status, focal deficit, or seizures can develop.

DIAGNOSIS is by brain CT or MRI. Small SDH may initially be missed on imaging. Restudy should be considered with any deterioration in function.

MANAGEMENT is often surgical, although some patients with small SDHs can be followed closely.

Epidural Hematoma

Epidural hematoma (EDH) is blood between the dura and bone. Cause is typically trauma. EDH is less common than SDH. Arterial bleeding is most common.

PRESENTATION is classically described as initial unconsciousness with an injury, followed by a lucid interval, then followed by a deterioration in mental status. However, many patients do not have a lucid interval.

DIAGNOSIS is considered in patients with marked encephalopathy following head injury or in patients who have had a deterioration in mental status.

MANAGEMENT is surgical. Neurosurgical consultation is recommended as soon as the diagnosis is considered since deterioration can be extremely rapid.

Subarachnoid Hemorrhage

Subarachnoid hemorrhage (SAH) is blood in the subarachnoid space. This can be seen after head injury or due to leak from vascular abnormality, most commonly an aneurysm.

PRESENTATION is most commonly with headache. Other symptoms can be diplopia, dizziness, visual disturbance, or mental status change. Less common findings can be motor or sensory deficit or seizure.

DIAGNOSIS is suspected with acute onset of headache, often described as the worst headache the patient has experienced. Good-quality CT brain shows subarachnoid blood in at least 90% of patients ultimately diagnosed as SAH. Imaging is most sensitive if performed within 6 hours from onset. If there is doubt, lumbar puncture (LP) can show blood in the CSF.

MANAGEMENT is complex and must involve neurosurgical consultation. Nimodipine is administered to reduce vasospasm. BP is treated to avoid hypertension or hypotension. Surgery for aneurysm may be needed. A ventricular drain may be needed if hydrocephalus develops.

Lobar Intracerebral Hemorrhage

Lobar intracerebral hemorrhage is less likely to be due to hypertension than hemorrhage in the basal ganglia or thalamus. Common causes include amyloid angiopathy, anticoagulation and other coagulopathies, vascular malformation, or recent thrombolytic therapy.

PRESENTATION depends on the location of the hemorrhage. Findings can be aphasia, hemiparesis, hemianopia, or other cerebral deficit. Most patients have headache and nausea. Drowsiness and confusion indicate progression of the hemorrhage. BP may be normal or elevated.

DIAGNOSIS is suspected when a patient presents with a stroke syndrome but also has headache. Nausea or altered mental status is supportive. Brain imaging with CT or MRI makes the diagnosis.

MANAGEMENT depends on size and location. Small hemorrhages can be followed. Large hemorrhages usually require medical management for increased ICP as outlined in Chapter 41. If the hemorrhage occurred in the setting of therapeutic anticoagulation, this should be reversed. A ventricular drain is sometimes placed when there is hydrocephalus or blood break-through into the ventricle. Surgical evacuation of the intraparenchymal blood is often considered, but there is little evidence for consistent efficacy. Therefore, surgery is usually reserved for life-saving evacuation of a lobar hemorrhage. Factor VIIa has been studied and there is promising data, but this is not in routine use at the time of this writing.

Cerebellar Hemorrhage

Cerebellar hemorrhage can develop from a variety of causes but hypertension is the most common etiology. Other causes can include vascular malformations, tumors, and amyloid angiopathy.

PRESENTATION is usually with acute but progressive onset of headache, nausea/vomiting, ataxia, and often vertigo. Ataxia is usually mainly noticed with gait but may be detectable in the extremity on exam if the bleed is in the cerebellar hemisphere. Dysarthria is common. Altered mental status can be followed by rapid deterioration.

DIAGNOSIS is suspected when a patient presents with abrupt onset of headache associated with vertigo and/or ataxia. Brain imaging with CT or MRI makes the diagnosis. As with all patients with intracranial hemorrhage, coagulation status should be checked.

MANAGEMENT is often surgical, in contrast to cerebral lobar hemorrhages. Surgery is typically performed urgently to reduce the risk of brainstem damage from compression or hydrocephalus. If surgery is delayed until there is brainstem neurologic deficit, the chance of recovery is reduced.

Basal Ganglia or Thalamus Hemorrhage

Basal ganglia or thalamus hemorrhage is commonly hypertensive. Development of bleeding from the putamen is most common of these.

PRESENTATION depends on locus of the hemorrhage:

- *Putamen hemorrhage* produces contralateral hemiparesis, often with headache and/or nausea.
- *Caudate hemorrhage* also produces hemiparesis and may produce altered mental status
- *Thalamic hemorrhage* produces contralateral sensory loss and, if there is extension of the blood, produces contralateral hemiparesis.

DIAGNOSIS is established on CT brain. Often the patient is considered for possible AIS, and hemorrhage is not clinically suspected.

MANAGEMENT is by control of BP, avoiding excessive lowering. Surgery is seldom advised; however, occasionally hydrocephalus may indicate the need for a ventricular drain.

Brainstem Hemorrhage

Brainstem hemorrhage is most common in the pons. The cause can be hypertension. Vascular malformation may contribute.

PRESENTATION is often with abrupt and irreversible unresponsiveness. Progression to coma over minutes suggests this diagnosis. Clues to diagnosis include absence of reflex ocular motor movements, upgoing plantar responses, and small but often reactive pupils.

DIAGNOSIS is suspected with acute onset of unresponsiveness and quadriparesis with loss of lateral eye movements. Diagnosis is confirmed by brain CT or MRI. Differential diagnosis is mainly brainstem ischemia.

MANAGEMENT is usually not surgical but supportive. While most patients have a poor outcome (functional debility or death), survivors can make a good recovery.

Evaluation and Management

Key steps in emergent evaluation and management of ICH are:

- Brief history
- Rapid focused exam

- CT brain stat
- Neurosurgical consultation, which should be stat if appears potentially surgical
- Medical stabilization

If there is critical mass effect that is not amenable to surgical decompression or a ventricular drain, medical management for increased ICP is considered, as discussed in Chapter 41.

Next steps in evaluation and management of ICH are:

- Determination of etiology of hemorrhage, if not already known
- Management of seizures, if present
- Management of autonomic dysfunction, if present
- Optimal BP control, appropriate to patients with ICH

Blood pressures are lowered to reduce the incidence of rebleeding, but should not be so low as to reduce perfusion pressure. Management can be difficult.

Sedation is generally avoided so that neurologic status can be monitored frequently. However, agitation, pain, or encephalopathy may require sedation. Also, hyperventilation to reduce ICP usually requires sedation if the patient is not already unconscious.

Management of brain edema as well as elevated ICPs in ICH patients should be approached by the utilization of hyperventilation, raising the head of the bed above 30 degrees, or hypertonic saline to achieve serum osmolarity capable of promoting the transfer of free water from the interstitial regions into the intravascular space. However, hypertonic saline should be used with caution. Mannitol has been used frequently, but there is no proven therapeutic benefit. Urgent neurosurgical evaluation for possible craniotomy may be needed in appropriate patients.[13]

Management of ICH including SAH:

- ED evaluation
  - CT of the head
  - Advanced life support
- Coagulopathy
  - Severe coagulopathies should be managed appropriately with platelets and other medical management.
  - Hemorrhages caused by vitamin K antagonists should be treated with reversal agents and patients should receive vitamin K.
- Deep vein thrombosis (DVT) prophylaxis
  - Pneumatic compression devices upon admission
- Glucose management
  - Hypoglycemia and hyperglycemia should be managed appropriately.
- Hypertension
  - Avoid hypertension or hypotension.
- Seizures
  - Clinical seizures should be managed properly.
  - Changes in neurological status should be evaluated by electroencephalography to look for subclinical seizures, in addition to brain CT.

- o Subclinical seizures should be managed as aggressively as clinical seizures.
- o Repeat brain imaging is recommended if seizures develop.
- Monitoring
  - o Patient should be monitored in the ICU or stroke unit staffed with dedicated stroke physicians and nurses.
- Neurosurgical evaluation with all ICH
  - o Urgent neurosurgical intervention with:
    - o Cerebellar hemorrhage with neurological deterioration
    - o Compression on the brainstem
    - o Developing hydrocephalus from ventricular obstruction
- Prevention of recurrent ICH
  - o Aggressive management of hypertension beginning at the onset of ICH
- Medical complications
  - o Dysphagia screen in all patients in an attempt to reduce pneumonia
- Rehabilitation/recovery
  - o Multidisciplinary rehabilitation

VASCULAR ABNORMALITIES
Cerebral Aneurysms

Unruptured intracranial aneurysms are often found incidentally. However, they also can cause focal neurological deficits due to compression of cranial nerves or other areas of the brain.

Management of unruptured aneurysms can vary from conservative monitoring to endovascular coiling or open surgical clipping. Neurosurgical colleagues should guide care and advice based of the most recent data.

Factors increasing mortality/morbidity in surgical intervention:

- Larger aneurysms
- History of ischemic cerebrovascular disease
- Patients over the age of 50
- Focal deficit/symptoms of the aneurysm

Arteriovenous Malformations

Arteriovenous malformations (AVMs) are abnormal tangles of arteries and veins that can occur either in the brain or the spinal cord. AVMs may be found incidentally and remain asymptomatic.

PRESENTATION can be with either focal symptoms such as seizures, intractable headaches, or some type of hemorrhagic presentation (SAH, intraparenchymal hemorrhage, or intraventricular hemorrhage).

DIAGNOSIS is can be made with or without hemorrhage. AVM may be an incidental finding on MRI or CT. In a patient with ICH, AVM is suspected when the hemorrhage is in a location not usually typical of hypertensive bleed or if imaging suggests an underlying structural lesion. CTA or MRA may reveal the AVM, but this might not be seen well until the region of hemorrhage is resolving. Angiography can be done to demonstrate an AVM.

MANAGEMENT is medical initially, treating any seizures, headaches, or mass effect from hemorrhage. Emergent surgery is usually not needed.

- Seizures are treated only if they develop; prophylactic treatment is not recommended if there have been no seizures.
- Headaches occasionally develop in the absence of identified hemorrhage and can have a migrainous character.
- There is controversy regarding when endovascular or surgical treatment is needed for AVMs. In general, procedures are more likely to be recommended for patients who have had a hemorrhage from the AVM and for younger patients with risk factors for rupture.

Cavernous Malformations

Cavernous malformations are dilated vascular spaces in the brain and/or the spinal cord. While the risk for bleeding is only about 0.5% annually, the risk of a recurrent hemorrhage is higher. Those located in the brainstem or subcortical regions often are associated with a higher risk of hemorrhage.

PRESENTATION can be with seizures or hemorrhage, but they are often incidental findings. Seizures are often difficult to control, especially those in the temporal lobe.

DIAGNOSIS is by brain MRI or CT. Hemorrhages caused by cavernous malformations often show multiple layers of hemosiderin on MRI that suggests prior subclinical hemorrhages.

MANAGEMENT of the seizures is outlined in Chapter 19. Treatment options for the malformation include stereotactic radiation or open surgery. However, those with a low risk of hemorrhage can be followed conservatively.

Dural Arteriovenous Fistulas

Dural arteriovenous fistulas are abnormal connections between dural arteries and a dural sinus. These fistulas can produce increased pressure and blood flow into the venous system of the CNS, which typically has a low pressure. This can lead to venous congestion with resulting ischemia or hemorrhagic infarction in the parenchyma. Draining veins can also rupture, leading to ICH, SAH, or subdural hematoma.

PRESENTATION can be with pulsatile tinnitus that may be heard using a stethoscope over the mastoid process, occiput, or the eye. Headache can develop when the fistula is associated with increased intracranial pressure. Dural arteriovenous fistulas in the spinal cord may lead to a chronic progressive painless myelopathy and/or radiculopathy. Some patients may present with paraplegia due to hemorrhage or infarction in the spinal cord. Valsalva or positional changes may worsen myelopathic symptoms.

DIAGNOSIS is suggested by apparent thickening of the dura on imaging. CTA/CT venography (CTV) or MRA/MR venography (MRV) may be able to demonstrate the lesion without angiography.

MANAGEMENT can be by surgery or endovascular embolization. Smaller lesions are more commonly treated by surgery. Larger and less accessible lesions are more commonly treated by embolization.

Carotid Cavernous Fistula

Carotid cavernous fistula is an abnormal communication between the carotid artery and the cavernous sinus. Cause can be traumatic or spontaneous.

PRESENTATION is typically with cranial nerve deficits corresponding to those located in the cavernous sinus—cranial nerves 3, 4, and 6 and the first two divisions of CN 5.

DIAGNOSIS of a dural intravenous fistula requires a high index of suspicion. Patients presenting with pulsatile tinnitus, abnormal flow voids on MRI, or unexplained brain/spinal cord edema should undergo angiography.

MANAGEMENT includes endovascular occlusion of the fistula, which at times may even allow reversal of long-standing deficits. Open surgery at times may be warranted.

Developmental Venous Anomaly

These lesions are typically asymptomatic and found incidentally. They often have a fingerlike enhancement on MRI. They may have a caput medusa appearance on cerebral angiography. Given their low risk of hemorrhage, in nonfocal patients, intervention/therapy is not usually warranted.

Arterial Dissections

Dissections of the carotid or vertebral arteries are a common source of stroke in the young. Most cases are associated with some type of identifiable trauma; however, they can be the result of apparently trivial events such as chiropractic manipulation, exercise, or sneezing/coughing episodes. Certain medical conditions can predispose patients to dissections, including:

- Ehlers-Danlos syndrome
- Fibromuscular dysplasia
- Marfan's syndrome
- Polycystic kidney disease
- Osteogenesis imperfecta
- Pseudoxanthoma elasticum

PRESENTATION depends on vessel affected:

- *Carotid dissection* often presents with pain in the anterolateral cervical and/or retro-orbital region. Cranial nerve abnormalities or Horner syndrome can be seen with carotid artery dissections, but are not always present.
- *Vertebral artery dissection* often presents with posterior head pain. Vertebral artery dissections commonly present with a lateral medullary syndrome due to ischemia in the posterior inferior cerebellar artery.

DIAGNOSIS is usually made by CTA, which often shows a flame-like appearance with a tapered narrowing of the artery. Double lumen and an intimal flap may also be seen. Conventional angiography is superior to CTA or MRA, but generally is used only if noninvasive studies are inclusive.

MANAGEMENT is often with dual antiplatelets (aspirin + clopidogrel) for 3 months then transitioning to monotherapy of clopidogrel along with statin therapy. Anticoagulation is still used for select high risk patients. However, the recent CADISS trial showed no difference in efficacy of antiplatelet and anticoagulant drugs at preventing stroke and death in patients with symptomatic carotid and vertebral artery dissection.[14]

Amyloid Angiopathy

Amyloid angiopathy is deposition of β-amyloid in the vessel walls thereby predisposing to hemorrhage. The most common result is lobar hemorrhages.

Amyloid angiopathy is suspected when a patient with hemorrhage is seen on imaging to have had multiple previous ICHs. This is best seen on MRI.

CEREBRAL VENOUS THROMBOSIS

Cerebral venous thrombosis (CVT) is occlusion of one or more of the cerebral veins and is an uncommon cause of infarct and/or hemorrhage. Occlusion of these veins typically points to an underlying hypercoagulable state, either from a genetic abnormality such as a protein C deficiency, or lupus anticoagulant, or a temporary hypercoagulable state from medications such as birth control or a pregnancy/puerperium state. CVT can also be an early sign of an underlying malignancy.

PRESENTATION is most commonly with headache along with focal weakness, aphasia, confusion/mental status changes, or seizure activity. Focal symptoms result from two different mechanisms: increased intracranial pressure due to impaired venous drainage or venous ischemia/infarction or hemorrhage.

DIAGNOSIS is easy to miss or be delayed. Patients presenting with severe headache with papilledema and diplopia (from a sixth-nerve palsy) without any other obvious explanation should be evaluated for CVT. Also, those who are pregnant or postpartum and/or those under the age of 50 presenting with either infarct and/or hemorrhage need consideration of evaluation of the cortical veins.

- *CT of the head without contrast* can be done emergently, which may show changes in the periphery suggesting increased pressure/edema along with hemorrhagic products and/or subacute infarct. Thrombosis can at times be visualized in the superior sagittal and/or transverse sinus.
- *MRI of the brain* can help clarify acute infarct and other possible areas of subtle hemorrhage.
- *MRV* can be done simultaneously with MRI and usually gives a clear view of the cortical venous system and areas of thrombosis.
- *CTV* with contrast can be used if MRV is not an option or does not offer a clear view of the venous system.

MANAGEMENT is typically with anticoagulation. Additional medications are used depending on whether complications such as seizures or increased ICP develop.

- *Anticoagulation* usually begins with IV low-molecular-weight heparin or heparin infusion, typically followed by transition to oral anticoagulants such as warfarin.

Anticoagulation should still be administered even if the patient has a hemorrhagic infarct due to CVT.[15]

- *Antibiotics* will be needed for those with otitis or mastoiditis and systemic infections (e.g., sepsis, meningitis).
- *Anticonvulsants* are recommended with the first seizure.
- Acetazolamide may be used for patients with symptoms of increased ICP. For those with refractory ICP, shunt placement, optic nerve fenestration, or decompressive craniotomy might be required.[16]

Cavernous Sinus Thrombosis

Cavernous sinus thrombosis is a special type of cerebral venous thrombosis that is usually related to facial, orbital, or sinus infection.

PRESENTATION is with headache first and subsequently cranial nerve deficits. Headache is usually in the upper face and peri-orbital region. Cranial nerve deficits are usually in the upper trigeminal distribution and/or involving ocular motor nerves. Associated findings can include fever, exophthalmos, and, with progression, cerebral deficits including mental status changes and meningeal signs.

DIAGNOSIS is suspected when a patient presents with headache and cranial nerve deficits. Brain imaging with MRI or CT is most sensitive if performed with contrast if cavernous sinus thrombosis is suspected. MRV is particularly sensitive to the venous abnormalities.

MANAGEMENT begins with antibiotics. Anticoagulant use is controversial but is likely not risky, so these are often used. Corticosteroids are often used to reduce the inflammatory response.

SPINAL INFARCTION

Spinal cord infarction is usually due to damage to the artery of Adamkiewicz, which comes off the thoracic aorta. The level of the damage varies between cases, but usually it is at about T10. Cause of the stroke can be atherosclerotic, aortic cross-clamping during surgery, or, less likely, vasculitis. Cervical spinal cord infarction rarely occurs but can be mistaken for transverse myelitis.

PRESENTATION is with acute neurologic deficit often with regional spine pain. Patients develop weakness and sensory change below the level of the lesion. Sensory involvement tends to spare position and vibration because of intact vasculature of the posterior columns (i.e., essentially, an anterior spinal artery infarction). There is also some preservation of light touch, although it is disturbed. Pain and temperature are significantly disturbed. The paralysis is initially flaccid, but becomes spastic.

DIAGNOSIS is suspected with acute onset of paralysis, especially with spine pain. No other etiology would be suspected to have as sudden an onset except perhaps vertebral collapse with acute compressive myelopathy. MRA or CTA of the aorta should be performed to look for dissection or occlusive disease.

MANAGEMENT is supportive. Management of adequate BP is key, avoiding hypotension that can exacerbate spinal ischemic just as it can with cerebral ischemia. There is no proven benefit of IV tPA or endovascular procedure for treatment of spinal infarction. Corticosteroids are often given to patients with myelopathy of uncertain cause but should be avoided when the etiology is believed to be ischemic. Secondary prevention with antiplatelets and statin are usually used unless surgery or anticoagulation is needed.

ROLE OF THE HOSPITAL NEUROLOGIST

Hospital neurologists spend much time in the ED evaluating potential strokes, especially at primary or comprehensive stroke centers.

Intake into the system happens in two ways. Most commonly, patients are seen on presentation to the ED. Less common, but increasing in proportion, are patients referred in from outside hospitals. Unfortunately some patients become ineligible to receive reperfusion therapy because of the time taken to evaluate the patient at the outside hospital. Early discussion with the hospital neurologist is essential for decisions about acute therapy:

- Does the patient meet criteria for IV tPA or endovascular therapy?
- If so, can tPA be initiated prior to transfer—so-called *drip-and-ship* scenario?
- If this is a time-critical scenario (e.g., tPA administration, endovascular candidate), can the patient be transferred by helicopter rather than by ground?
- If the patient is not a candidate for acute reperfusion therapy, is there reason to justify transfer?

Some referral hospitals tend to defer transfers if there is no emergent treatment for which transfer is needed. However, outside providers often consider acute stroke care out of their comfort zone, and, in these cases, transfer is reasonable even if there is not a specific intervention that will be performed.

17 Infectious Diseases

Karl E. Misulis, MD, PhD and
E. Lee Murray, MD

CHAPTER CONTENTS

- Overview
- Meningitis
  - Viral Meningitis
  - Bacterial Meningitis
  - Fungal Meningitis
- Encephalitis
- Viral Myelitis
- Prion Encephalopathies
  - Creutzfeldt-Jakob Disease
  - Variant CJD and Bovine Spongiform Encephalopathy
- Brain Abscess
- Herpes Zoster and Post-herpetic Neuralgia
  - Herpes Zoster
  - Post-herpetic Neuralgia
- Neurosyphilis
- Human Immunodeficiency Virus
  - Dementia
  - Neuropathy
  - Toxoplasma
- Progressive Multifocal Leukoencephalopathy
- Endocarditis
- Whipple Disease
- Lyme Disease
- West Nile Virus
- Zika Virus

OVERVIEW

Infectious diseases are a common cause of hospital neurology consultation either because infection has directly involved nervous structures or patients with infection have developed a neurologic condition.

Neurologic complications of sepsis were discussed in Chapter 11. Detailed discussion of cerebrospinal fluid (CSF) analysis and interpretation is presented in Chapter 40.

MENINGITIS

Meningitis is most commonly first seen in the ED; hospital-acquired meningitis is rare in the absence of instrumentation. The most common cause is viral, with bacterial being less common, and fungal being quite rare and usually seen in an immunocompromised host.

Symptoms of meningitis depend on etiology, but the classic triad is fever, headache, and neck pain. Chronic meningitis will not be expected to have all of these, and non-bacterial meningitis may not be associated with fever. Altered mental status is common with meningitis of any cause.

Meningeal signs: Signs of meningeal inflammation depend on etiology. Meningeal signs are more often absent than present, but they are still commonly evaluated.

- *Kernig sign*: Supine patient has hip and knee flexed, then the knee is straightened so that the foot points upward. Sign is positive if there is resistance to straightening of the knee.
- *Brudzinski sign*: Supine patient has neck passively flexed to the chest. Sign is positive if there is reactive flexion of the hip.
- *Neck rigidity* is the most important of these signs. This is decreased mobility of the cervical spine because of muscle rigidity. This is often tested by attempts at active or passive flexion of the neck to the chest.

Viral Meningitis

Viral meningitis has many possible pathogens. The most common are enteroviruses, responsible for about 85% of viral meningitides, followed by herpes simplex virus 2 (HSV2). A list of encephalitides that are likely to be seen includes:

- Enterovirus (e.g., coxsackievirus, echovirus)
- HSV, usually type 2
- Varicella zoster virus (VZV)
- Western equine virus
- West Nile virus
- St. Louis virus
- California encephalitis virus
- La Crosse virus
- Lymphocytic choriomeningitis virus
- HIV

Routes of infection are varied and depend on the specific agent. Some are seasonal, with the common enteroviruses predominating in summer and early fall.

PRESENTATION is with a constellation of symptoms that can include headache, neck pain, nausea, and vomiting, usually with fever. Rash and photophobia can occur. Prodromal symptoms with malaise and myalgias can occur. Encephalopathy can occur, but seizures are uncommon.

DIAGNOSIS is suspected when patients present with headache and fever, especially with mental status change. Blood WBC is usually increased. CSF analysis makes the diagnosis.

Computed tomography (CT) or *magnetic resonance imaging (MRI) brain* is often done. It is obligatory if encephalopathy or seizure develops. Contrast enhancement can show meningeal enhancement.

CSF findings:

- *CSF appearance*: Usually clear
- *Opening pressure*: Normal or mildly elevated
- *WBC*: Usually in the range of 10–1,000 cells/µL, usually lymphocytic but may be polymorphonuclear early
- *Glucose*: usually normal but may be reduced in HSV encephalitis
- *Protein*: Usually mildly elevated
- *Polymerase chain reaction (PCR)*: May be positive for selected viruses, including HSV, VZV, West Nile virus (WNV), enterovirus
- *Cultures and smears*: Seldom revealing for viral meningitis

Electroencephalogram (EEG) can be normal or show diffuse slowing. Periodic discharges can be seen with HSV encephalitis but would not be expected with meningitis.

MANAGEMENT is supportive for most viral meningitides. Most are self-limited disorders. The main opportunity is treating meningitis due to HSV and HIV, and for treating patients in whom the meningitis might be bacterial.

- *HSV meningitis* is treated with acyclovir.
- *HIV meningitis* is treated with antiretroviral agents.
- *Cytomegalovirus (CMV) meningitis* in immunocompromised patients is treated beginning with ganciclovir.

Bacterial meningitis may be suspected at the time of presentation because there is an overlap in CSF WBC counts, and not all patients with bacterial meningitis have low glucose. *Empiric therapy*[1] may be given as if the patient had bacterial meningitis:

- Vancomycin + either ceftriaxone or cefotaxime
- Ampicillin is added if listeria is suspected.

Dexamethasone is routinely used for patients with bacterial meningitis; if there is concern about a bacterial cause at the time of initial evaluation, then administration is recommended. A common protocol is dexamethasone 10 mg IV q6h for 4 days.

Bacterial Meningitis

Bacterial meningitis is much more acute than viral meningitis for most patients. Important organisms include:

- *Strep pneumoniae* (Pneumococcal meningitis): Most common
- *Haemophilus influenzae*: Less common since vaccine
- *Neisseria meningitidis* (meningococcal meningitis): Especially with high-density housing (e.g., college dorms)

- *Listeria monocytogenes*: Especially in alcoholics; immunosuppressed; pregnant; chronic diseases such as hepatic and renal failure, and diabetes; and elderly
- *Gram-negative bacilli*: Especially after neurosurgical procedures, immunosuppressed, elderly (e.g., *Escherichia coli*, *Klebsiella pneumoniae*)
- *Staphylococci*: Especially after head injury, neurosurgical procedure, shunts
- *Group B Streptococcus*: with immunocompromised state, alcoholism, pregnancy, hepatic or renal failure, pregnancy

PRESENTATION is with various combinations of fever, headache, nausea/vomiting, and neck pain, stiffness, or rigidity. Rash is common with meningococcal meningitis. Symptoms can be subtle initially, especially with an immunocompromised state. With more severe meningitis, cerebral symptoms may develop—delirium, confusion, progressing to seizures and/or coma. Cranial nerve palsies can occur.

DIAGNOSIS is suspected by headache with signs of inflammation such as fever or increased blood WBC. Diagnosis is confirmed by lumbar puncture (LP).

- Patients with sinuses as a source may have active sinusitis at the time of presentation, and this should be looked for using sinus CT.
- Brain imaging with CT or MRI should be done emergently and prior to the LP if there are signs of encephalopathy, cranial nerve palsy, or seizure. If none of these is present, LP can be done as soon as meningitis is considered so CSF can be obtained prior to urgent administration of antibiotics.

CSF findings:

- Appearance is clear or cloudy depending on cell count.
- Opening pressure is elevated.
- WBC is typically in the thousands with bacterial meningitis, although levels down into the low 100s can be seen. Polymorphonuclear predominance favors bacterial etiology.
- Protein is usually elevated.
- Glucose is typically low, and very low levels signify a poor prognosis.

MANAGEMENT begins with empiric therapy immediately after suspicion of bacterial meningitis. Antibiotics are usually ordered as soon as meningitis is suspected and given as soon as the LP is completed. If there must be a delay in LP because of pending imaging, logistics, or otherwise, then antibiotics are given immediately. Consultation with infectious disease is recommended since local antibiograms differ and recommendations made here may be replaced by updated information since publication.

Empiric therapy for suspected bacterial meningitis at the time of writing is as follows:

- Most patients
  - Vancomycin + either ceftriaxone or cefotaxime
  - Ampicillin is added if:
    - *Listeria* is suspected on the basis of disorders listed at the beginning of this section
  - Pregnancy

- Post-neurosurgery, penetrating injury, or CSF shunt
  - Vancomycin
  - Plus either:
    - Cefepime, or ceftazidime, or meropenem

Doses depend on a number of factors including size, age, and comorbid conditions, so please consult published prescribing information. Organism-specific therapy is guided by identification and sensitivities; our infectious disease colleagues should be consulted for assistance.

Steroids have become part of standard therapy for bacterial meningitis. A standard dose is dexamethasone 10 mg IV q6h for 4 days.

Intrathecal antibiotics are sometimes considered for patients who have had recent neurosurgery or instrumentation and who have not responded to IV antibiotics.

Some patients with severe bacterial meningitis develop *cerebral edema* with risk for herniation. Standard measures for increased intracranial pressure (ICP) are commonly given (Chapter 41).

Seizures are treated with standard antiepileptic drugs (AEDs), usually parenteral, including fosphenytoin, valproate, or levetiracetam. Midazolam or propofol can be given for status epilepticus.

Fungal Meningitis

Fungal meningitis is uncommon in immunocompetent patients. *Cryptococcus neoformans* is the most common organism. Other notable agents are *Aspergillus, Histoplasma capsulatum, Blastomyces,* and *Coccidioides immitis.*

PRESENTATION is usually subacute to chronic with cognitive changes. Headache and fever often occur, but this is not invariable. Deficits can include ataxia, weakness of extremities, and occasionally cranial nerve palsies, especially with cryptococcal meningitis.

DIAGNOSIS is usually considered when a patient with confusion and/or ataxia has negative imaging and basic lab studies. Since most cases are immunocompromised, this history is helpful.

Brain imaging with CT or MRI often shows hydrocephalus, especially with cryptococcal meningitis. Contrast reveals meningeal inflammatory change in many patients.

CSF findings:

- Opening pressure: Increased, usually 20–30 cm H_2O, but may be normal
- Appearance: Clear or cloudy
- WBC: 10–500 cells/μL
- Glucose: Reduced
- Protein: Increased

Definitive identification of organism can be established by CSF analysis including smears, cultures, and special testing. Cryptococcal antigen in CSF has high sensitivity and specificity.[2]

MANAGEMENT of cryptococcal meningitis is usually with amphotericin B in patients without AIDS. Flucytosine may be added, which can reduce the amount of amphotericin needed. Patients with AIDS are started on treatment with amphotericin B + flucytosine but then are treated with fluconazole. Increased ICP is a common in cryptococcal meningitis and, if untreated, can lead to severe neurological deficits. Evidence has shown that therapeutic lumbar punctures on a daily basis can lead to improved survival.[3]

ENCEPHALITIS

Encephalitis is usually viral but can be prion or autoimmune. Prion diseases are given their own subheading later in this chapter. We discuss viral encephalitis here.

Viral encephalitis can be caused by a wide variety of agents. Some of the most common include HSV, VZV, influenza virus, enteroviruses, and lymphocytic choriomeningitis virus. The arbovirus family of encephalitides includes WNV, Japanese, Eastern and Western equine, Venezuelan, California, and St. Louis virus. In addition, encephalitis can be caused by measles virus, mumps virus, or rabies virus.

PRESENTATION is commonly with altered mental status, which can be a depressed level of consciousness or behavioral disorder. Fever and headache are common but not invariable. Neck pain and meningeal signs suggest a meningeal component to the infection, *meningoencephalitis*. Encephalitis can be associated with symptoms of myelopathy indicating *myelitis* or *encephalomyelitis*. Few symptoms are specific to defined etiologies, but focal deficits and seizures favor HSV.

DIAGNOSIS is suspected with headache, fever, and neck pain. Neurologic symptoms strongly suggest the diagnosis including confusion, focal motor deficits, and seizures.

Brain imaging with CT or MRI is performed urgently to look for abscess or other structural abnormality giving similar symptoms. HSV encephalitis often has temporal signal change indicating edema and perhaps hemorrhage best seen on MRI.

LP is performed if there is no sign of risk of herniation, such as hydrocephalus, cerebral edema, or brainstem edema. CSF findings are as follows:

- Opening pressure is usually modestly increased.
- WBC is increased in CSF, usually at least 100 WBC/μL, and can be as high as 1,000. Higher levels raise concern for bacterial infection.
- Glucose is usually normal; however, it is commonly reduced in lymphocytic choriomeningitis.
- Protein is usually mildly elevated.
- PCR can be performed for many types of encephalitis including HSV, VZV, CMV, arboviruses, equine viruses, WNV, and Epstein Barr virus (EBV), as well as for a host of nonviral infections. Availability differs between institutions.

EEG is abnormal in most patients with encephalitis. Polymorphic slowing with a mixed frequency is common. Spikes, which can be focal or generalized, can be seen in many types. Periodic lateralized epileptiform discharges (PLEDs) suggest HSV.

MANAGEMENT mainly includes antiviral therapy, especially for HSV encephalitis. Since in the ED the diagnosis of HSV encephalitis can be suspected but often not certain, patients who might have HSV encephalitis should be started on an antiviral agent and then the treatment altered depending on subsequent results. Note that HSV PCR may be negative especially early in the course of the disease.

- *Acyclovir* is administered immediately on suspicion of HSV encephalitis, adjusted for renal function, and continuation is dependent on results of the lab tests.
- *Ganciclovir* is used for CMV encephalitis but with variable success.
- *Corticosteroids* have been tried, as with bacterial meningitis, but there is no consensus and this is still under study.
- *Anticonvulsants* are used for patients with seizures and include the usual parenteral meds: fosphenytoin, valproate, or levetiracetam. Sometimes, the seizures can be very difficult to control, and lacosamide can be tried.
- *Osmotic agents* are occasionally used for patients with increased ICP with cerebral edema.

VIRAL MYELITIS

Viral myelitis can be from a variety of agents.[4] Some of the most important include HSV, VZV, CMV, EBV, HIV, WNV, echovirus, and, recently, even a report of myelitis with Zika virus.[5] For many of these, systemic symptoms are associated. But generally, the pattern of clinical findings is insufficient to determine a precise etiologic diagnosis. Some clinical scenarios are as follows:

- WNV can produce headache, fever, GI distress, and rash prior to development of flaccid weakness.
- HSV, especially HSV-2, can produce an ascending myelitis that begins with sensory and sphincter disturbance, then progressive weakness.[6]
- HIV can produce a progressive painless myelopathy, usually late in the course when other complications such as dementia or opportunistic infection have developed. A myelitis with acute HIV infection is rare but has been reported.[7]

Postviral myelitis develops as well and can present with subacute myelopathy usually without prodromal symptoms. Additional information is found in Chapter 22.

PRION ENCEPHALOPATHIES

Prion diseases are rare but important causes of encephalopathy. Patients with prion diseases are often initially considered to possibly have a chronic neurodegenerative disorder. Discussion of prion diseases in a text can be problematic because these diseases can be infectious, inherited, or sporadic.

Hospital neurologists will occasionally see *Creutzfeldt-Jakob disease* (CJD), but the other disorders are not expected in the hospital setting. *Kuru* is not expected in most of our regions of practice and is not discussed here.

Creutzfeldt-Jakob Disease

CJD is also called *subacute spongiform encephalopathy*. Cases can be sporadic or transmitted by medical procedures. There may be a familial predisposition.

PRESENTATION is classically with dementia, myoclonus, and ataxia, but the most common initial presentation is confusion often with psychiatric features such as hallucinations and behavioral change. Progression is over weeks to months. Development of myoclonus is later in the disease course, with spontaneous and stimulus-sensitive myoclonus. Startle can develop. Cerebellar ataxia affects gait and appendicular movements. Other symptoms can include seizures and visual disturbance.

DIAGNOSIS is considered when a patient with cognitive decline has accompanying ataxia and myoclonus. Clues may be rapid decline and myoclonus. Myoclonus might be overlooked early, especially if it is restricted, for example to the fingers. Of the studies listed here, we often have to repeat the EEG in order to see classic findings suggestive of CJD. However, we seldom recommend brain biopsy since there is no disease-modifying therapy.

- *Imaging* with CT brain may be unrevealing. MRI often shows areas of increased signal on diffusion signal in the cortical ribbon and/or increased T2 signal in the lenticular nucleus.
- *CSF* is usually normal, but the protein may be mildly increased. CSF may show the 14-3-3 protein, which is supportive but not definitive.
- *EEG* classically shows periodic sharp waves, which is an appearance strongly suggestive of CJD; however, this is not perfectly specific and is not universally present; repeat study may be needed to see this.
- *Pathology* of the brain at the time of biopsy or autopsy is the definitive test.

MANAGEMENT is generally supportive; there is no specific treatment for CJD. Myoclonus and seizures are treated with standard medications, especially valproate, levetiracetam, or clonazepam.

Prevention is key, which includes proper handling of body fluids, surgical instruments, and other exposed materials. The Centers for Disease Control (CDC) website has detailed recommendations on infection control practices.[8]

Variant CJD and Bovine Spongiform Encephalopathy

Variant CJD (vCJD) and *Bovine Spongiform Encephalopathy (BSE)* are related conditions and transmissible prion diseases. BSE, otherwise known as *mad cow disease*, was identified in cattle. After the BSE epidemic in United Kingdom, surveillance for prion disease revealed a disorder that looked similar to CJD but with some important differences.

PRESENTATION is similar to that of CJD but tends to affect younger patients and has a slower progression. Patients with vCJD are usually less than 40 years of age and commonly less than 30 years. Dementia, ataxia, and later myoclonus develop. Behavioral changes develop as with sporadic CJD.

DIAGNOSIS should not be suspected in the United States; sporadic CJD would be much more likely. Since there is no disease-modifying therapy for vCJD, we often do most of the studies mentioned here but seldom do a brain biopsy.

- *MRI brain scans* may show characteristic findings in the thalamus that are not seen with CJD and can help with differentiation.
- *EEG* often does not show the periodic pattern seen in CJD. Diffuse slowing is more typical.

- *CSF* may show the 14-3-3 protein and other markers, but these are not specific for vCJD. CSF is otherwise normal and much less likely to show these markers than sporadic CJD.
- *Pathology* is definitive for some patients, but, unfortunately, specimens are commonly negative.

MANAGEMENT is supportive. There are no disease-modifying treatments. Seizures and myoclonus are treated with standard drugs.

BRAIN ABSCESS

Brain abscess can be bacterial, fungi, or parasitic. Typically, patients present with symptoms necessitating imaging, and an enhancing lesion is identified; the question then becomes "Is this is abscess or tumor?" Sites of origin can include contiguous spread and distant spread. Subacute bacterial endocarditis (SBE) can result in stroke or abscess formation, but stroke is statistically more likely. Sinus origin most likely affects the frontal and temporal lobe. Ear origin produces abscesses most likely in the cerebellum. Distant sites, such as cardiac and pulmonary, can produce abscesses anywhere. Endocarditis is especially likely to produce multiple abscesses.

Many organisms can produce brain abscess, but some of the most important include:

- *Streptococcus*: Sinus, dental, ear, endocarditis
- *Bacteroides*: Especially sinus and dental
- *Staphylococcus*: Especially with endocarditis or neurosurgery
- *Enterobacteria*: Especially ear and neurosurgical
- *Pseudomonas*: Especially ear, neurosurgical
- *Aspergillus*: Especially in immunosuppressed
- *Toxoplasma*: Especially with HIV

PRESENTATION is classically headache, fever, and focal symptoms referable to the abscess. However, this constellation is present in a minority of patients. Headache is the most common symptom, followed by cognitive deficits and focal neurologic signs. Fever is inconstant. Other symptoms can include nausea, vomiting, and seizures. Exam can show cognitive change and focal deficits of almost any localization.

DIAGNOSIS is suspected when a patient presents with a headache and focal deficits, and imaging shows a mass lesion.

- *Imaging* of the brain is performed urgently and shows a focal lesion that enhances with a ring-like character. MRI is superior to CT. When this is seen, the main differential diagnosis is tumor. If the initial scan is unenhanced, the differential diagnosis is broader and includes stroke or other low-density structural lesions. Early in the stage of cerebritis, CT may show only lucency and little enhancement. Later, a more definite capsule forms that has a more typical appearance. MRI may show high signal on T2 and fluid-attenuated inversion recovery (FLAIR) with the edema. Contrasted MRI might not show significant enhancement very early, so restudy is needed if there is a diagnostic question.

- *Lab* studies usually show an increase in WBC even in the absence of fever. Blood cultures may show positive growth, but absence of growth does not rule out abscess as a diagnosis.
- *CSF* is usually not obtained because of the risk of herniation with mass lesion. If there is little mass effect, LP can be performed although it is usually not needed. Protein is usually increased. Glucose is usually normal. WBC is often but not invariably increased, although not as elevated as with bacterial meningitis. Opening pressure may be normal or increased.
- *Echocardiogram* is often done if there is concern over a cardiac source.
- *Sinus imaging* is usually performed unless there is another obvious source.
- *Aspiration and/or biopsy* of an accessible lesion is usually done.

Identification of the infectious source is not possible in 15–20% of patients.

MANAGEMENT begins before there is a complete diagnosis. Suspicion of brain abscess from presentation and imaging triggers the institution of high-dose antibiotics. Blood cultures should be drawn before the antibiotics are started if possible.

Surgery is usually more diagnostic than therapeutic, but if there is significant mass effect, single or even repeated aspirations can be performed. Open drainage is advocated by some clinicians. Early in the stage of cerebritis, before a complete abscess has formed, surgery might not be performed emergently so antibiotics are administered without delay.

Antibiotics are given urgently. *Empiric therapy* depends on the suspected source. Recommendations are changing, so consult the latest literature and guidelines. Duration of antibiotic therapy depends on abscess size, whether it was at the cerebritis stage, and if there was surgical drainage.

Steroids can have a deleterious effect on medical therapy by reducing antibiotic effectiveness, so corticosteroids are used mainly when significant edema with mass effect demands treatment.

HERPES ZOSTER AND POST-HERPETIC NEURALGIA

Herpes zoster produces *shingles* or reactivation of the VZV, causing pain in one nerve root or cranial nerve distribution. Predisposing factors include immunocompromised state such as cancer or HIV and advanced age, although it often occurs with none of these issues. Cranial nerves affected are often CN 5 and CN 7.

Herpes Zoster

PRESENTATION usually begins with skin sensitivity in one dermatome, followed by sharp dysesthetic pain, often lancinating. Rash develops in the area, ultimately becoming vesicular, which, along with the limited distribution, gives a characteristic appearance.

Ramsay Hunt syndrome is herpes zoster of the geniculate ganglion and presents with CN 7 palsy with pain and vesicles in and around the ear.

Herpes zoster ophthalmicus is involvement of the trigeminal ganglion, producing pain and rash around the eye extending to the forehead.

MANAGEMENT of herpes zoster and subtypes is with antivirals such as famciclovir plus common medications for neuropathic pain, especially gabapentin. Herpes zoster ophthalmicus may require topical corticosteroids, as directed by ophthalmology.

Prevention of herpes zoster is offered by vaccine, which is recommended to patients starting at age 60 years.

Post-Herpetic Neuralgia

Post-herpetic neuralgia is persistent pain in some patients with herpes zoster that remains after the skin manifestations have resolved. By definition, the pain has to outlast the herpes zoster by 3 months.

PRESENTATION is with sharp shooting or stabbing pain in the region of the recent herpes zoster.

MANAGEMENT is with typical medications for neuropathic pain.

NEUROSYPHILIS

Neurosyphilis is a spectrum of manifestations of syphilis. Neurosyphilis has three stages. Meningitis may develop in secondary syphilis, but neurologic complications are most common in tertiary syphilis.

PRESENTATION depends on the type of neurologic complication:

- *Asymptomatic neurosyphilis* can be a mild meningitis that resolves. About 5% of these progress to more advanced neurosyphilis without treatment.
- *Meningovascular neurosyphilis* presents with headache and neck pain, cognitive change, and visual disturbance. Myelopathy can develop.
- *Parenchymatous neurosyphilis* is also called *general paresis* and develops years after initial infection. Findings include cognitive changes, which can be behavioral and/ or frank dementia. Focal signs and seizures may be seen.
- *Tabes dorsalis* develops many years after initial infection. There is degeneration of the posterior columns and nerve roots. Findings include ataxia, neuropathic pain, and incontinence. The Argyll Robertson pupil is seen at this stage—pupil constriction to accommodation but not to light.

DIAGNOSIS is considered in a patient with meningitis or encephalopathy, especially when syphilis serology of blood or CSF returns abnormal. MRI may show no significant abnormalities or inflammatory or ischemic changes. CSF shows a mild pleocytosis and increased protein.

MANAGEMENT should be guided by infectious disease colleagues since this is a long-term process. Antibiotics are prescribed for the patient, but additionally sex partners should be approached about evaluation and treatment. Treatment of neurologic complications is symptomatic (e.g., anticonvulsants for seizures or neuropathic pain).

HUMAN IMMUNODEFICIENCY VIRUS

Hospital neurologists are commonly involved in care of patients with HIV relative to some commonly encountered neurologic manifestations:

- Cryptococcal meningitis
- Dementia

- Neuropathy
- Toxoplasmosis

Less common complications encountered include myelopathy, myopathy, and polyradiculopathy.

Dementia

Dementia develops in many patients with HIV. HIV-associated dementia and opportunistic infections are of principal concern.

HIV-associated dementia is neuronal degeneration due to the virus. Presentation is with cognitive decline, sometimes with behavioral abnormalities. Other neurologic manifestations of HIV may be present, including sensory and motor deficits. Diagnosis is suspected with the cognitive disturbance with no other cause being identified. Brain imaging with MRI or CT is performed to look for opportunistic infection. CSF analysis may be needed. Management depends on antiretroviral therapy. Cholinesterase inhibitors and memantine have not been shown to be effective, although there has been limited study.

Opportunistic infections can produce cognitive deterioration, with a presentation that can be a rapidly progressive dementia. This is in the differential diagnosis of all HIV patients with dementia. Focal signs may occur depending on type and location of the infection. Diagnosis is by brain imaging with MRI or CT. Management is of the underlying infection, as determined by our infectious disease colleagues.

Neuropathy

Multiple neuropathic syndromes can develop. These are distinguished by symptomatology, stage of disease at which they occur, and clinical findings. The most important are discussed here.

Distal symmetric polyneuropathy is the most common neuropathy, affecting at least 35% of patients with HIV.[9] Sensory symptoms predominate, with pain and hypersensitivity. Diagnosis depends on recognition of neuropathy symptoms, electromyography (EMG), and nerve conduction studies (NCS) to characterize the neuropathy as a distal sensorimotor polyneuropathy, and rule-out of other causes. There is no specific test for this neuropathy, so other causes must be eliminated including diabetes, vitamin deficiency, or toxic neuropathy (e.g., from medication or ethanol). Management is treatment of the neuropathic pain, usually with tricyclic antidepressants (TCAs) and/ or AEDs. Vitamin B_{12} supplementation may be helpful even in the absence of documented deficiency because of reduced B_{12} utilization.

Inflammatory neuropathies have been reported in patients with HIV, although the relative incidence is not clear compared to patients without HIV. The diagnostic approach to possible acute inflammatory demyelinating polyneuropathy (AIDP) and chronic inflammatory demyelinating polyneuropathy (CIDP) is the same as for patients without HIV. Management is usually with IV immunoglobulin (IVIg) or plasma exchange.

Progressive lumbosacral plexopathy is seen mainly in patients with more advanced HIV/AIDS disease but is less common recently because of aggressive antiretroviral therapy. It is due to CMV and typically affects bilateral lumbosacral plexuses. Presentation is with leg weakness, often bilateral, which can progress to complete paralysis, with bowel and bladder incontinence. Sensory symptoms are minor, with paresthesias but without significant sensory loss. Reflexes are suppressed and usually absent. Diagnosis is suspected because of the progressive leg weakness. Differential diagnosis includes inflammatory neuropathy or cord or cauda equina lesion. Clues to this disorder are the relative absence of arm involvement with marked leg weakness, areflexia, sphincter disturbance, and motor predominance. CSF shows pleocytosis, usually polymorphonuclear with elevated protein. CSF can be analyzed for CMV. Management is with ganciclovir and/or foscarnet, and most clinicians treat with suspicion before a certain diagnosis has been made.

Mononeuropathy multiplex typically occurs in patients with established symptomatic HIV infection or AIDS. Presentation is with dysfunction of any combination of peripheral and cranial nerves. Motor and sensory symptoms develop. Diagnosis is suspected by the multifocal symptoms. This differs from distal symmetric polyneuropathy by the asymmetric involvement and motor deficits. And it differs from inflammatory neuropathies by the asymmetry and relative preservation of reflexes. It differs from lumbosacral plexopathy by the upper extremity and possibly cranial nerve involvement and absence of sphincter and total leg involvement.

Toxoplasmosis

Toxoplasmosis is a parasitic infection that is usually asymptomatic but can have neurologic manifestations, especially in immunosuppressed patients and children with congenital acquisition. Presentation of CNS toxoplasmosis is typically with headache and cognitive change, with focal findings representative of the localization of the lesions. Diagnosis is suspected in a patient with HIV who has intracranial enhancing mass lesions, especially with a ring-enhancement. MRI brain with contrast is most sensitive. CSF is analyzed for a range of infections and usually shows a modest lymphocytic pleocytosis with some elevation in protein. In a typical clinical scenario, these findings are usually sufficient to warrant toxoplasmosis treatment without biopsy. Management is per our infectious disease colleagues. If the patient undergoes empiric toxoplasma therapy without improvement in the lesions, then biopsy should be considered.

PROGRESSIVE MULTIFOCAL LEUKOENCEPHALOPATHY

Progressive multifocal leukoencephalopathy (PML) is an infectious disorder due to reactivation of the JC virus. It is typically seen in immunosuppressed patients, especially HIV, cancers, transplant patients, and, from the perspective of neurologists, patients with multiple sclerosis and related disorders who are on certain immunosuppressant drugs.

PRESENTATION is with focal symptoms and signs, such as weakness, incoordination, visual loss, and dominant or nondominant hemisphere findings. Cognitive deficits can occur with extensive disease. Multifocal symptoms can occur.

DIAGNOSIS is suspected when focal symptoms develop in a patient at risk, mainly immunosuppressed. Brain imaging with MRI shows areas of increased signal on T2 and FLAIR imaging with a patchy diffuse character very different from a typical mass lesion. Contrast usually does not produce enhancement. CSF analysis may show JC virus DNA on PCR. Biopsy is usually not needed.

MANAGEMENT in patients on immunosuppressive therapy is to remove the offending agents. Patients on natalizumab may also be treated with plasma exchange to remove remaining drug. Patients with HIV are treated with aggressive antiretroviral therapy.

Patients on immunosuppressive therapy and HIV appropriately treated may develop *immune reconstitution inflammatory syndrome* (IRIS), which can worsen symptoms. This is discussed in more detail in Chapter 22.

ENDOCARDITIS

Endocarditis is usually bacterial and related to a host predisposition to infection, which can include prosthetic heart valve, IV drug abuse, or other vascular instrumentation. *Staphylococcus* and *Streptococcus* are the most common organisms, although others may occur, including fungi. Noninfectious endocarditis can occur.

PRESENTATION of neurologic complications of endocarditis is usually with transient ischemic attack (TIA) or cerebrovascular accident (CVA) but can be infectious aneurysm; intracranial hemorrhage, which can be from aneurysm or not; and meningitis. Seizures can occur.

DIAGNOSIS is suspected especially when a patient with a stroke syndrome is found to have a heart murmur. Petechiae and splinter hemorrhages are supportive. Blood cultures are performed. Brain imaging with MRI or CT shows focal defects. Echo confirms the embolic source.

MANAGEMENT is by antibiotics. Anticoagulation is avoided because of the risk of hemorrhage. Valve repair may be needed.

Patients at risk of endocarditis require antibiotic prophylaxis including some patients with congenital heart disease, previous endocarditis, and prosthetic heart valves.

WHIPPLE DISEASE

Whipple disease is due to infection with *Tropheryma whippelii*. Symptoms are usually intestinal and musculoskeletal, but neurologic manifestations can occur. This is commonly considered but rarely diagnosed.

PRESENTATION is most commonly with diarrhea, arthralgias, and fever. Neurologic manifestations can include dementia, delirium, frontal-lobe dysfunction, meningoencephalitis, seizures including status epilepticus, cerebellar ataxia, supranuclear vertical gaze palsy, and pyramidal or extrapyramidal findings.

DIAGNOSIS is made by biopsy, usually of the small bowel. Neurologists may consider the diagnosis when a patient presents with neurologic deficits with diarrhea and arthralgias. Oculomasticatory myorhythmia is characteristic of Whipple disease; there are smooth convergent/divergent eye movements associated with synchronous contractions of the masseter. A supranuclear vertical gaze can be seen in these patients.

MANAGEMENT is with antibiotics. If biopsy is negative yet the presentation is typical, treatment is often administered.

LYME DISEASE

Lyme disease is a tick-borne infection with *Borrelia burgdorferi*. There are regional concentrations, especially from the northeastern United States to the Midwest. However, it can be acquired in a more extensive region.

PRESENTATION is with erythema migrans, a characteristic rash with initially a red center but then an expanding margin with darker indurated center. Lyme disease can become disseminated early with new lesions that do not have the indurated center.

Neurologic involvement can be:

- Bell palsy
- Meningitis
- Encephalitis

The meningitis has an aseptic appearance with usually only a modest lymphocytic pleocytosis. Bell palsy can be bilateral.

Late after Lyme disease, patients may present with cognitive change associated with the more common arthralgias. This is a controversial area.

DIAGNOSIS is suspected by the typical rash. Serology can be confirmatory, but, when suspected, treatment should not wait for positive serologies. Neurologic evaluation is requested when a patient has headache or cognitive change. If acute CNS infection is suspected, then brain imaging and LP should be performed. We are also occasionally asked to consult for presumptive chronic Lyme disease; this should be handled in the outpatient setting once we have ruled out acute illness in the hospital setting.

Treatment is with antibiotics early in the course. Our task is to ensure that the acute illness has been treated appropriately.

WEST NILE

Of those who develop WNV, only a small percentage will developed neuroinvasive disease. The rapid onset of flaccid paralysis in conjunction with encephalopathy should raise suspicion for WNV. However, flaccid paralysis can occur without overt signs of meningitis or encephalitis.

Symptoms include, but are not limited to headache, fever, meningeal signs, and photophobia. Extrapyramidal symptoms (rigidity, bradykinesia, and postural instability) are common. Paralysis can occur quite rapidly, often as early as 48 hours after symptom onset.

Given the clinical presentation, WNV can have a similar presentation to AIDP. CSF examination along with electrodiagnostic testing can help decipher the two entities, as clarified by Leis and Stokic.[10]

- Onset of deficits with WNV is typically during the acute phase of infection rather than delayed as with AIDP.
- WNV is often asymmetric whereas AIDP is usually symmetric
- WNV is more likely to produce sphincter disturbance whereas AIDP is more likely to produce sensory symptoms and deficits.
- CSF in WNV often shows pleocytosis whereas it is usually acellular in AIDP.
- EMG & NCS in WNV can show axonal changes whereas AIDP is demyelinating.
- WNV is often associated with CNS deficits, e.g. encephalopathy, myelopathy.

ZIKA

Recently, Zika virus has been associated not only with microcephaly in newborns,[11] but also with AIDP and acute disseminated encephalomyelitis (ADEM). This is a field that is rapidly expanding. The CDC publishes updates ahead of peer-reviewed publications.[12]

18 Cognitive Disorders

Howard S. Kirshner, MD and
Karl E. Misulis, MD, PhD

CHAPTER CONTENTS

- Overview
- Acute and Subacute Cognitive Disorders
  - Delirium
  - Metabolic Encephalopathy
  - Transient Global Amnesia
  - Syncope
- Chronic Cognitive Disorders
  - First Recognition of Dementia During Hospitalization
  - Hospitalization of the Patient with Dementia
  - Alzheimer's Disease
  - Dementia with Lewy Bodies and Parkinson Disease with Dementia
  - Vascular Dementia
  - Frontotemporal Dementia
- Mild Cognitive Impairment
- Management of Hospitalized Patients with Dementia

OVERVIEW

Dementia is usually evaluated and managed in the outpatient arena, but hospital-based neurologists often deal with patients with dementia. These may be either patients with dementia whose condition is exacerbated by concurrent illness and hospitalization, or patients with hospital-acquired delirium in whom there is a suspicion of dementia. Patients with dementia are less likely to return to home care following hospitalization.

ACUTE AND SUBACUTE COGNITIVE DISORDERS
Delirium

The differential diagnosis and presentation of delirium in the hospital setting were discussed in Chapter 5. This discussion of the management of hospitalized patients with dementia overlaps that of Chapter 5. Patients more likely to develop delirium in the hospital are those with advanced age, dementia, and sensory deprivation (visual/hearing loss). Patients are also predisposed by sleep deprivation in the hospital caused by the disturbances of ongoing care (medications, presence of equipment and lines).

PRESENTATION is with acute to subacute cognitive change that can be hyperactive or hypoactive.

DIAGNOSIS is suspected when a patient develops confusion, agitation, or lethargy. Brain imaging for stroke, edema, or other structural etiology is often appropriate. Labs should include examination for increased WBC, for urinary tract infection (UTI), and for metabolic disorders including renal, hepatic, and perhaps thyroid dysfunction. If there is concern over a malnourished or an alcoholic state, then studies should include thiamine levels; on suspicion, we consider giving thiamine without laboratory or historical confirmation.

MANAGEMENT is difficult. We try to avoid sedative-hypnotics if possible. Nonpharmacological therapy can include sitters, minimizing interventions at night to maintain sleep, and a quiet environment. Some patients are reassured by a few personal items from home, such as pictures.

Metabolic Encephalopathy

Metabolic encephalopathy is commonly encountered in hospital neurology practice. This was discussed in Chapter 5, but is detailed further here.

PRESENTATION is usually with confusion or lethargy, but delirium with agitation can occur. Focal findings are not expected and would point to a pre-existing lesion or another acute diagnosis.

DIAGNOSIS is established by absence of other causes and identification of responsible cause(s); we usually find metabolic encephalopathies to be multifactorial. Imaging is needed, magnetic resonance imaging (MRI) of the brain is preferable to computed tomography. Electroencephalogram (EEG) shows diffuse slowing, often with a polymorphic appearance. CSF analysis may be needed if there are inflammatory markers or seizures. Among the causes we often identify are:

- Renal insufficiency: New or worsening
- Hepatic failure: New or worsening
- Electrolyte abnormality
- Sepsis/Systemic inflammatory response syndrome (SIRS)
- Urinary tract infection
- Pneumonia
- Medication (e.g., cefepime); or altered metabolism increasing levels of an old medication (e.g., phenytoin with renal failure)
- Withdrawal state, from substance which was stopped or reduced (e.g. benzodiazepine, ethanol)

MANAGEMENT is by correction of the defects, if possible. Withdrawal of any offending medications is recommended if possible.

Transient Global Amnesia

Transient global amnesia (TGA) is the acute onset of short-term memory difficulty without other findings. Cause is uncertain but may be related to migraine or vascular disease; there may be multiple causes for the same presentation.

PRESENTATION is with acute onset of memory loss from the onset forward; in other words, *antegrade*. Patients are often aware of the deficit and anxious because of it. They may function relatively normally during the event (e.g., driving without incident). Exam is otherwise normal.

DIAGNOSIS is suspected when a patient presents with acute memory loss and the absence of encephalopathy or focal signs. The awareness and anxiety suggests TGA rather than psychogenic amnesia. The otherwise normal demeanor and cognitive function in other areas differentiates TGA from toxic, metabolic, and infectious encephalopathies. Imaging with MRI is preferential to CT and is usually normal, but occasionally there is restricted diffusion in the hippocampus on one or both sides. EEG is normal or shows mild nonspecific slowing, but there have been reports of epileptiform discharges; we believe this is rare, and TGA is typically not a seizure.

MANAGEMENT is supportive. The symptoms resolve within hours, usually less than 12 but almost always less than 24 hours. If vascular risk factors are identified during the evaluation, these are addressed even though the link to the presentation is uncertain.

Syncope

Syncope was discussed in Chapter 5 regarding differential diagnosis, which is expansive. Here, we discuss a few selected syncopal disorders seen in hospital practice. Syncope can be recurrent and lead to serious injury, so we advise patients with syncope that if they feel presyncopal to lower their head to the floor; we have seen multiple patients with damage or death due to injury from syncope.

Neurocardiogenic syncope: Also called *vasovagal syncope*, is drop in blood pressure usually triggered by an event such as fright or a bowel movement. If recurrent, avoiding precipitating events may help. If autonomic insufficiency is suspected, this should be evaluated with autonomic testing.

Cough syncope: This condition presents with syncope precipitated by coughing fits, most commonly seen in patients with COPD. Association with cough might not be recognized by the patient and should be asked about. Clonic activity is common and raises the concern for seizures. Treatment is focused on the cough.

Micturition syncope: Micturition causes hypotension, particularly when standing, resulting in syncope. Patients usually are aware of the trigger and learn to sit while urinating.

CHRONIC COGNITIVE DISORDERS
First Recognition of Dementia During Hospitalization

Patients with dementia have an increased incidence of hospital-acquired delirium, so it is expected that a significant proportion of patients with delirium have historical evidence to suggest pre-existing incipient dementia or mild cognitive impairment.

DIAGNOSIS of dementia is similar to that in the outpatient arena, with brain imaging (MRI is preferable to CT) and basic labs including thyroid function tests, B_{12} level, and other studies as indicated. EEG is usually not needed, but hospitalized patients with prominent mental status change should have EEG performed to look for nonconvulsive seizure activity. Lumbar puncture (LP) should be considered when the patient has a subacute or acute change in mental status that is not explained by labs or imaging findings.

Neuropsychological testing is commonly performed in the outpatient arena, but this is not best performed when the patient is confused in the hospital. It is better to perform the neuropsychological testing as an outpatient, after the patient has improved to a baseline. Unfortunately, many patients with delirium have residual cognitive impairment after the illness.[1-2]

Hospitalization of the Patient with Dementia

Patients with dementia are hospitalized at a greater rate than are people without dementia of similar age. This is likely due to comorbid conditions that predispose to dementia including hypertension, diabetes, obesity, congestive heart failure, and other concurrent disorders. Potential for exacerbation of dementia and hospitalization psychosis should be anticipated and prepared for.

Patients with a baseline Mini-Mental State Exam (MMSE) score of 24 or less have the greatest risk for development of delirium in the hospital, which suggests early dementia is the major risk factor.[3]

The prescription of sedative-hypnotics should be avoided if possible, and management should rely on nonpharmacological therapy where possible. Unfortunately, although the literature is replete with opinions that neuroleptics and related agents are never needed, this is not the case. While these agents are certainly overused, judicious use when other nonpharmacological measures have failed is appropriate. Haloperidol (especially IM) and lorazepam are both effective, but it is not clear that the combination works better than either alone. Oral haloperidol carries a high risk of extrapyramidal reactions and parkinsonism in elderly patients, and lorazepam can exacerbate confusion. Newer, atypical antipsychotic agents such as quetiapine and olanzapine are often used, especially in nighttime doses.

Alzheimer Disease

Alzheimer disease (AD) is the most common dementia, responsible for at least half of cases. Vascular risk factors predispose to AD. These include obesity, diabetes, hypertension, hyperlipidemia, atrial fibrillation, obstructive sleep apnea, and stroke. This blurs the distinction between AD and vascular dementia.

PRESENTATION begins with memory loss, confusion, and judgment errors. Noncognitive deficits are not expected early in the disease. With advanced AD, ambulation, continence, and swallowing are affected.

- Patients with AD usually have a history of preclinical decline. This may be mild cognitive impairment (MCI), as discussed later.
- Stages of AD are important for treatment and clinical advice. In general, patients are less responsive to treatment with advanced disease. However, since these medications do not cure or otherwise alter the course of the disease, early treatment is not essential; they have mainly symptomatic benefit. A commonly used system features seven stages, but three stages suffice for most clinical decision-making.[4]

Stages of Alzheimer Disease

- *Mild*
  - ○ Episodes of memory loss, some difficulty with comprehension and expression of language; mood change is common
  - ○ Able to do most personal activities.
  - ○ Many are able to attend to legal and financial activities, but the time will come when they cannot.
  - ○ Can have symptomatic improvement in response to cholinesterase inhibitors.
- *Moderate*
  - ○ Memory difficulty extends to well-known people and places, persistently abnormal.
  - ○ May have delusions and increasing behavioral abnormalities.
  - ○ Assistance needed for legal and financial tasks.
  - ○ Can respond to cholinesterase inhibitors and/or memantine.
- *Severe*
  - ○ Marked confusion and memory loss; verbal function is limited or absent. Delusions and hallucinations are common.
  - ○ Ultimately, difficulty with ambulation, continence, and then swallowing.
  - ○ Assistance is needed for almost all tasks.
  - ○ May respond to memantine and/or cholinesterase inhibitors.

Global Deterioration Scale

The Global Deterioration scale developed by Reisberg et al. (1982) can be used to evaluate a patient's current status or the progression of AD:

- 1: No complaints of cognitive difficulty and no objective deficits
- 2: *Age Associated memory impairment.* Subjective complaints of memory impairment but no objective deficits
- 3: *Mild cognitive impairment.* Objective deficits, although mild; impaired performance on complex tasks and more pervasive memory deficit
- 4: *Mild dementia.* Deficits in recall of personal history; more marked deficits with impaired concentration, calculations, and complex tasks
- 5: *Moderate dementia.* Needs assistance for many tasks but usually continent and can do self-care; disorientation, impaired recall of personal historical details, continues to know much valid personal history
- 6: *Moderately severe dementia.* Marked memory difficulty, often not remembering close family; unaware of current news and often personal events. Mood and personality changes may include anxiety, agitation, or obsessions. Delusions and hallucinations are common.
- 7: *Severe dementia.* No functional memory; language is also nonfunctional with little or no speech. Ultimately, loss of ambulation, continence, and eventually swallowing occur; predisposition to aspiration.

DIAGNOSIS is suspected with progressive memory deficit in an elderly patient with no other neurologic symptoms. Imaging may show no abnormalities early in the course. Ultimately, MRI or CT brain show atrophy. Positron emission tomography (PET), either fluorodeoxyglucose for regional hypometabolism or an amyloid ligand for diagnosis of amyloid deposition in AD, can be helpful diagnostically, but these are usually not done on an inpatient basis. Neuropsych testing shows characteristic deficits but is seldom performed during hospitalization. Spinal fluid analysis for tau and A-beta amyloid content can be helpful in diagnosis but is also not usually done in the hospital.

Differential diagnosis is broad, but clinical diagnosis is usually accurate even without studies. Vascular dementia usually manifests focal signs, often with a stepwise deterioration, and the vascular lesions are evident on MRI. Dementia with Lewy bodies (DLB) shows parkinsonism, as well as rapid fluctuations in mental status, early visual hallucinations, and REM sleep behavior disorder. Frontotemporal dementia produces prominent frontal-lobe/behavioral symptoms or progressive aphasia early in the course, typically has an earlier age of onset, and sometimes has a more rapid progression than AD. Cognitive changes with aging and MCI require neuropsych testing to evaluate.

MANAGEMENT of AD in hospitalized patients begins with re-evaluation if the diagnosis if not established. Because of exacerbation of mental status during hospitalization and concurrent illness, behavioral management is needed, and sometimes sedatives or antipsychotics might be considered, although they should be avoided if possible (see the discussion under "Delirium").

Medications specifically for AD include:

- *Cholinesterase inhibitors*: Donepezil, rivastigmine, galantamine
- *NMDA-receptor antagonist*: Memantine

Indications approved by the US Food and Drug Administration (FDA) are differentiated by stage of disease:

- *Mild*: Donepezil, rivastigmine, galantamine
- *Moderate*: Donepezil, rivastigmine, galantamine, and memantine
- *Severe*: Donepezil, rivastigmine, and memantine.

So far, the medications used are only proved effective in improving symptoms, mainly improving short-term memory, although improvements in behavior have also been reported. None has been proved to slow the progression of the degeneration.

Vascular risk factor management may be able to slow the progression of AD. Physical exercise has a clear benefit, and mental exercises may also be effective.

Assessment of response to treatment is difficult. Although some patients will exhibit a true improvement, many more have a decrease in their rate of clinical deterioration compared to untreated patients. This is the province of the outpatient arena and is not discussed further here.

Dementia with Lewy Bodies and Parkinson Disease with Dementia

DLB is characterized by dementia with features of Parkinson disease. The cognitive disturbance develops before the motor deficits. However, patients with onset of the motor symptoms more than 1 year prior to the cognitive symptoms are diagnosed as having *Parkinson disease with dementia* (PDD).

PRESENTATION includes confusion, often with visual hallucinations early in the course. Motor difficulties include impaired coordination and stiffness. Patients are predisposed to orthostatic hypotension, syncope, and REM sleep disorder. Exam shows dementia with hallucinations and attention deficits early in the course. Motor deficits of parkinsonism are predominantly rigidity and bradykinesia rather than tremor.

DIAGNOSIS usually begins with imaging. MRI brain is preferable to CT brain. Routine labs are usually normal. Levels of B_{12}, thyroid function, and rapid plasma reagin (RPR) may be appropriate.

Differential diagnosis is broad. Some of these include:

- *Alzheimer disease*: No parkinsonism
- *Frontotemporal dementia*: No parkinsonism, early behavioral change
- *Vascular dementia*: Focal signs not seen with AD; step-wise progression may be seen.
- *Progressive supranuclear palsy (PSP)*: Rigidity and eye movement abnormalities
- *Normal pressure hydrocephalus (NPH)*: Gait difficulty without rigidity
- *Corticobasal syndrome (CBS)*: Limb apraxia with parkinsonism

DLB is differentiated from AD and FTD by the parkinsonian symptoms and early hallucinations. DLB is differentiated from NPH and vascular dementia by imaging and follow-up studies. DLB is differentiated from CBS and PSP by a different presentation of the motor symptoms.

MANAGEMENT is largely symptomatic. No treatments have been proved to slow the progression of the disease.

- *Hallucinations and delusions*: Neuroleptics are sometimes ordered, but especially the older agents can markedly exacerbate motor symptoms and even the newer antipsychotic agents can worsen parkinsonism. Recent clinical data support the use of cholinesterase inhibitors for the noncognitive psychotic symptoms and behavioral aberrations. Rivastigmine has been specifically tested and approved for PDD.
- *Motor symptoms* might respond to dopaminergic agents, but this is not universal. Dopamine agonists may be more effective than carbidopa/levodopa preparations, but they can cause increased confusion and orthostatic hypotension. Anticholinergic agents should be avoided because of the potential for worsening cognition.
- *Cognitive deficits* are mainly treated with cholinesterase inhibitors. Memantine may also be effective.

Vascular Dementia

Vascular dementia can be due to one or multiple infarcts of almost any etiology. About a third of patients with presumed vascular dementia have coexistent Alzheimer pathology identified at autopsy. Vascular risk factors predispose to AD also.

PRESENTATION of vascular dementia is usually cognitive deterioration in the setting of a history of known cerebrovascular disease or risk factors for stroke. Either a single stroke or multiple strokes may have occurred. Features of vascular cognitive impairment and dementia include prominent impairment of executive function, attention, and concentration, as well as focal cognitive signs such as aphasia or alexia related to focal areas of infarction. Isolated memory loss is much more typical of AD than vascular dementia.

DIAGNOSIS is by clinical presentation and imaging showing significant cerebrovascular disease, especially single or multiple strokes. MRI brain is the preferred imaging modality; contrast is not needed unless mass lesion or inflammatory component is suspected.

Vascular dementia can be divided into subtypes:

- *Multi-infarct dementia*: Multiple sequential and/or simultaneous infarcts affecting cortical neurons and connections
- *Single-infarct dementia*: Cognitive deficit from single infarcts especially in the parietal region, anterior cerebral artery distribution/frontal lobes, thalamus, posterior cerebral artery territory with hippocampal infarction
- *Lacunar syndrome*: Multiple subcortical infarctions, small-vessel disease
- *Binswanger disease*: Diffuse white matter disease due to lipohyalinosis of small arteries and fibrinoid necrosis of larger arteries
- *CADASIL*: Subcortical infarctions due to defect on chromosome 19; suspected with multiple infarcts in a patient without significant risk factors other than family history. This disorder is most notable for confluent white matter lesions, which characteristically affect the anterior temporal poles.
- *Cerebral amyloid angiopathy*: Recurrent cerebral hemorrhages and microhemorrhages, usually in the elderly. There is an overlap between vascular amyloid and AD.

MANAGEMENT of the vascular component of these causes of cognitive decline is discussed in Chapter 16. No specific treatment for the cognitive disturbance has been developed; however, there is evidence that some patients may response favorably to cholinesterase inhibitors, so this is reasonable to try, especially with the overlapping pathology already discussed. Pentoxifylline may be helpful, with significant improvement in patients with multi-infarct dementia in one study.[5]

Frontotemporal Dementia

FTD is a family of disorders where degeneration is regional to the frontal and temporal lobes, in contrast to AD, where the atrophy affects the hippocampi and parietal lobes early. Some patients present with early symptoms; these are predominantly behavioral, whereas others present with early onset of language deficits. *Pick's disease* was the term used for FTD with a specific pathologic finding of Pick bodies, but FTD is the clinical diagnosis used for the behavioral form of this family of disease, as well as being an umbrella term for this family. *Primary progressive aphasia (PPA)* and *semantic dementia* are forms with prominent language deficits at presentation.

PRESENTATION: The behavioral form of FTD is much less common than AD, but is the most common entity in this group. FTD presents with frontal lobe dysfunction prior to development of memory deficit. Some patients have predominantly disinhibited and impulsive behavioral change; others are more apathetic. Common other findings including affective disturbance with depression or anxiety. Cognitive and language changes come later in the course, in the behavioral variant FTD.

Primary progressive aphasia has three forms: progressive nonfluent aphasia, semantic dementia, and logopenic progressive aphasia. These are considered individually in Table 18.1.

FTD with early behavioral deficit is most suspected when patients with dementia have a history of disinhibition and personality change predating the memory decline. The diagnosis is harder to make with personality change without cognitive deterioration, and definitive diagnosis may need to wait for clinical progression.

DIAGNOSIS: Evaluation includes imaging, since the pathology is focal. Primary progressive aphasia must be differentiated from other structural causes of language difficulty, especially tumor and vascular disease. Neuropsych testing is helpful.

MANAGEMENT: Options for FTDs are quite limited. Selective serotonin reuptake inhibitors (SSRIs) can be helpful for behavioral symptoms. In some patients, cholinesterase inhibitors aggravate the behavior disorder, although in some there may be a memory benefit. Memantine has been anecdotally reported to help cognition in FTD, but supportive controlled data are lacking.

MILD COGNITIVE IMPAIRMENT

MCI is characterized by cognitive decline out of proportion to expected cognitive changes with aging yet not to the point of interfering with daily functioning. This is the province of the outpatient neurologist and is not considered here further other than to restate that patients with MCI have an increased risk for hospital delirium.[6]

Table 18.1 Frontotemporal dementias (FTDs)

Disorder	Features
Frontotemporal dementia with predominant behavioral features	*Early*: Personality change, disinhibition, impulsive behavior, or alternatively apathy
	Later: Memory difficulty, loss of speech
Primary progressive aphasias (PPA)	
Progressive nonfluent aphasia	*Early*: Expressive more than receptive aphasia, word finding difficulty, anomia, paraphasic errors
	Later: Cognitive deficits
	This variant of FTD is often a tauopathy.
Semantic dementia	Fluent aphasia with word finding difficulty, anomia, associative visual agnosia; the key feature of semantic dementia is loss of single word meaning.
	Later: Behavioral changes
	This variant is often related to a progranulin mutation and accumulation of TDP42.
Logopenic progressive aphasia	Prominent word-finding difficulty, difficulty with repetition, slow speech
	Cognitive and behavioral deficits develop more than in the other PPAs.
	This variant is usually a focal presentation of Alzheimer's disease.

MANAGEMENT OF HOSPITALIZED PATIENTS WITH DEMENTIA

Patients with dementia commonly have an exacerbation of confusion, and this can develop into frank delirium. Features of particular concern include psychosis and sleep–wake cycle abnormalities. These are exacerbated by the unfamiliar surroundings, concurrent illness, medications (especially narcotic analgesics, tranquilizers, anticholinergic agents), and potential for sleep deprivation due to ongoing medical care.

Behavioral management can often be helped by having family in the room with proper coaching to use a nonaggressive style. Sitters may be needed if family is not available. Familiar objects in the room can help—a pillow from home, pictures of loved ones—but dangerous objects should be eliminated. A regular day/night regimen should be followed as much as possible, although circadian rhythm is usually disturbed.

Psychiatric consultation may be needed and can help with medication selection.

Medications that are often used include haloperidol (Haldol) with alternative neuroleptics being the atypicals, including especially quetiapine (Seroquel), olanzapine (Zyprexa), and risperidone (Risperdal).[7] Risperidone can exacerbate rigidity in patients with Parkinson disease and DLB, and patients with the latter can be particularly sensitive to any of these agents.

19 Seizures and Epilepsy

Bassel W. Abou-Khalil, MD and
Karl E. Misulis, MD, PhD

CHAPTER CONTENTS

- Overview
  - Spectrum of Clinical Seizures
  - Differential Diagnosis of Seizures
  - Symptomatic Seizures
- Epilepsy
  - New-Onset Seizure
  - EEG Findings
  - AED Choice
- Seizure Clusters
- Status Epilepticus
  - Convulsive Status Epilepticus
  - Nonconvulsive Status Epilepticus
- Pregnancy
- AED Discontinuation
- Safety Issues
- Sudden Unexplained Death in Epilepsy

Seizure evaluation and management is a core function of the hospital neurologist. Most patients with seizures can be evaluated on outpatient basis, and admission purely for diagnosis of a single seizure is usually not needed. However, we do admit individuals in whom we fear an underlying cause that deserves rapid attention, if there is a prolonged postictal state, or if a patient fails to return to baseline.

OVERVIEW
Spectrum of Clinical Seizures

Classifications of seizures evolve, but generalized and focal seizures continue to be broad categories of interest at initial presentation. The International League Against Epilepsy (ILAE) classification of epilepsies is presented later in this chapter in the section entitled "EPILEPSY." The clinical description in the list presents the seizure types most commonly seen in the hospital setting:

- *Generalized tonic-clonic seizure*
  - Generalized motor activity usually with generalized tonic posturing then clonic activity. This is usually followed by limp unresponsiveness and labored

respiration at termination. There is no focal motor activity at onset. However, some asymmetry, including forced head turning at onset, could still be consistent with a generalized onset.

- *Focal seizure evolving to a bilateral, convulsive seizure*
  - o Focal seizure leading to bilateral motor activity, usually with tonic then clonic activity (but there could be preceding clonic activity). The transition usually includes tonic or clonic activity and forced head turning contralateral to the side where seizures start. The postictal state is similar to what is seen with a generalized onset tonic-clonic seizure.
- *Focal motor seizure without evolution to generalized tonic-clonic activity*
  - o Focal motor activity, usually clonic but could be tonic or dystonic in appearance. The term is usually used for seizures that do not affect consciousness.
- *Focal seizures with impairment of consciousness or awareness (complex partial seizures or discognitive seizures)*
  - o These may start with an aura or with altered awareness/consciousness. There could be total loss of awareness and responsiveness or only subtle confusion or slowing of responses. There may be motor manifestations such as lip smacking/chewing motions (with temporal involvement), fumbling/picking motions, and dystonic posturing of one or more extremities.

Differential Diagnosis of Seizure

The differential diagnosis of clinical seizures includes *epileptic seizures* versus *nonepileptic psychogenic events* versus *nonepileptic physiological events. Syncope* is the most common physiological event in the differential diagnosis.

- Epileptic seizure
  - o Seizures can vary considerably in clinical manifestations. If seizure is captured on electroencephalogram (EEG), there will be an associated ictal discharge, but EEG changes may not be seen with a focal motor seizure with preserved awareness. Diagnosis is supported by abnormal interictal EEG, but interictal abnormality is not necessary.
- Nonepileptic psychogenic events (also called nonepileptic psychogenic seizures or pseudoseizures)
  - o Atypical clinical features (below).
  - o EEG during an episode is normal or only shows movement and muscle artifact. Long-term recording is sometimes needed.
- Syncope
  - o Commonly associated with multifocal myoclonus and even with tonic posturing. Myoclonus is usually of short duration, less than 15 seconds.
- Movement disorder (tremor, myoclonus, asterixis, hemiballismus)
  - o Movement disorders with positive motor manifestations can be mistaken for seizure if episodic or episodically worse (e.g., myoclonus from metabolic derangement, paroxysmal dyskinesia). Negative myoclonus can also be seen with toxic-metabolic encephalopathy, most commonly hepatic. Acute onset of a hemiballismus from infarction can also be mistaken for seizure.

Table 19.1 Differentiation of epileptic seizure from psychogenic nonepileptic event

Feature	Epileptic seizure	Psychogenic nonepileptic seizure
Motor activity	Unilateral or bilateral synchronous.	Often alternating or asynchronous extremity motions, forward pelvic thrusting, large amplitude side-to-side head motions
Consciousness	May be partially or totally preserved with focal seizures, completely lost with generalized tonic-clonic seizures.	May be responsive during generalized convulsive seizure. May resist eye opening while unresponsive.
Eye exam	Usually pupillary dilation. Eyelids passive. No resistance to eye opening.	Normal or dilated pupils. Often difficult to examine because of forced eye closure or upturning of the eyes. Almost always some resistance to passive eye opening.
Continence	Incontinence often occurs with generalized seizure	Incontinence often reported but uncommon on examination after an event. This is not a helpful differentiating historical feature.
EEG	Electrographic seizure activity but may be at least partly obscured by movement artifact.	Normal or muscle/movement artifact. May be difficult to rule-out electrical seizure if muscle artifact dominates the EEG or if there is prominent rhythmic artifact.
Prolactin level	Often elevated briefly after generalized tonic-clonic seizures.	Normal.
Provocation	Usually unprovoked, but can be provoked by injury, stroke, brain infection, and, in patients with epilepsy, can be triggered by stress, illness, sleep deprivation, and certain medications.	Often precipitated by stressful situation.

Differentiation of epileptic seizure from psychogenic nonepileptic event is crucial and often difficult (see Table 19.1).

Hospital neurologists are often asked to differentiate seizure from syncope (see Table 19.2).

Table 19.2 Differentiation of seizure from syncope

Feature	Seizure	Syncope
Motor activity	Longer duration, more that 15 seconds.	Brief multifocal myoclonus, lasting less than 15 seconds.
Position	No positional provocation.	Upright posture or sitting, if there is an orthostatic component.
Appearance	Normal color, flushed, or cyanotic with long-duration.	Pale at onset.
Post-episode appearance	Often lethargic and confused for minutes	Post-episode disorientation is brief, if present at all.
Vital signs	Often tachycardic and hypertensive during and shortly after the episode.	Hypotensive during the episode but normotensive or even hypertensive after.
Prolactin level	Often briefly elevated after a generalized tonic-clonic seizure and to a lesser extent after a focal seizure involving the temporal lobe.	Often elevated after syncope; this is not a differentiating feature.

Vital signs are particularly problematic, since the report is frequently given that BP was normal or elevated after syncope is over. Determining timing and patient status at the time of the vital signs is key.

Prolactin levels are not as helpful as we would like, partly because of the brief time of elevation and the multitude of other reasons for prolactin elevation. Prolactin does not help in the distinction of seizure and syncope because it can be increased after both. Prolactin is usually not increased with psychogenic nonepileptic seizures unless elevated for another reason. Meds that can give elevated prolactin levels include select antipsychotics, antidepressants, antihypertensive meds (e.g., verapamil), opiates, and H_2 antagonists.[1]

The summary statement of the *Therapeutics and Technology Assessment Subcommittee* reports that elevated prolactin measured 10–20 minutes after a seizure can be an adjunct in differentiating generalized tonic-clonic and complex partial seizure from psychogenic nonepileptic seizure.[2]

Symptomatic Seizure

The epilepsies will be discussed in detail in the section entitled "EPILEPSY." Here, we are considering seizures, which are symptomatic of another medical condition in hospitalized patients. Features of some important symptomatic seizures are shown in Table 19.3.

Table 19.3 Symptomatic seizures

Disorder	Type	Elements
Trauma	Closed head injury	Seizures occur acutely and/or remotely from the injury. Acute seizures are less likely to result in long-term seizure disorder. Late seizures predict development of epilepsy.
	Penetrating injury	Acute seizures are common in this setting, and recurrence is very frequent; the risk of epilepsy is increased 580 times
Infection	Encephalitis	*HSV*: Seizures and encephalopathy with febrile presentation.
	Meningitis	Seizures can occur with meningitis but less so than with encephalitis.
	Sepsis	Seizures with sepsis must have CNS infection ruled-out, but the seizures are usually secondary—medications, vascular.
	Prion disease	Seizures may occur with myoclonus and dementia
Autoimmune encephalitis	Limbic encephalitis	*Anti-NMDA receptor encephalitis*: seizures with psychiatric symptoms, often with ovarian teratoma
Anti-voltage-gated potassium channel-complex antibody encephalitis: may start with very brief facio-brachial dystonic seizures. May be associated with hyponatremia, episodic bradycardia, neuromyotonia, increased sweating
Other limbic encephalitides (anti-GABA$_B$ receptor, anti-AMPA receptor, anti-GAD, onconeural antibody encephalitis)
Limbic encephalitis can be a paraneoplastic condition, most commonly with small cell lung cancer
Metabolic	Electrolyte	Hypernatremia: Weakness, lethargy, seizures, coma.
Hyponatremia: Nausea, vomiting, encephalopathy, seizures, respiratory failure.
	Glucose	Hyperglycemia: focal seizures are common
Hypoglycemia: autonomic symptoms with confusion, agitation, tremor, generalized convulsive seizure.
	Hepatic	Acute failure: Confusion, inattention, delirium, tremor, asterixis, lethargy, coma. Seizures may occur but are not the most prominent finding.
	Renal	Confusion, encephalopathy, tremor, myoclonus, asterixis, seizures, which may be generalized or focal.

(continued)

Table 19.3 Continued

Disorder	Type	Elements
Medications and toxins	Antibiotics	Multiple antibiotics can trigger seizures in individuals with low seizure threshold (e.g., cefepime, meropenem).
	Chemotherapeutics	PRES can develop from some chemotherapies producing seizures and encephalopathy.
	Antiepileptics	Seizures can be a manifestation of toxicity with several seizure medications in patients with epilepsy, particularly phenytoin. Tiagabine may trigger nonconvulsive status epilepticus in individuals who do not have epilepsy.
Neoplastic disease	Brain tumors	Low-grade brain tumors can present with seizures. The risk of recurrence is very high, and these patients can be considered to have epilepsy. High-grade tumors are less likely to present with seizures; focal symptoms are more common.
	Metastases	Seizures with known cancer can be from metastases, but also consider medications and metabolic causes.
	Non-neurologic tumors	*Limbic encephalitis*: These may present with seizures, most commonly focal from the temporal lobe, but there is often associated memory deficit or psychotic features.

EPILEPSY

Most of the difficulty with seizure diagnosis is differentiation of epileptic from nonepileptic events, as discussed earlier. When a condition is determined to be epileptic, then differentiation into types is important for treatment selection and prognosis.

Spectrum of Seizure Manifestations

Seizure signs and symptoms include motor manifestations, automatisms, sensory phenomena, experiential phenomena, autonomic signs, and symptoms. These are summarized here.

Symptoms and signs of seizures:

- Motor
  - *Elementary*: Tonic, clonic, dystonic, versive, myoclonic, negative myoclonus, atonic
  - *Complex*: Automatisms; can be oro-alimentary (e.g., lip smacking, chewing)
  - *Manual*: Can be de novo or perseveration, manipulative; e.g., picking/fumbling with objects such as clothes, or nonmanipulative such as rhythmic hand movements which are not clonic), pedal (involving foot), gelastic (laughing), dacrystic (crying)

- Sensory
  - *Elementary*: Flashing lights, tones, tingling or numbness, olfactory, gustatory
  - *Complex*: Visual or auditory hallucinations or distortion of perception
- Experiential
  - *Affective*: Fear, euphoria, sadness
  - *Dysmnesic*: Déjà vu, jamais vu
  - *Cognitive*: Altered memory, perception, or executive function
- Autonomic
  - *Subjective*: Nausea, epigastric sensation, feeling hot
  - *Objective*: Pallor, flushing, vomiting

Seizure classification can be performed in a few ways. The most common structure is that developed in 1981 by the ILAE, summarized in Table 19.4.

Table 19.4 Seizure classification

Seizure type	Subtype	Features
Partial seizures	Simple partial seizures	Focal seizures without disturbance of consciousness. Could be motor, sensory, autonomic, psychic, or a combination.
	Complex partial seizures	Focal seizure with impairment of consciousness or awareness.
	Partial evolving to secondarily generalized seizures	Focal seizure evolving to generalized seizure. Often focal motor or versive.
Generalized seizures	Typical absence seizures	Sudden arrest of activity, simple automatisms. No aura, no postictal manifestations.
	Atypical absence seizures	Sudden loss of awareness, May have slower recovery. Motor manifestations may be greater, e.g. Myoclonic, tonic, or atonic.
	Myoclonic seizures	Brief myoclonic jerks usually without disturbance of consciousness.
	Clonic seizures	Rhythmic's shaking of the extremities
	Tonic seizures	Stiffening of the extremities, often with flexion of the neck and upward gaze.
	Tonic-clonic seizures	Initial tonic phase followed by a clonic phase.
	Atonic seizures	Sudden loss of tone of the head or whole body.
Unclassified epileptic seizures		

Most generalized seizures seen in hospital practice are tonic-clonic. Generalized tonic seizures without a clonic component are usually seen in patients with extensive pre-existing neurologic deficit. There may be some subtle jerks at the end of the seizure.

Partial seizures have a varied semiology depending on the locus of discharge:

- Frontal
  - Cephalic aura is most common.
  - *Motor Cortex*: Focal clonic or tonic-clonic activity
  - *Supplementary area*: Posturing, especially proximally
  - *Cingulate and orbito-frontal*: Complex partial seizure with gestural automatisms
- Temporal
  - *Mesial*: Epigastric sensation or memory-based experience followed by motor arrest, staring, often with oro-alimentary and/or extremity automatisms; may be ipsilateral manipulative automatisms with contralateral dystonic posturing
  - *Lateral*: Auditory aura followed by facial twitching
- Parietal
  - Somatosensory experience, usually marching. Objective manifestations reflect spread to frontal lobe (contralateral posturing, clonic activity, head and eye deviation), or temporal lobe (staring, immobility, oro-alimentary automatisms).
- Occipital
  - Elementary visual hallucination; objective manifestations include blinking, eye deviation, usually contralateral. May spread to frontal or temporal regions with associated manifestations.

New-Onset Seizure or First Unprovoked Seizure

New-onset seizure is a common cause for neurology consultation especially in the ED. Krumholz[3] recently authored the AAN Guidelines for management of a first unprovoked seizure in adults. Relevant data is summarized as follows:

- *Risk of seizure recurrence*:
  - Patients are advised that the risk of recurrence is greatest in the first 2 years and is approximately 21–45%.
- *Factors indicating an increased risk of subsequent seizure*:
  - Prior brain insult
  - Epileptiform abnormalities on EEG
  - Brain imaging showing significant abnormality
  - Nocturnal seizure
- *Effects of antiepileptic drug (AED) use from the start rather than waiting for second seizure*:
  - Likely reduces the incidence of seizures by about 35% during the first 2 years, but may not improve quality of life
  - Does not seem to reduce recurrence rates at 3 years and greater
  - Adverse effects of AEDs can be seen in 7–31% of patients, although most are mild and reversible.
- *Recommendations on whether to use AED immediately*:
  - Individualized based on patient situation and preferences, in addition to the recurrence risk just described.

Some may consider the AAN recommendations to be a bit soft regarding definitive advice regarding AED use, but, for this decision, patient situation and preference are key. For example, patients who will be driving or who have jobs for which the implications of a second seizure are severe often elect to be on an AED. On the other hand, a student who will be on campus and not in need of a car likely will decide to forego immediate AED therapy.

EEG Findings

EEG findings are summarized in the reference portion of this book, Chapter 40, and in Table 19.5.[4]

There are also normal and abnormal EEG patterns that can look epileptiform but are not necessarily associated with seizures. Details of these patterns are beyond the scope of this book. Interested readers are referred to the *Atlas of EEG, Seizure Semiology, and Management* (Oxford University Press, 2013).[5]

Table 19.5 Electroencephalogram (EEG) findings in seizures

Seizure type	Ictal EEG Features
Simple partial seizure	Most often no definite EEG change is noted. Focal ictal discharge may be seen
Complex partial seizure	Focal ictal discharge, especially with temporal lobe seizures, but ictal discharge may rapidly become widespread. Routine scalp recordings often do not show ictal discharge when the seizure is of orbitofrontal or medial frontal/parietal origin
Primarily generalized tonic-clonic seizure	Generalized spike-and-wave or fast spike discharges at onset, with decreasing frequency during the event. Muscle artifact usually masks the EEG. The muscle artifact pattern is usually confluent during the tonic phase, but develops pauses of progressively increasing duration during the clonic phase. Postictal attenuation then slow activity.
Secondarily-generalized tonic-clonic seizure	Focal ictal discharge which then spreads to become a generalized discharge. The pattern of muscle artifact after generalization is similar to what is seen with the primarily generalized tonic-clonic seizure
Absence seizure	2.5 to 4 per second spike-and-wave discharge which arises out of an otherwise normal background and without postictal abnormalities. Often provoked by hyperventilation.
Atypical absence seizure	Slow spike-and-wave discharge of <2.5 Hz.
Myoclonic seizure	Single or brief serial irregular generalized spike-and-wave or polyspike-and-wave discharge.
Nonepileptic psychogenic event	There is either a normal EEG appearance or muscle and movement artifact which obscures the recording. No postictal slow activity.

AED Choice

We generally recommend not prescribing AEDs in an adult with a single unprovoked seizure if brain imaging and EEG are normal. The risk of seizure recurrence in that setting is approximately 25%. However, if the seizure is severe or if a second seizure could endanger the patient's career or livelihood, it is reasonable to start an AED.[6] A seizure provoked by a rapidly reversible process, such as metabolic derangement or drug exposure, will not require long-term treatment. However, when the seizures are repetitive, short-term treatment is needed, at least until the underlying cause has been removed. The duration of this short-term therapy could be a few days in the case of a metabolic derangement such as hyponatremia, or a few months for a longer process such as acute disseminated encephalomyelitis (ADEM) or posterior reversible encephalopathy syndrome (PRES).

Some patients with epilepsy have symptoms that are infrequent or mild enough that treatment is not needed, but these are clearly in the minority. As with all patients with epilepsy, these patients must be advised of safety issues and specific driving limitations, in keeping with regulations and accepted practice in your area.

Numerous AEDs are available, but some are not practical in the hospital setting. Medications that require a slow titration (e.g., lamotrigine, topiramate, or tiagabine) are not considered when attempting to achieve rapid seizure control.[7]

Recommendations for consideration for AEDs are found in Table 19.6. Note that not all of these are FDA-approved indications, but there is study evidence to suggest that these are viable options.

Table 19.6 Antiepileptic drugs for selected seizure types

Disorder	Features
Partial-onset epilepsy	Carbamazepine, phenytoin, valproate are old drugs approved for initial monotherapy. Among the new drugs, oxcarbazepine, topiramate, lacosamide, eslicarbazepine are FDA approved for initial monotherapy. Good evidence also exists for lamotrigine, levetiracetam, and gabapentin.
Primary generalized absence epilepsy	Ethosuximide is usually the first drug. If generalized motor seizures coexist then valproate is a better option. Lamotrigine is less effective overall, but should be considered in the place of valproate if pregnancy is possible.
Generalized tonic-clonic seizures	Valproate is usually the first drug to be used for men. For women of child-bearing potential, lamotrigine or levetiracetam should be used first.
Juvenile myoclonic epilepsy	Valproate is the most effective agent, and remains the drug of choice for men. Levetiracetam is FDA approved as adjunctive therapy but may be effective as monotherapy. Lamotrigine is effective against generalized tonic-clonic seizures and may be effective against myoclonic seizures, but may exacerbate myoclonic seizures in some individuals. One of these latter two should be considered in women of child-bearing potential. Topiramate or zonisamide are also alternatives therapies.

Specifics of up-to-date prescribing information should be obtained from the manufacturers. In addition, information on these and all meds can be obtained from the government website dailymed.nlm.nih.gov, as well as from several commercial sites.

SEIZURE CLUSTERS

Seizure clusters (also referred to as acute repetitive seizures and serial seizures) are a common reason for presentation to the ED.[8] They are defined as closely grouped seizures of any type, recurring over minutes to a couple of days, and exceeding baseline seizure frequency. Recovery should occur between seizures; otherwise, this is the condition of *status epilepticus* (SE). However, seizure clusters may evolve into status epilepticus if not treated aggressively. Clusters of mild seizures, such as simple partial seizures or mild complex partial seizures, can be treated with oral benzodiazepines (lorazepam 1–2 mg or diazepam 5–10 mg). More severe clusters require other modes of administration, most commonly with benzodiazepines. Acceptable modes of administration include intravenous administration of lorazepam (1–4 mg), intramuscular administration of midazolam (10 mg) or diazepam (0.2 mg/kg up to 20 mg), or rectal administration of diazepam (0.2 mg/kg) (all adult doses). For patients with recurrent seizure clusters, home treatment by caregivers may obviate the need for ED visits and hospitalization.

STATUS EPILEPTICUS

SE is defined as recurrent seizures without recovery between events or seizure lasting 30 minutes or longer. Any seizure type can develop into status epilepticus, but the most severe and most serious form is *generalized convulsive status epilepticus* (GCSE), which can evolve from focal seizure activity or from generalized seizure activity.

Convulsive Status Epilepticus

SE, particularly GCSE, is a medical emergency. For GCSE, 30 minutes is the time limit before irreversible neuronal injury may begin if seizure activity is not controlled. Most self-limited generalized convulsive seizures resolve within 2 minutes, and it is now recognized that after 5 minutes of continuous generalized convulsive seizure activity it becomes highly unlikely that the seizure will stop spontaneously. Hence, this has become the practical definition of GCSE, and treatment should begin by 5 minutes: do not wait until 30 minutes have passed.[9] Complex partial seizures should be treated within 10–15 minutes.

First-line treatment is a benzodiazepine, preferable lorazepam. It is recommended to use an effective dose from onset. The recommended dose of lorazepam is 0.1 mg/kg, not to exceed 10 mg IV. Unless there is a rapidly reversible cause for epilepsy, a second-line agent is needed, even if the SE is controlled. Traditionally, this has been fosphenytoin at a dose of 20 mg/kg. However, there is mounting evidence that valproate is equally effective, used at a dose of 30 mg/kg. If seizure activity is improving but is not controlled, it is reasonable to give an additional 10 mg/kg of fosphenytoin or 10 mg/kg of valproate. However, if seizures continue, the next step should be general anesthesia with midazolam or propofol. Pentobarbital can also be used, but it is associated with greater incidence of hypotension and slower recovery after seizure control; thus, it is reserved for situations where general anesthesia has to be continued for longer than one day. When SE persists despite general anesthesia or recurs after withdrawal of anesthetics, it is considered *super-refractory*.

In such instances, a variety of approaches could be considered, including the use of ket-amine infusion (1.5 mg/kg every 5 minutes up to 4.5 mg/kg or seizure termination, then infusion starting with 1.2 mg/kg/hour), or large doses of topiramate (500 mg b.i.d.) by nasogastric tube, or IV methylprednisolone for presumptive autoimmune etiology.[10]

The management of SE usually occurs in parallel with investigation using lab stud-ies, but seizure management takes precedence over imaging and lumbar puncture (LP). If the patient does not have a diagnosis of epilepsy, then the etiologic diagnosis must be established. Emergent imaging, usually with computed tomography (CT) is performed because patients are usually not sufficiently stable for magnetic resonance imaging (MRI). EEG should be performed urgently if possible, particularly in a patient who does not begin to wake up after clinical seizure activity has stopped. In such cases, nonconvulsive status epilepticus (NCSE) could evolve from GCSE. LP may be needed but might have to be delayed until the patient is stable and the SE controlled. If LP is indicated for suspected meningitis or encephalitis but delayed, coverage with antimi-crobial therapy should be administered.

Even in patients with known epilepsy, continuous EEG monitoring should be con-sidered if available. Some bedside ICU monitors have inputs for EEG although with a restricted number of channels.

Protocols for management of SE are found in Table 19.7. These are based on Vanderbilt's protocols and are discussed in more detail in the *Atlas of EEG, Seizure Semiology, & Management.*[11]

Table 19.7 Management of generalized convulsive status epilepticus

Time frame	Procedures
0–15 min	Place IV. Blood for studies. Normal saline at TKO. If glucose low: 1 amp D50 + start second IV with D5NS
	Thiamine 100 mg IVP if D50 given or malnourished or alcoholic.
	If actively seizing:
	Lorazepam 10 mg IV at <2 mg/min.
	Fosphenytoin 20 mg/kg; max rate 150 mg/min, slower if AV block or hypotensive.
	Do not use fosphenytoin if SE is due to a metabolic cause unlikely to respond to phenytoin.
	Concurrent phenytoin use is not a contraindication to this treatment.
15–60 min	If seizures are decreasing after fosphenytoin load:
	Additional fosphenytoin 10 mg/kg
	If seizures are continuing and intubation is required:
	Thiopental (with succinyl choline if necessary)
	Consider additional dose of fosphenytoin 10 mg/kg.
	For continuing seizures post-intubation:
	Midazolam 0.3 mg/kg slow IV, may repeat at 5 min intervals × 3, then
	Midazolam infusion 2 μg/kg/min, increase by 1 μg/kg/min every 15 min until seizure activity stops.
	or
	Propofol 1–2 mg/kg, then 2–10 mg/kg/h
	or

Table 19.7 Continued

Time frame	Procedures
	Pentobarbital 5 mg/kg loading dose (to achieve burst suppression on EEG with interburst intervals of approx. 7 sec); repeat load as necessary to max of 15 mg/kg, then 1–3 mg/kg/h maintenance dose × 6–12 h; re-evaluate patient.
After 60 min	EEG if patient has not awakened.
	Identify etiology of SE: Imaging with CT or MRI, LP if indicated with a treatment plan.
	Treat hyperthermia if present
	Bedside glucose for patients still seizing
	Check phenytoin level.
	Maintenance AEDs if indicated.

Nonconvulsive Status Epilepticus

NCSE refers to SE that is not associated with convulsive motor activity. The term applies to complex partial or absence SE and also to patients in coma who have electrographic evidence of seizure activity without the associated convulsive component.[12,13]

The diagnosis of NCSE requires EEG confirmation because the clinical manifestations are often nonspecific. They may include impaired cognition, subtle twitching of the face or limbs, unresponsiveness with eyes open, head or eye deviation, automatisms, or altered behavior. While some EEG patterns are diagnostic of electrographic SE, other patterns (such as lateralized or generalized periodic discharges) should be considered intermediate patterns along the interictal–ictal continuum, and the diagnosis has to take into consideration both clinical and EEG criteria. Table 19.8 summarizes the key criteria for EEG diagnosis of NCSE.

In the treatment of complex partial SE with partially preserved responsiveness, it is best to avoid depressing the level of consciousness. After an initial dose of lorazepam, nonsedating IV medications should be used, including fosphenytoin, valproate, levetiracetam, and lacosamide. General anesthesia should be avoided if at all possible.

Table 19.8 EEG criteria for nonconvulsive status epilepticus in patients without prior epileptic encephalopathy such as Lennox-Gastaut syndrome[14]

1	Repetitive spikes, polyspikes, sharp waves, spike-and-wave, or sharp-and-slow-wave discharges recurring at >2.5 Hz
2	Repetitive spikes, polyspikes, sharp waves, spike-and-wave, or sharp-and-slow-wave discharges, recurring at <2.5 Hz with associated clinical manifestation + Clinical improvement after IV benzodiazepines, or increase in EEG reactivity and normalization of EEG background activity
3	Rhythmic waves at >0.5 Hz with increase in voltage and change in frequency at onset, evolution in pattern with change in frequency by >1 Hz or change in location, decrementing termination (voltage or frequency), responding clinically or electrographically (increased reactivity and appearance of normal background EEG activity) to treatment with IV benzodiazepines

Table 19.9 Management of complex partial status epilepticus

Time frame	Procedures
0–30 min	IV. Normal saline at TKO
	Continuous EEG in progress.
	Lorazepam 1–2 mg IV at <2 mg/min
	One of the following:
	Fosphenytoin 20 mg/kg IV. Max rate of 150 mg/min.
	or
	Levetiracetam 20 mg/kg IV
	or
	Valproate 30 mg/kg IV
	or
	Lacosamide 400 mg IV
30–60 min	If seizure activity continues, cross over to another agent
	Fosphenytoin 20 mg/kg IV
	or
	Levetiracetam 20 mg/kg IV
	or
	Valproate 30 mg/kg IV
	or
	Lacosamide 400 mg IV
Late treatment	Continue to sequence nonsedating AEDs, avoiding excessive sedation.
	Avoid general anesthesia as long as possible.

It is crucial to treat the etiology of SE in parallel with the treatment of the seizure activity. For example, an immune etiology requires immunological therapy (IV methylprednisolone, IV immunoglobulin, or plasma exchange) See Table 19.9.

Generalized absence SE can be treated with lorazepam IV and/or valproate IV.

NCSE in a patient in coma often has a more serious prognosis, particularly when the etiology is hypoxic ischemic injury. The outcome depends on the etiology as well as treatment of seizure activity.

PREGNANCY

Management of AEDs during pregnancy is complex. In general, valproate should be discontinued if possible as soon as pregnancy is identified, with transition to an alternative agent. Although early gestational effects have already taken place, later exposure during pregnancy also places the child at risk, including the risk of lower IQ.

Women of child-bearing potential should generally be given alternatives to teratogenic agents, if possible. If a woman is specifically interested in becoming pregnant, then she should be given the opportunity to change to a safer agent and consider discontinuation of AEDs if clinically appropriate, e.g. seizures controlled for more than 2 years, or for mild seizure types such as absence or myoclonic. At the least, simplification of regimen is considered.

Prenatal folic acid and multivitamins should be given to all women who become pregnant and are on AEDs. It is preferable to start supplements before conception.

AED levels should be closely monitored because of changes in metabolism and volume of distribution. In particular, lamotrigine has a considerable increase in clearance during pregnancy and almost always requires dose adjustment.

Seizures in pregnancy are discussed in additional detail in Chapter 27.

AED DISCONTINUATION

AED discontinuation is considered after a time of seizure freedom. This is the province of the outpatient neurologist, except that we are sometimes asked whether AEDs can be discontinued because a medical condition might be related to the medication.

In general, AED discontinuation is considered after about 5 years in adults. Note that some patients taken off seizure medications who have recurrent events may not have immediate and total control with reinstitution of their previous regimen.

SAFETY ISSUES

Driving laws differ significantly between states. The time from an unprovoked seizure to resumption of driving varies from 3 months to 1 year with 6 months being the most common recommendation. Consult local laws for guidance.

SUDDEN UNEXPLAINED DEATH IN EPILEPSY

The risk of sudden death is increased at least 20-fold in young-adult patients with uncontrolled epilepsy. The sudden death is usually not related to trauma, drowning, or toxicological or anatomical causes, hence the term *sudden unexplained death with epilepsy* (SUDEP). The risk is increased especially with tonic-clonic seizures and with noncompliance.

Discussion of SUDEP with patients and families should be encouraged so that they are prepared for the eventuality and also as a tool to promote compliance.

20 Headache

E. Lee Murray, MD and
Karl E. Misulis, MD, PhD

CHAPTER CONTENTS

- Overview
- Migraine
  - Clinical Disorders
  - Acute Therapy
  - Preventive Therapies
  - Medication Overuse Headache
- Cluster
- Pseudotumor Cerebri
- Trigeminal Neuralgia
- Temporal Arteritis
- Reversible Cerebral Vasoconstriction Syndrome

OVERVIEW

Most headaches are managed in an outpatient setting. However, patients with severe headache, intractable headache, or headache with atypical features will present to the ED and might be admitted.

Proposed criteria for admission:[1]

- Prolonged unrelenting headache with associated symptoms, such as nausea and vomiting, hindering daily activities
- Severe dehydration
- Concern for a possible secondary etiology, such as infection (abscess or meningitis) or an acute vascular process (stroke, subarachnoid hemorrhage, aneurysm, vasculitis)
- Status migrainous with dependence on opiates or other analgesics, barbiturates, triptans, or ergots
- Need for detoxification
- Intractable headache that requires dihydroergotamine (DHE)
- Treatment with medications with potential side effects requiring monitoring

When laying out a potential treatment plan, it is important to investigate reasons for worsening headache. It is also important to develop and agree to a realistic treatment goal at the time of admission. Most patients will not be headache-free at the time of discharge.

The possible causes of refractory headache are multiple:

- Incorrect diagnosis
- More than one headache type
- Medication overuse headache
- Medication induced headache
- Noncompliance
- Concomitant medical issues causing headache
- Wrong therapeutic choice for headache type
- Inadequate therapeutic trial

Unrealistic expectations from the patient's perspective (expecting total headache freedom) can also make headache seem "refractory" when indeed therapies have been beneficial.

Most headaches encountered on an inpatient basis are migrainous in nature. Differential diagnosis and appropriate workup should be considered, and these are detailed in Chapter 10.

MIGRAINE

Migraine patients seen in the ED or inpatient setting can be administered meds not available on an outpatient basis. Treatments address pain, associated nausea and vomiting, and, if possible, underlying precipitating factors.

Patients with medication overuse headache should be withdrawn from the offending medications, if possible, and started on preventative therapy.

Clinical Disorders

Migraine is clinically subdivided on the basis of associated symptoms. Common clinical features include headache, which can be unilateral, regional, or holocephalic. Character is often throbbing but can be steady, and there may be a sharp component to the pain. Associated symptoms that support the diagnosis of migraine include nausea or vomiting, photophobia, phonophobia, and possibly an aura.

Migraine with Aura

Migraine with aura or *classic migraine* is a typical migraine preceded by an aura of neurologic symptoms. Common symptoms include:

- Visual: Scintillating scotoma or field defect
- Sensory: Numbness or tingling on one side
- Brainstem: Vertigo, ataxia

There are other potential auras, such as confusion or language difficulty; these are less common, but when they occur, they are likely to be seen in the ED.

Typical of the aura is "marching" of the symptoms. The visual defects move across the visual field. Sensory symptoms march through the limb. If more than one symptom is manifest, they are often not synchronous, transitioning from predominance of one modality to another within a single episode. This temporal evolution helps to differentiate migraine aura from stroke.

DIAGNOSIS is usually clinical, but, with the aura, patients may come to the ED for evaluation of possible stroke. If there is no history of prior migraine or aura, then neurologic evaluation will be needed. Magnetic resonance imaging (MRI) of the brain with MR angiography (MRA) is appropriate.

MANAGEMENT is in common with migraine, in general, with abortive therapy for patients with acute migraine. Preventative therapy is used when frequency and severity make even effective abortive therapy insufficient.

Migraine without Aura

Migraine without aura or *common migraine* has the same general character as migraine with aura, but there is no aura. Also, migraine without aura is more likely to be bilateral.

DIAGNOSIS is clinical, and, in the absence of neurologic symptoms, appearance in the ED and necessity for diagnostic studies is less. However, severe headache when it first occurs may trigger evaluation for subarachnoid hemorrhage or other serious pathology.

MANAGEMENT is as for other migraines, described in the following sections.

Hemiplegic Migraine

Hemiplegic migraine presents with an aura of unilateral paralysis. The weakness usually develops prior to the headache. Hemiplegic migraine is often familial.

Complicated Migraine

Complicated migraine is an otherwise typical migraine headache in which there is prolonged neurologic deficit. The deficits usually start before the headache and outlast the headache by at least several hours or a day.

Migraine Equivalent

Migraine equivalent is a term commonly used for neurologic symptoms that have the character of an aura but without headache. Therefore, this is in the differential diagnosis of acute focal symptoms and signs.

DIAGNOSIS is suspected when a patient has deficit that marches, as is typical with an aura.

Migrainous Infarction

Migrainous infarction is acute ischemic stroke in the setting of a migraine headache. The neurologic deficit thought initially to be aura persists. MRI shows acute ischemia.

DIAGNOSIS is usually initially suspected as being migraine-with-aura or hemiplegic-migraine or perhaps complicated-migraine, depending on the stage of the symptoms at the time of ED presentation. MRI shows acute ischemia.

Acute Therapy

Approaches to management of migraine are *abortive therapy* and *preventative therapy*. Attention to medical issues is of particular importance for migraine patients seen in the ED or hospitalized. Often, patients are dehydrated, and replacement of fluids can be an important part of management. Acute therapy includes

- Analgesics
- NSAIDs
- Triptans
- Ergots

Analgesics suffice for many people, especially young individuals. Acetaminophen and aspirin are most commonly used. Opiate analgesics are avoided except for rescue therapy. A common reason for analgesic ineffectiveness is underdosing, but excessive dose or frequency can predispose to adverse effects and worsening headache.

NSAIDs seem to be effective for many patients, although data are incomplete. Commonly used agents include naproxen, ibuprofen, diclofenac, and ketoprofen. These are used alone or in combination with a triptan.

Caffeine is used as an adjunct to at least analgesics and is effective for some patients.

Triptans are a cornerstone for migraine management. These are used alone or in combination with NSAIDs, and there are preparations with these in combination. Patients may respond to one agent and not to others. Among the most commonly used are sumatriptan, rizatriptan, almotriptan, zolmitriptan, naratriptan, frovatriptan, and eletriptan. None of these stands out far above the others. Route of administration may be a point of preference since sumatriptan is the only one available as an injection. Sumatriptan and zolmitriptan are available as intranasal spray. Triptans should be avoided if there is persistent neurologic deficit, and they are not typically given for hemiplegic or basilar migraine.

Valproate is often used by the hospital neurologist when the patient has refractory migraine necessitating ED visit or hospitalization. A serum pregnancy test in females of reproductive age and liver function studies should be obtained prior to infusion.

DHE is commonly used for migraine, although we tend to avoid its use in patients with neurologic deficit in association with suspected migraine. Also, DHE should not be given with triptans. DHE can be given repeatedly up to 3 mg/day and 6 mg/week. There are published protocols for dosing that exceeds this dose and variant dosing schemes.[2-4] Contraindications to DHE include pregnancy and a history of cerebrovascular disease or uncontrolled hypertension.

Chlorpromazine can be helpful and is used especially in the ED. Pretreatment with diphenhydramine or benztropine is common

Occipital nerve blocks should be considered as a possible treatment modality in those patients with headaches and neck pain or unilateral headache. Bilateral occipital blocks can be beneficial in chronic headaches.

Selection of specific agents from these possibilities is individualized, and patient-specific factors can affect selection. The hospital neurologist typically sees patients in the ED who have often failed oral meds. Orr and colleagues recently reported an analysis of multiple parenteral meds commonly given in the ED.[5] The consensus of the authors identified best evidence supporting IV metoclopramide and prochlorperazine and subcutaneous sumatriptan. Other meds had support of efficacy but of a lesser degree. They discouraged the use of morphine and hydromorphone.

Preventive Therapies

Preventive oral therapies should be started as an inpatient to assess tolerability and also to push the dosage to a potential therapeutic dose.

Patients who are experiencing more than 15 headache days per month or having frequent headaches that interfere with daily activity, including work or school, should be considered for daily preventive therapies.

Several classes of medications can be used, and medical comorbidities can aid with selection. The following comorbidities may suggest specific options to consider:

- *Epilepsy*: Topiramate, valproate, zonisamide, gabapentin
- *Insomnia*: Amitriptyline, nortriptyline, protriptyline
- *Hypertension*: Propranolol, verapamil
- *Musculoskeletal pain*: Amitriptyline, nortriptyline, protriptyline, gabapentin
- *Overweight*: Topiramate, zonisamide
- *Underweight*: Valproate

Lifestyle issues can greatly affect migraine frequency. Among the issues that may help to reduce the frequency and severity of migraine are:

- *Hydration*: Not dehydrated but not water-intoxicated
- *Sleep*: Not too much or too little
- *Caffeine*: Avoid excessive use, and avoid caffeine withdrawal.
- *Judicious medication use*: Watch out for development of medication overuse headache. Avoid taking meds for several days in a row.
- *Watch for food triggers*: This is controversial but, for some people, chocolate, wine, cheese, nitrates, and nitrites may exacerbate migraine.

Medication Overuse Headache

Patients with medication overuse headache should be withdrawn from the offending medications. Some medications, such as butalbital, must be tapered.

CLUSTER

Cluster headache is a type of vascular headache that is more common in males than females, unlike migraine. Age of onset can be from 20 to 50 years.

PRESENTATION is with typically short unilateral peri-orbital steady headaches, lasting from 30 to 180 minutes, and with a quick time to peak onset. Nightly occurrence is common, which disturbs sleep patterns as well as causing disturbing pain. Associated symptoms can be nasal congestion or conjunctival injection. The episodes often cluster—occurring regularly for a period of weeks—then disappear for months or longer.

DIAGNOSIS is clinical. Cluster is differentiated from migraine by the orbital/peri-orbital distribution, brief duration, male predominance, and clustering. Patients with cluster are often quite anxious during the headache, in contrast to patients with migraine. Imaging is normal and usually not needed.

MANAGEMENT is with many of the same meds used for migraine. As with migraine, medication overuse headache can be seen in cluster patients. The most common medications that serve as a genesis for medication overuse headaches include oral triptans, acetaminophen, and opiate receptor agonist analgesics.[6]

- *Abortive therapies*
  - o *Oxygen*: Inhaled oxygen, 100% at 10–12 L/min for 15 minutes is an effective, safe treatment of acute cluster headache.
  - o *Triptans*: Sumatriptan 6 mg subcutaneous, sumatriptan 20 mg intranasal, or zolmitriptan 5 mg intranasal are effective in the acute treatment of cluster headache. Three doses of zolmitriptan in 24 hours are acceptable. There is no evidence to support the use of oral triptans in cluster.
  - o *DHE*: 1 mg IM is effective in the relief of acute cluster attacks. Longer periods of treatment may need to be employed, similar to that outlined for migraine.
  - o *Lidocaine*: Topical lidocaine nasal drops (often 4% lidocaine) can be used to treat acute cluster attacks. The patient lies down with the head tilted backward toward the floor at 30 degrees and turned to the side of the headache.
- *Preventive therapies*
  - o *Verapamil* is considered the first-line therapy in prevention of cluster headache. Baseline EKG should be obtained. Typical starting dose is 80 mg three times daily; thereafter, the total daily dose is increased in increments of 80 mg every 10–14 days. EKGs should be obtained during the titration.
  - o *Lithium carbonate* is used at a dose of 600–900 mg per day in divided doses. Lithium levels should be followed along with thyroid function studies and renal function.
  - o *Anticonvulsants: Topiramate,* and *gabapentin* are useful in the prevention of cluster attacks.
  - o *Prednisone* is often given to abort a cluster while other preventative therapies are being instituted and escalated.

PSEUDOTUMOR CEREBRI

Pseudotumor cerebri also is called *idiopathic intracranial hypertension* (IIH). However, we recommend using the term pseudotumor cerebri because it is in common clinical use by non-neurologists. This condition causes reduced CSF resorption of unknown etiology; increased venous pressure may be a cause for some patients either from reduced available venous vasculature or increased arterial pressure.

PRESENTATION is usually with headache and papilledema. Ocular motor deficit can produce diplopia, most commonly CN 6 palsy, giving horizontal diplopia. Brain imaging is unremarkable.

DIAGNOSIS is considered when a patient presents with headache and papilledema. This is most common in young women, especially with increased body mass index. Brain imaging is best with MRI rather than CT and is typically normal. Some patients will have an *empty sella*, which is best seen on MRI, but this is not a specific finding. Lumbar puncture (LP) usually shows marked increase in CSF opening pressure; when pseudotumor cerebri is suspected, removal of CSF sufficient to lower the pressure is often recommended. Headache often transiently improves after the LP.

MANAGEMENT often begins with CSF drainage followed by weight loss, which helps many patients. Since weight reduction is often unsuccessful or only transient, medical treatment with acetazolamide is often offered.

- *Lumbar puncture*: CSF is removed and opening pressure measured. This has diagnostic and therapeutic benefit.
- *Medical therapy: Acetazolamide*, a carbonic anhydrase inhibitor is often used first-line for medical management, although it should not be given to patients with an allergy to sulfa drugs. *Furosemide, zonisamide,* and *topiramate* are alternatives.
- *Surgical therapy* includes optic nerve fenestration, lumboperitoneal shunt, or, less likely, ventriculoperitoneal shunt.
- *Ophthalmology consultation* is recommended for all patients.

TRIGEMINAL NEURALGIA

Trigeminal neuralgia is a prototypic neuropathic pain with symptoms from large-fiber involvement. Compression of CN 5 by a branch of the basilar artery is commonly implicated, causing inflammation of the nerve.

PRESENTATION is with paroxysms of pain in a trigeminal distribution, usually V2 or V3. V1 is affected only rarely. The pain is brief and electric or stabbing. The pain is activity-dependent, often triggered by local cutaneous stimulation (a trigger region) or talking or chewing. The pain seldom occurs during sleep.

DIAGNOSIS is suspected with episodic unilateral facial pain in the absence of motor deficit. MRI is unremarkable. Trigeminal neuralgia can be misdiagnosed as hemifacial spasm if there is wincing, although this is typically mild. Unilateral headache in the elderly suggests consideration of temporal arteritis, but this is a steady temporal-region pain without the electric component. Cavernous sinus lesion can produce trigeminal pain, but ocular motor abnormalities are expected. Multiple sclerosis can cause trigeminal neuralgia, although usually in younger patients, and this would only rarely be the only manifestation.

MANAGEMENT usually begins with medical trials including especially baclofen or anticonvulsants. Some of the anticonvulsants used are oxcarbazepine, carbamazepine, or phenytoin, and alternatives could be gabapentin or pregabalin. Local capsaicin can be used for a trigger region. Surgery can be performed if patients fail medical therapy.

TEMPORAL ARTERITIS

Temporal arteritis (TA) is an inflammatory disorder that extends beyond the temporal artery. *Giant cell arteritis* is a more accurate name and is used by many authors, but most of our non-neurology colleagues use the term *temporal arteritis* in routine practice. Most patients are at least 50 years old.

PRESENTATION is with headache, which is classically in one temporal region, associated with tenderness and thickening of the temporal artery. Accompanying the headache are systemic inflammatory symptoms with malaise, fatigue, and possible fever. Pain extends to the neck and shoulders in many patients. Jaw claudication (pain in the jaw muscles with chewing) is an important although inconstant finding. Visual loss can develop progressing to blindness, but, more commonly, there are more minor visual symptoms of blurring or scotoma prior to frank loss of vision. Urgent treatment is essential to reduce the risk of progression of visual loss.

DIAGNOSIS is considered when a patient over the age of 50 years develops headache. Since not all patients have a classic presentation, this cannot be used to rule out the diagnosis (e.g., some patients have more generalized headache or occipital headache). The erythrocyte sedimentation rate (ESR) is increased, usually markedly but not invariably. Temporal artery biopsy is recommended for most patients in whom TA is considered. However, treatment should begin on suspicion prior to getting biopsy results.

MANAGEMENT begins with corticosteroids, usually prednisone 40–60 mg/day with gradual tapering, although prolonged treatment is often used. Intravenous methylprednisolone may be used if there are visual symptoms, often 1,000 mg/day for 3–5 days. Aspirin is recommended for patients if they are not already on an antiplatelet agent.

REVERSIBLE CEREBRAL VASOCONSTRICTION SYNDROME

RCVS is an uncommon and likely under-diagnosed cause of acute thunderclap headache. The hospital neurologist may see RCVS where the provisional diagnosis is acute ischemic stroke or subarachnoid hemorrhage.

Recurrent thunderclap headache is a common presentation. Focal deficits can develop with clinical and imaging findings of infarction and/or hemorrhage in a minority.

Emergent evaluation is indicated. Vasoconstriction can be demonstrated on CTA or MRA or catheter angiography.

Management is supportive. Calcium channel blockers have been tried with little supportive evidence. Other stroke risk factors should be addressed.

21 Neuromuscular Disorders

E. Lee Murray, MD and
Veda V. Vedanarayanan, MD, FRCPC

CHAPTER CONTENTS

- Overview
- Peripheral Nerve
  - Acute Inflammatory Demyelinating Polyneuropathy
  - Acute-Onset Chronic Inflammatory Demyelinating Polyneuropathy
  - Chronic Inflammatory Demyelinating Polyneuropathy
  - Multifocal Motor Neuropathy
  - Mononeuropathies
  - Idiopathic Brachial Plexitis
  - Diabetic Lumbosacral Plexopathy
  - Mononeuritis Multiplex
  - Hereditary Neuropathy with Pressure Palsies
- Neuromuscular Junction
  - Myasthenia Gravis
  - Lambert Eaton Myasthenic Syndrome
  - Botulism
  - Tick Paralysis
- Muscle
  - Muscles, Weakness, and Laboratory Studies
  - Rhabdomyolysis
  - Critical Illness Neuromyopathy
  - Inflammatory Myopathies
  - Muscular Dystrophies
  - Periodic Paralysis
  - Metabolic and Endocrine Myopathies
- Motoneuron Degeneration
  - Amyotrophic Lateral Sclerosis
  - Progressive Muscular Atrophy
- Neuromuscular Respiratory Failure

OVERVIEW

Neuromuscular disorders may be encountered as known chronic conditions that are exacerbated by a hospital stay, be the principal reason for admission, or develop during a prolonged hospitalization.

PERIPHERAL NERVE
Acute Inflammatory Demyelinating Polyneuropathy

Acute inflammatory demyelinating polyneuropathy (AIDP) or *Guillain-Barré syndrome* (GBS) is an immune-mediated peripheral neuropathy with an acute to subacute, monophasic course that typically reaches maximal symptomatology at 3–4 weeks. Most cases present as an inflammatory demyelinating pathology; however, axonal variants do exist.

AIDP is often associated with a preceding illness. The most common are:

- *Campylobacter jejuni*
- Cytomegalovirus
- Upper respiratory tract infections
- Hepatitis

PRESENTATION is typically with progressive generalized weakness, which at times leads to respiratory compromise and dysautonomia. Weakness usually starts in the lower extremities; however, some cases will begin in the upper extremities or all four extremities simultaneously. Most patients will present with reduced or absent reflexes; however, reflexes may be preserved for several days after onset. Severe cases can progress to respiratory insufficiency necessitating ventilatory support. Dysautonomia is common especially with severe disease.

DIAGNOSIS is suspected with progressive weakness and especially with associated reduced or absent tendon reflexes.

- *Brain and spine imaging* are unrevealing and often not necessary. However, if CNS demyelination or primary spinal cord pathology is considered, magnetic resonance imaging (MRI) of the brain and/or spinal cord may be needed.
- *Electromyography and nerve conduction studies (EMG/NCS)* typically show evidence of demyelinating features, including prolongation or absence of F-waves, reduced velocities, and evidence of temporal dispersion when viewing the compound motor action potential (CMAP) wave forms. Very early in the course, EMG/NCS studies might be normal. Prolonged or absent late responses (F-waves and/or H-reflexes) are the earliest finding on electrodiagnostic testing.
- *CSF* findings include albuminocytologic dissociation—elevation in CSF protein without an elevation in CSF WBC. However, elevation in the CSF WBC can be seen in patients with AIDP associated with HIV. There can be a delay in the elevation of protein of up to 2 weeks. Therefore, if there remains a clinical question, repeat CSF examination may be warranted.

MANAGEMENT usually begins with hospital admission; patients who are diagnosed with AIDP should be maintained in the hospital for close monitoring until it has been determined that the course of the disease has reached a plateau or has begun to improve. Weakness can progress rapidly, leading to profound paralysis, respiratory insufficiency, and/or autonomic dysfunction with cardiovascular complications requiring emergency intervention. Telemetry is recommended.

- *ICU* monitoring should be considered for all patients with any signs of respiratory distress, a forced vital capacity of less than 20 mL/kg, severe bulbar palsy, or significant dysautonomia.
- *General medical care* includes deep vein thrombosis (DVT) prophylaxis; monitoring for infection and skin breakdown, especially in those with severe motor dysfunction; nutritional support; and regular bowel care to prevent the development of an adynamic ileus.
- *Immunotherapy: Plasmapheresis* or *IV immunoglobulin* (IVIg) can be used in patients with AIDP. Immunotherapy shortens the recovery time and lessens long-term disability. There is no evidence that one treatment modality is superior to the other. Decisions on which therapy to pursue depend on concomitant medical issues, contraindications, availability at the treating facility, and patient preference. Corticosteroids have been shown to not be effective in AIDP and should not be used. Typical dosing for IVIg is 0.4 g/kg/day for 3–5 days. Plasma exchange is typically carried out for a total of 3–5 exchanges.[1]
- *Pain*: Patients typically may develop fairly severe neuropathic pain. Typical neuropathic pain medications including gabapentin, pregabalin, duloxetine, or tricyclic antidepressants can be beneficial.
- *Therapy:* Involvement of occupational and physical therapy early in the course can also hasten recovery. Speech therapy is also warranted, especially in those with significant bulbar symptoms, to promote safe swallowing.
- *Autonomic involvement*: Along with respiratory compromise, autonomic dysfunction in AIDP can be life-threatening. Patients should be monitored closely so life support measures can be put in place if needed. Autonomic dysfunction is seen more often in the demyelinating forms than in the axonal variants. Autonomic changes can be:
  o Bradycardia or tachycardia
  o Orthostatic hypotension
  o Paroxysmal hypertension
  o Anhydrosis and/or diaphoresis
  o Urinary retention
  o Facial flushing
- *Hyponatremia* can be seen in AIDP and is usually due to the syndrome of inappropriate antidiuretic hormone (SIADH) and natriuresis. The treatment differs; both require replenishment of sodium but SIADH needs fluid restriction, and, natriuresis requires intravascular volume expansion.[2]

Axonal Variants

Axonal variants are less common in Western countries than demyelinating forms. Axonal types are more often seen in Asian populations.

Acute motor axonal neuropathy (AMAN) is often preceded by *Campylobacter jejuni* infection. Presenting clinical features and overall disease progression are very similar to

AIDP. Since this is predominantly axonal, reflexes can be preserved. Electrodiagnostic testing shows axonal changes rather than prominent demyelination.

Acute motor and sensory axonal neuropathy (AMSAN) is a more severe variant of AIDP. It is characterized by involvement of both sensory and motor fibers with significant axonal degeneration. Recovery is often delayed or incomplete. Electrodiagnostic testing reveals involvement of both motor and sensory responses with denervation noted on needle electromyogram (EMG).

Acute-Onset Chronic Inflammatory Demyelinating Polyneuropathy

Acute-onset chronic inflammatory demyelinating polyneuropathy (A-CIDP) presents similarly to AIDP. This is CIDP but with a more rapid onset. Approximately 16% of patients with CIDP present acutely.[3]

PRESENTATION is with typical AIDP initially, then there is regression after initial improvement with immunotherapy.

DIAGNOSIS is suspected when a patient with AIDP has worsening after initial response to therapy. Differentiating AIDP from A-CIDP is important because those with A-CIDP variant will require continued long-term treatments.

Patients with A-CIDP are more likely to have the following features:

- Prominent sensory signs
- Sacral sparing

Patients who did not progress to A-CIDP are more likely to have the following features:

- Autonomic disturbance
- Facial weakness
- Severe motor signs
- Require ventilatory support
- Identified antecedent illness

MANAGEMENT of A-CIDP is as for CIDP.

Chronic Inflammatory Demyelinating Polyneuropathy

CIDP is a demyelinating neuropathy similar to AIDP but with a more protracted course. Patients have a progressive course over more than 4 weeks.

PRESENTATION is with weakness and sensory deficit with decreased or absent reflexes. There is usually no identified antecedent illness. Autonomic and respiratory difficulties are not expected. Cranial nerve abnormalities are uncommon.

DIAGNOSIS is suspected in a patient with progressive weakness and sensory disturbance and reduced or absent reflexes.

- Imaging of the brain and spine is unremarkable and seldom needed.
- CSF shows findings similar to AIDP with increased protein and no increase in WBC.
- NCS shows demyelinating polyneuropathy. Multifocal conduction block is strongly supportive of the diagnosis.

- EMG shows no denervation early in the course. Late in the course, denervation may be seen in a minority of patients.

MANAGEMENT is similar to AIDP with response to IVIg or plasma exchange. In addition, corticosteroids are effective for CIDP whereas they are not for AIDP. Patients often respond best to one treatment, so if there is no response to a particular modality, one of the others should be considered. Treatment options include the following:

- Prednisone is often given at 60–80 mg/day for several weeks then tapered as tolerated. While this is effective and used first-line by many clinicians, the deleterious effects of long-term corticosteroids are of concern.
- IVIg is an excellent alternative to prednisone and used as first-line treatment by some, especially if comorbid conditions make corticosteroid treatment risky (e.g., diabetes). Initial treatment is usually for 3–5 days, but follow-up doses are needed at intervals dictated by response and relapse.
- Plasma exchange is effective and is comparable to prednisone and IVIg in response rate, but because of the logistics of performing plasma exchange (frequency and duration of treatments, vascular access) this is seldom used first-line for CIDP.

Multifocal Motor Neuropathy

Multifocal motor neuropathy (MMN) is an inflammatory demyelination restricted to motor nerves. In other respects, it is similar to CIDP.

PRESENTATION is with progressive weakness, often starting in one limb but then becoming more extensive. Although this is not a motoneuron degeneration, fasciculations can occur, but since the motoneurons are relatively preserved, there is not the marked atrophy of amyotrophic lateral sclerosis (ALS).

DIAGNOSIS is suspected with progressive weakness without corticospinal tract signs. EMG and NCS show conduction block. Anti-GM1 antibodies can be seen.

MANAGEMENT is most commonly with IVIg. Cyclophosphamide is also used.

Mononeuropathies

Most mononeuropathies are diagnosed in the outpatient setting, but some acute presentations may be encountered in the hospital. Some of the important mononeuropathy scenarios are as follows:

Radial neuropathy: Compression produces weakness of the wrist and finger extensors with resultant wrist drop. Triceps weakness may be seen. This presentation may trigger admission because of concern over monoplegia from stroke. Without careful exam, wrist instability may give the perception of finger flexor weakness, whereas with stabilization of the wrist, full strength of median- and ulnar-innervated muscles can be demonstrated. Classically, this is seen in alcoholics who become somnolent while resting their arm in a position vulnerable to radial palsy.

Peroneal neuropathy: Weakness of the tibialis anterior is most prominent, producing deficit in foot dorsiflexion. This can be hospital-acquired since the peroneal nerve is susceptible to compression at the fibular neck, making prolonged bedrest a risk for peroneal palsy. The lesion may be higher because if the sciatic nerve is compressed, the peroneal division seems more susceptible to compression damage.

Sciatic neuropathy: Weakness of the peroneal or tibial divisions can produce deficits in foot dorsiflexion or plantar flexion and may additionally affect the knee flexors. Potential causes of damage include hip or knee fractures or surgery, pelvic fractures, and, less likely, injections.

Femoral neuropathy: Weakness of the knee extensors is most evident. Common causes include pelvic surgery and bleeding into the region of the nerve or plexus (e.g., from surgery or arterial puncture).

Diabetic amyotrophy: Damage to the lumbosacral plexus from diabetes produces pain and weakness most prominent in the quadriceps but also involving other L2–L3 innervated muscles. Superimposed polyneuropathy may produce deficits beyond this distribution. This may trigger hospitalization because of concern over possible stroke, especially anterior cerebral artery infarction, which can produce unilateral leg weakness without arm involvement. Proximal distribution of the deficits and regional pain support the correct clinical diagnosis.

Ulnar neuropathy: Intrinsic weakness of the hand from ulnar neuropathy is common in diabetics but is unlikely to trigger hospital admission or consultation.

Median neuropathy: Deficits of hand function from lesions of the median nerve at the wrist (carpal tunnel syndrome) or higher are uncommon in hospital practice. Diagnosis is assisted by careful examination of median-, ulnar-, and radial-innervated muscles to distinguish median neuropathy from a central lesion.

Herpes zoster and post-herpetic neuralgia: Reactivation of the varicella zoster virus produces pain in a single nerve root distribution and is associated with vesicular rash. This can be followed by prolonged neuropathic pain. This is discussed in Chapter 17.

Idiopathic Brachial Plexitis

Idiopathic brachial plexitis or *neurogenic amyotrophy* (also known as *Parsonage-Turner syndrome*) is an idiopathic attack on the brachial plexus. This is often believed to be an inflammatory autoimmune process that presents in a multifocal distribution. Neurogenic amyotrophy is often used as a preferred term because it is not clear that the pathology is consistently in the plexus.

PRESENTATION typically is with a fairly acute onset of pain in the shoulder then weakness and numbness in the shoulder girdle and arm. The weakness can be remarkably focal. Most patients experience a plateau of symptoms fairly quickly, with a slow resolution.

DIAGNOSIS is suggested by rapid onset of shoulder pain and arm weakness that does not fall into one radicular distribution. Electrodiagnostic studies may often be normal initially due to the acute onset. CSF may show a mild pleocytosis. Differential diagnosis includes an acute radiculopathy or a traumatic injury to the shoulder and/ or brachial plexus.

MANAGEMENT includes physical therapy along with symptomatic neuropathic pain therapies.

Diabetic Lumbosacral Plexopathy

Diabetic lumbosacral plexopathy or *diabetic amyotrophy* is a lumbar radiculoplexopathy affecting the lower extremity.

PRESENTATION is with pain in the back, hip, and upper leg. Weakness develops in proximal muscles, particularly quadriceps and iliopsoas. Symptoms often develop after an epoch of significant weight loss.

DIAGNOSIS is suspected with proximal pain and weakness in a patient with known diabetes. Hgb A1C is often measured to assess diabetic control. MRI of the lumbar spine and plexus can look for structural causes of plexopathy. EMG may show denervation, especially in these proximal muscles and additionally often shows a coexistent peripheral neuropathy.

MANAGEMENT begins with optimal glucose control. Physical therapy is helpful. No medications have become standard therapy; there is some evidence for immunotherapy, but this is not proved and not recommended for most patients.[4]

Mononeuritis Multiplex

Mononeuritis multiplex is dysfunction of multiple individual nerves. The most common cause is diabetes. There are many other causes including polyarteritis nodosa, sarcoidosis, Lyme disease, HIV, Wegener granulomatosis, and hereditary neuropathy with liability to pressure palsies.

PRESENTATION is with deficits affecting multiple individual nerves, typically asymmetric. Almost any nerve can be affected. Typical findings include wrist drop, foot drop, and/or a cranial neuropathy.

DIAGNOSIS is suspected with asymmetric individual peripheral nerve deficits (e.g., ulnar and peroneal).

- *EMG with NCS* can show conduction blocks in individual nerves; however, studies may be normal early in the course.
- *Serological studies* investigating a broader autoimmune process should be obtained.
- *Nerve biopsy* can be helpful in diagnosing vasculitis and should be considered prior to initiation of powerful immunosuppressive therapies such as cyclophosphamide.

Hereditary Neuropathy with Pressure Palsies

Hereditary neuropathy with pressure palsies (HNPP) is an autosomal dominant condition that results in reduced levels of the normal PMP22 protein.

PRESENTATION is with episodes of pressure palsies affecting almost any nerves. Deficits are caused by compression, which can be mild and brief. Motor and sensory deficit are typical, but pain is uncommon. The deficit can be brief or persistent.

DIAGNOSIS is suspected when a patient reports episodes of pressure palsies in various nerve distributions. EMG and NCS usually show mild neuropathic changes. The principal differential diagnosis is peripheral neuropathy with secondary predisposition to pressure palsies, but, in this case, the EMG abnormalities would be more severe and the clinical manifestations of polyneuropathy would be more marked.

MANAGEMENT is supportive, with advice on methods to reduce pressure palsies, including avoiding static positions, cushioning, and adequate nutrition to avoid predisposition to palsies from deficiency.

NEUROMUSCULAR JUNCTION

Disorders of the *neuromuscular junction* (NMJ) seen in the hospital include *myasthenia gravis* (MG), *Lambert-Eaton myasthenic syndrome*, *botulism*, and *tick paralysis*.

Myasthenia Gravis

MG is an autoimmune disease in which, for most patients, antibodies target the nicotinic acetylcholine receptor at the NMJ, and this results in fatigable weakness. Muscle-specific tyrosine kinase (MuSK) antibodies are seen in some of the otherwise seronegative patients.

PRESENTATION is with fatigable weakness that can be purely ocular or systemic. Ocular manifestations include diplopia and ptosis. There are no sensory symptoms. Bulbar function is affected in many patients and can be a reason for hospital admission; it can be associated with neck flexor weakness. Respiratory support is needed for some patients in myasthenic crisis.

DIAGNOSIS is considered in patients with weakness, especially when accompanied by ptosis and other ocular motor abnormalities. Studies that are helpful in making the diagnosis include:

- *Acetylcholine receptor (AChR)* antibodies: Binding antibodies are used to support the clinical diagnosis.
- *Anti-striational muscle antibodies*: Often positive in patients who do not have MG, so these are of less value diagnostically.
- *MuSK antibodies*: Positive in some patients with otherwise negative antibody studies.
- *EMG with repetitive nerve stimulation (RNS)*: Sensitive for showing the NMJ defect by a decremental response to low frequencies of stimulation. If MG or other NMJ defect is suspected, this should be indicated specifically in the electrodiagnostic order.
- *Edrophonium test* is the administration of this cholinesterase inhibitor while watching an objective motor deficit such as ptosis. This is still used but less extensively because of improvements in serological testing and the relative insensitivity of the technique.
- *Ocular cooling* is placement of an ice pack on the eyelids; this can result in temporary improvement in ptosis. This has the same limitations as the edrophonium test and is used but not universally.

Hospital status: Most patients seen in an inpatient setting have an established diagnosis of MG and are already taking appropriate medications. Noncompliance with medications, infection, or physiologic stressors can result in an exacerbation of the disease. Therefore, a patient presenting with an exacerbation should be evaluated for systemic conditions such as infectious processes, especially respiratory infections, and electrolyte discrepancies. Any new medication should also be considered as a potential exacerbating factor.

Medications that could lead to an exacerbation:

- *Antibiotics*: Macrolides, fluoroquinolones, aminoglycosides, tetracycline, and chloroquine
- *Antidysrhythmic agents*: Beta-blockers, calcium channel blockers, quinidine, lidocaine, procainamide, and trimethaphan
- *Antipsychotics*: Phenothiazines, sulpiride, atypicals antipsychotics
- *Cardiovascular*: Propranolol, quinidine, verapamil, beryllium, statins
- *Miscellaneous*: Phenytoin, lithium, chlorpromazine, muscle relaxants, levothyroxine, adrenocorticotropic hormone (ACTH), and, paradoxically, corticosteroids

New medications that are not list here and correspond with a myasthenic exacerbation should be considered as a potential causative source.

Autoimmune thyroid disorders can be seen in those with myasthenia and should be evaluated and treated.[5]

MANAGEMENT begins with medical stabilization. Patients who seem to be at risk for respiratory or other bulbar compromise should be admitted to the ICU.

- *Cholinesterase inhibitors* increase the availability of acetylcholine at the neuromuscular junction.
- *Immune modulating agents* are used in almost all patients. For patients with fairly mild disease, escalating doses of *prednisone* or similar corticosteroid is often used. For more severe disease or corticosteroid intolerance, treatment with either *IVIG* or *plasma exchange* should be considered. Note that transient worsening of weakness after beginning corticosteroid therapy can occur and requires monitoring during institution and dose escalation. Steroid-sparing agents such as azathioprine or mycophenolate mofetil can be considered in patients with poor tolerance to corticosteroids and/or in those who continue to have significant symptoms despite other therapies.

Severe Exacerbations of MG

Severe exacerbations of myasthenia gravis including *myasthenic crisis* may present dramatically and should be considered an emergency. Findings can include:

- Facial weakness
- Severe neck flexion weakness
- Jaw weakness
- Nasal voice
- Weak cough
- Severe generalized weakness
- Absent gag reflex
- Respiratory distress

The hallmark of myasthenic crisis is respiratory failure. Patients experiencing severe respiratory and/or bulbar compromise may need to be electively intubated. Aspiration pneumonia may develop in those who have had difficulties clearing secretions.

Cholinergic Crisis

Treatment options for MG include the use of cholinesterase inhibitors. However, excessive cholinergic activity can lead to a cholinergic crisis. This may have a similar presentation as an organophosphate poisoning, which at times can cause generalized muscle weakness, wheezing, respiratory failure, and diaphoresis. Given the similar symptoms to MG, a cholinergic crisis may be difficult to distinguish from a potential myasthenic exacerbation.

Typical presentation of a cholinergic crisis includes miosis and the mnemonic SLUDGE syndrome: Salivation, Lacrimation, Urinary incontinence, Diarrhea, Gastrointestinal upset and hypermotility, Emesis.

Lambert-Eaton Myasthenic Syndrome

Lambert-Eaton Myasthenic syndrome (LEMS) is also termed *myasthenic syndrome*, although we do not prefer the latter name because the clinical appearance and immunology is different from myasthenia. This is an autoimmune disorder where antibodies work against voltage-gated calcium channels (VGCC). This is often considered a paraneoplastic syndrome. but many patients with LEMS do not have and do not develop cancer. This is discussed in detail in Chapter 25.

Botulism

Botulism is due to neuromuscular blockade by the toxin of *Clostridium botulinum*. Source of the toxin can be from bacteria in food or in wounds. Food is usually contaminated due to improper canning, especially in the home. Wound contamination can be seen with extensive lesions such as burns.

PRESENTATION is with progressive weakness. If the source is food, GI complaints often precede the neuromuscular deficits. If the source is a wound, there is a history of very recent injury, such as trauma or burn. Weakness usually develops within 12–36 hours for food-borne botulism, although longer and shorter intervals can develop depending on toxin dose. Wound botulism has a longer incubation period, several days to a week or more. Associated symptoms can be dry mouth, vomiting, and diarrhea along with cranial nerve involvement. Descending paralysis is then seen and continues to progress to involve respiratory muscles.

DIAGNOSIS is clinical initially and is suspected with progressive weakness with a history of either suspect ingestion and GI distress or a significant wound. Toxin assay is available and can be run on serum or stool. Contemporaneous diagnosis of suspected botulism in a different person with a possible related exposure is supportive. EMG shows low-voltage motor unit potentials with an incremental response to repetitive stimulation.

MANAGEMENT is supportive. Respiratory support is critical. When the diagnosis is suspected, possible development of botulism in others has to be considered and queried. Antitoxin is available from the Centers for Disease Control (CDC) for symptomatic patients.

Tick Paralysis

Tick paralysis is typically caused by *Dermacentor* tick, which releases the toxin in its saliva when it has been attached for several days.

PRESENTATION is with generalized weakness progressing to flaccid paralysis. Other symptoms include ataxia and nystagmus. There are no sensory findings. Reflexes are typically absent. Respiratory compromise can occur in severe cases.

DIAGNOSIS is suspected with progressive paralysis. Differential diagnosis considered includes MG, AIDP, and botulism. Diagnosis is supported by finding the tick, particularly in hair. There are no specific laboratory findings.

MANAGEMENT is by removal of the tick. This typically results in improvement within hours to a few days.

MUSCLE

The vast majority of muscle diseases present with a subacute or chronic progression and therefore are not commonly seen in the hospital setting. However, a limited number of inflammatory, toxic/metabolic, and genetic disorders can lead to acute and severe muscle weakness requiring hospitalization and, at times, critical care management

Muscles, Weakness, and Laboratory Studies

Pattern of Muscle Weakness

Pattern of weakness can narrow the differential diagnosis.

- *Limb-girdle*: Most common pattern of weakness; nonspecific
- *Prominent distal weakness*: myotonic dystrophy, inclusion body myositis, Miyoshi myopathies
- *Neck extensor weakness*: Polymyositis, muscular dystrophy, inclusion body myositis
- *Early respiratory involvement*: Severe polymyositis, acid maltase deficiency
- *Predominant pharyngeal and ocular*: Mitochondrial, oculopharyngeal dystrophy

Muscle Enzymes

Typical serological testing for suspected muscle disease includes creatine phosphokinase (CPK), aldolase, and lactate dehydrogenase (LDH). Elevations in CPK do not always indicate muscle disease. African-Americans tend to have higher normal values of CPK, especially men.

Nonmyopathy etiologies of elevated CPK include:

- Connective tissue disorders
- Cardiac disease
- Electrolyte disturbances (hyponatremia, hypophosphatemia, hypokalemia)
- Thyroid dysfunction
- Hyperparathyroidism
- Kidney disease
- Malignancy
- Medications (statins, isotretinoin, beta-blockers)
- Toxins (cocaine, heroin, ethanol)
- Muscle trauma, crush injuries

Myoglobinuria

Myoglobinuria is usually indicative of rhabdomyolysis and the destruction of muscle tissue. Typically, patients have muscle weakness along with exceptionally dark urine. Potential causes of myoglobinuria include:

- Trauma/Ischemia
  - Seizure/Status epilepticus
  - Crush injuries
  - Electrical shock
- Acquired myopathies
  - Inflammatory myopathies
  - Infections
- Metabolic myopathies
  - Malignant hypothermia
  - Neuroleptic malignant syndrome
  - McArdle syndrome
- Toxins/Drugs
  - Statins
  - Alcohol
  - Snake venom
- Environmental
  - Heat stroke
  - Heavy exercise
- Muscular dystrophies

Rhabdomyolysis

Rhabdomyolysis is seen in the hospital setting from a variety of causes. Most common are trauma, status epilepticus, immobility (unrelieved muscle compression), and toxic/metabolic. In the ED, rhabdomyolysis in association with ethanol intoxication and abuse is often seen.

Medications that can lead to myopathy or rhabdomyolysis include:

- Amiodarone
- Chloroquine
- Colchicine
- Statins
- Corticosteroids
- D-Penicillamine
- Zidovudine (AZT)
- Propofol
- Isotretinoin
- Lithium
- Cyclosporine
- Streptokinase
- Vinca alkaloids

PRESENTATION is with muscle pain that can be regional or generalized, depending on etiology. Muscles become tender and are often swollen. Fever may develop. Myoglobinuria may be noted and is the first clue to the diagnosis.

DIAGNOSIS is suspected with muscle pain and/or swelling with tenderness. Lab shows increased CPK. Additional study with EMG and imaging is often not needed with acute rhabdomyolysis.

Rhabdomyolysis can also be the initial presentation of an underlying muscle pathology such as McArdle syndrome or other glycogen storage abnormalities, carnitine palmitoyltransferase deficiency, malignant hyperthermia, or neuroleptic malignant syndrome.

Inflammatory and paraneoplastic myopathies often do not lead to rhabdomyolysis; however, excessive muscle breakdown leading to rhabdomyolysis can be seen in anti-signal recognition particle (SRP) myopathy, anti-MAS antibody inflammatory myopathies, or in fulminant paraneoplastic dermatomyositis or acute necrotizing paraneoplastic myopathy.

MANAGEMENT of rhabdomyolysis includes aggressive hydration to prevent acute renal failure. This may require the use of mannitol and loop diuretics, along with urinary alkalization. Consultation with critical care and nephrology should be considered.

Critical Illness Neuromyopathy

Critical illness neuromyopathy (CIN) is development of flaccid weakness along with failure to wean from the ventilator in the ICU. This is particularly common in patients with prolonged hospitalization. CIN can be critical illness axonal polyneuropathy or critical illness myopathy, therefore the term neuromyopathy is used. More than 50% of patients with severe sepsis and multiorgan failure who have been ventilated for more than 72 hours can develop CIN. Patients can be awake and may be able to communicate by eye blink or head nod, but they have little or no movement of the extremities. Patients who have received corticosteroids and/or neuromuscular blocking agents are predisposed to CIN.

PRESENTATION is with weakness in extremity muscles, usually sparing facial and ocular muscles. Deep tendon reflexes are usually absent or depressed but may be present in pure critical illness myopathy. Sensory examination is often difficult to accurately obtain. Often, CIN is not considered unless mental status is sufficiently preserved to make evident the disconnect between mental status and strength.

DIAGNOSIS is suspected when a patient in the ICU has marked weakness and decreased tone. EMG/NCS can be performed, but often are fraught with technical complications from electrical interference in the ICU, edema that is often seen in ICU patients, and inability for ICU patients to be able to cognitively activate muscle.

NCS and EMG: Common electrodiagnostic findings in critical illness polyneuropathy include low CMAP and sensory (SNAP) amplitudes with conduction velocities within normal range or mildly reduced. Critical illness myopathy will show spontaneous insertional activity with fibrillations and positive sharp waves with or without myopathic motor units.[6] Prolonged CMAP duration has been suggested as the earliest sign of critical illness myopathy.[7]

MANAGEMENT is supportive. There is no specific treatment. A careful examination is needed to rule out any cortical or spinal structural anomalies or toxic or metabolic abnormalities. Some studies suggest early and aggressive treatment of hyperglycemia along with early mobilization.

Inflammatory Myopathies

Inflammatory myopathies may be idiopathic, associated with a connective tissue disorder, or paraneoplastic. *Polymyositis* is most often seen in adulthood, whereas *dermatomyositis* may be seen in both pediatric and adult populations. *Inclusion body myositis* typically presents after the age of 50 and usually has a chronic presentation.

Polymyositis

Polymyositis usually develops in patients at or approaching middle age.

PRESENTATION is typically with a progressive limb-girdle pattern of weakness and is usually symmetrical. Weakness usually develops over weeks to months. Despite the inflammatory nature of the pathology, the muscles are generally not painful or tender. Shortness of breath can occur with involvement of respiratory and bulbar muscles, but this is rare. Cardiac involvement can result in conduction defects/arrhythmias, dilated cardiomyopathy, congestive heart failure (CHF), or myocarditis. Dysphasia commonly occurs due to weakness of the oropharynx and facial muscles.

DIAGNOSIS is suspected with progressive weakness in the absence of sensory involvement. Labs, EMG, and, ultimately, muscle biopsy make the diagnosis.

- CPK values are typically significantly elevated; however, they can rarely be normal. Patients with interstitial lung disease often correlate with anti-Jo-1 antibodies.
- EMG usually reveals spontaneous activity.
- NCS may show low-amplitude CMAPs. Sensory responses should be normal in the absence of other neuropathic diseases.
- Echocardiogram may show a reduced ejection fraction.
- Muscle biopsy shows inflammatory changes but because the pathology is focal, multiple specimens may need to be submitted for diagnosis.

Dermatomyositis

Dermatomyositis is usually an idiopathic disease process; however, with increasing age there is an increasing association with cancer. The malignancies most commonly associated with dermatomyositis include ovarian, breast, lung, and gastric/colon cancers, and Hodgkin lymphoma.

PRESENTATION is typically with proximal weakness associated with a heliotrope rash. Skin changes are often noted on the knees and elbows, at the base of the neck, and upper chest. This "shawl sign" worsens with sun exposure. Close examination at the base the fingernails reveals telangiectasia-like changes.

MANAGEMENT of polymyositis and dermatomyositis is very similar. High-dose corticosteroids are typically considered first-line therapies. Poor response to prednisone or comorbidities such as diabetes mellitus that limit the use of corticosteroids may require use of steroid sparing agents such as azathioprine, methotrexate, or mycophenolate. High-dose IVIg can also be used.

Treatment options include:

- Prednisone
- Methylprednisolone IV for severe disease, then prednisone.
- Azathioprine
- Mycophenolate mofetil
- Methotrexate
- Intravenous immunoglobulin
- Cyclophosphamide

Muscular Dystrophies

Muscular dystrophies (MD) are usually not diagnosed in the hospital setting. However, patients with MD can be admitted for complications of their weakness or comorbid conditions. These are a group of inherited myopathies. Specifics will not be discussed here because of our focus on hospital neurology, but some of the important types are briefly discussed. There are many more not discussed here.

- *Duchenne dystrophy*: X-linked, affecting mainly males. Starts in childhood with progression to disability and death by early adulthood. Clinical findings are proximal leg weakness, toe-walking, pseudohypertrophy of the calves, and marked elevation in CPK.
- *Becker dystrophy*: Similar to Duchenne but with later onset and longer survival. Also X-linked. CPK levels are elevated but less so.
- *Limb-girdle dystrophy*: Group of disorders rather than a single disease. Autosomal recessive inheritance. Weakness is mainly in proximal muscles of the upper and lower extremities. CPK is not markedly elevated.
- *Fascioscapulohumeral dystrophy (FSH)*: Autosomal dominant disorder. Clinical findings include weakness of the face, neck, and proximal upper body. CPK is usually normal.

These and related disorders are usually diagnosed as outpatients with clinical exam, laboratory studies including muscle enzymes, NCS and EMG, and, ultimately, muscle biopsy for most patients. Treatment is purely supportive for most; however, Duchenne dystrophy may respond to corticosteroids.

Hospital implications: We most often see patients with MD who have complications of their weakness. This is most often seen in Duchenne dystrophy when a young adult is admitted because of cardiac or respiratory issues. There is no specific role for the neurologist in these conditions other than ensuring that the diagnosis is correct and advising the patient, care team, and family regarding expectations and options.

Periodic Paralyses

Periodic paralyses are a group of disorders that produce episodic paralysis. Potassium levels can be increased, decreased, or normal.

- *Hypokalemic periodic paralysis*: Episodes of weakness especially on awakening, after a meal, or after exercise; duration is hours to even days.
- *Hyperkalemic periodic paralysis*: Episodes of paralysis often after exercise; duration is usually an hour or less.

- *Normokalemic periodic paralysis*: Episodes of paralysis lasting longer, like hyperka-lemic, but with normal potassium

PRESENTATION to the hospital neurologist is usually with episodic weakness with decreased tone, but with preservation of consciousness and respiratory function.

DIAGNOSIS is considered when a patient presents with episodes of paralysis. If the potassium is abnormal, this may trigger additional consideration.

MANAGEMENT depends on the type. Hypokalemic and normokalemic are treated routinely with dichlorphenamide or acetazolamide. The hyperkalemic type has brief episodes and may also be treated with dichlorphenamide for prevention, and the patient may be given IV calcium gluconate to terminate an acute attack.

Metabolic and Endocrine Myopathies

Systemic endocrine and metabolic derangements can lead to acute/subacute muscle weakness. Hypokalemia and hypophosphatemia are known culprits.

Hyper- and hypothyroidism along with hyperparathyroid can cause myopathic changes. Patients with hypothyroidism may also have mental slowing and hair loss, along with thick skin. Weakness is typically proximal and often associated with pain. Delayed reflexes may be noted. In contrast, hyperthyroid myopathic patients often have brisk reflexes with significant elevations in CPK.

MOTONEURON DEGENERATION
Amyotrophic Lateral Sclerosis

ALS comprises upper and lower motoneuron degeneration affecting any skeletal mus-cles. Most cases are sporadic.

PRESENTATION is with progressive weakness that is initially asymmetric but ulti-mately becomes generalized. Bulbar muscle involvement develops. There are no sensory findings. Exam often shows extensor plantar responses and hyperreflexia. Fasciculations may be seen.

DIAGNOSIS is suspected with progressive weakness with corticospinal tract signs. Imaging is usually preformed for the rostral extent of the deficit: for example, if the patient has bulbar symptoms, then an MRI of the brain is performed; if the patient has multilevel upper and lower motoneuron signs, then MRI of the cervical spine at a minimum is per-formed. EMG documents the denervation and can visualize the fasciculations.

MANAGEMENT is largely supportive. Riluzole is often offered; this may reduce the progression thereby improving survival by up to 3 months. Patients must know that riluzole does not halt progression or improve function. Soon after the diagnosis has been confirmed, the topics of tube feedings and ventilatory support should be discussed

Progressive Muscular Atrophy

Progressive muscular atrophy is degeneration of the lower motoneurons producing muscle weakness and atrophy. The distinction from ALS is blurred since some patients at autopsy will show upper motoneuron degeneration.

PRESENTATION is with progressive weakness and wasting without corticospinal tract signs. Fasciculations are seen.

DIAGNOSIS is suspected by weakness and fasciculations without corticospinal tract signs. EMG shows denervation and can document the fasciculations. Main differential diagnosis is multifocal motor neuropathy (MMN), an autoimmune disorder; serology and NCS differentiate this in that MMN would have conduction block not seen with progressive muscular atrophy.

MANAGEMENT is supportive. No medication alters the progress of the disease.

NEUROMUSCULAR RESPIRATORY FAILURE

Neuromuscular respiratory failure can present in patients with or without a known neuromuscular disease. Myasthenic crisis is a classic presentation in which the diagnosis is known. However, occasionally, a neuromuscular etiology is not identified until failure to wean from a ventilator is recognized. Respiratory failure can occur due to weakness of the diaphragm and/or weakness of the bulbar musculature.

Etiologies of neuromuscular respiratory weakness can be divided into those with a primary neurological process, such as MG or AIDP, and those with neuromuscular weakness secondary to a systemic process, such as CIN.

- Neuromuscular junction
  - Myasthenia gravis
  - Organophosphate poisoning
  - Lambert-Eaton myasthenic syndrome
  - Snake venom
  - Botulism
- Anterior horn
  - West Nile
  - Motoneuron disease
  - Poliomyelitis
- Peripheral nerve
  - AIDP
  - Critical illness neuropathy
  - Toxins (e.g., hydroxychloroquine)
  - Paraneoplastic syndromes
  - Vasculitis
  - Phrenic nerve injury
- Muscle
  - Critical illness myopathy
  - Inflammatory myopathy
  - Rhabdomyolysis
  - Toxins
  - Metabolic myopathy (e.g., acid maltase deficiency)

Discovering the etiology of neuromuscular respiratory failure has prognostic implications. Those in whom no etiology can be found have a poor long-term prognosis.

Diagnostic testing includes forced vital capacity and maximal inspiratory and expiratory pressures.[8] Chest x-ray and arterial blood gases should be done to evaluate for possible pulmonary processes such as pneumonia and atelectasis. The presence of lobar atelectasis or severe pneumonia lowers the threshold for initiating mechanical ventilation.

22 Demyelinating Diseases

Karl E. Misulis, MD, PhD and
E. Lee Murray, MD

CHAPTER CONTENTS

- Overview
- Multiple Sclerosis
  - Overview of MS
  - First Diagnosis of MS in the Hospital
  - Exacerbation of MS
  - Complication of MS
  - Complication of MS Therapy
- Neuromyelitis Optica
- Acute Disseminated Encephalomyelitis
- Optic Neuritis
- Transverse Myelitis

OVERVIEW

The hospital neurologist is often consulted to coordinate the evaluation and management of a host of demyelinating diseases. Among the most common scenarios are:

- Deficits that may be a new diagnosis of multiple sclerosis (MS), acute disseminated encephalomyelitis (ADEM), or neuromyelitis optica (NMO)
- Visual loss that may be optic neuritis
- Myelopathy that may be transverse myelitis or NMO
- Treatment of MS exacerbation
- Abnormal magnetic resonance imaging (MRI) suggestive of demyelinating disease

MULTIPLE SCLEROSIS

MS is a common diagnosis for outpatient and inpatient neurology care. The hospital neurologist's responsibilities for patients with MS usually revolves around one of the following:

- Neurologic presentation in a patient not previously known to have MS
- Exacerbation of MS
- Complication of MS
- Complication of MS therapy

A detailed discussion of comprehensive MS management is beyond the scope of this text and will not be discussed here. Here, we concentrate on the implications of MS for hospital neurology practice.

Overview of MS

MS usually presents in relative youth, from childhood to middle age with an average age at diagnosis of about 30 years.

PRESENTATION can be with almost any central neurologic deficit, but most common are visual loss, diplopia, gait and/or limb ataxia, paraparesis, or hemiparesis. Onset can be subacute, developing over hours to days.

DIAGNOSIS is suspected when a patient seen in the hospital or ED with neurologic deficit has either multifocal deficits, history of a subacute progression, or history of previous attacks of neurologic deficit. Relatively young age supports the diagnosis.

- *MRI brain* is performed and shows areas of increased signal on T2 and fluid attenuated inversion recovery (FLAIR). There are defined criteria that have undergone revision.[1]
- *CSF* is most helpful if it shows oligoclonal bands. There may be a mild pleocytosis and mild elevation in protein. Because of liberalization of MRI criteria, CSF is not universally evaluated.
- *Evoked potentials* have historically been used for identification of lesions, but this is less used now, especially in a hospital setting.

The diagnosis of MS is divided into categories based on clinical history and lesion identification on tests such as MRI and evoked potential:

- *Definite MS*: Two or more attacks + two or more test-identified lesions
- *Probable MS*: Either single attack + multifocal test-identified lesions, or a single identified lesion + two or more attacks
- *Clinically isolated syndrome (MS)*: A single attack typical of MS without test evidence of another lesion

Location of the lesions is implicated in the criteria. The criteria from the working group cited earlier indicate that, for identification of spatially distinct lesions, there should be at least two lesions that are in separate CNS arenas—periventricular, juxtacortical, infratentorial, and spinal cord.

When the disorder is believed to be MS, there are subdivisions:

- *Relapsing-remitting*: Episodic attacks with no progression between them
- *Secondary progressive*: Progressive phase after years of relapsing-remitting
- *Primary progressive*: Progressive disease from the onset

MANAGEMENT in the hospital setting begins with treatment of an acute attack. Then, disease-modifying therapy can be introduced, but we often do not start this therapy in the hospital since office follow-up for care coordination and monitoring is required.

Acute attack: Whether a first attack or a relapse, corticosteroids are used. IV administration is usually used first, and then oral is typically used for subsequent attacks.

After the high-dose administration, a taper is sometimes used. Regimens that have been used include :

- Methylprednisolone 1 g/day IV × 3–5 days
- Prednisone 1,000 mg/day PO × 3–5 days
- Dexamethasone 160 mg/day PO × 3–5 days

Disease-modifying therapy is used especially for relapsing-remitting MS and is often offered to patients who do not meet criteria but are felt to potentially be at high risk for MS. Detailed discussion is beyond the scope of this book. There are numerous medications approved for disease-modifying therapy, just a few of which are interferons, glatiramer, natalizumab, mitoxantrone, fingolimod, and dimethyl fumarate Others have been released and more are in development. All of these are approved for relapsing forms of MS, mitoxantrone is also used for select patients with secondary progressive MS.

First Diagnosis of MS in the Hospital

PRESENTATION in the hospital setting is usually with significant motor or visual deficit. Paraparesis, hemiparesis, diplopia, and monocular or binocular visual loss would be the most likely ED presentations.

DIAGNOSIS is more or less difficult depending on the type. Objective neurologic deficit with typical MRI lesions is most common. If the MRI findings are absent or equivocal, then diagnosis is less certain.

Optic neuritis (ON) is covered later. However, when a patient presents to the hospital with ON and is found to have historical and/or imaging evidence of MS, treatment of the acute event with high-dose corticosteroids is routine. Disease-modifying therapy is offered after acute hospitalization.

Tumefactive MS is an MS lesion that has the appearance of a tumor.[2] This is a difficult diagnostic dilemma. Some possible clinical scenarios include:

- *Enhancing mass lesion without other lesions in a patient not known to have MS*: Biopsy will often be needed. However, if the lesion might be MS and biopsy is difficult or impossible because of location or other factors, then a course of high-dose corticosteroids can be considered. Caution is required since some tumors can regress with corticosteroids, alone (e.g., lymphoma).
- *Enhancing mass lesion with other lesions suggestive of MS*: If CSF is positive, treatment may be attempted without biopsy, but if there is failure to resolve the lesion, then biopsy is needed.
- *Enhancing mass lesion in a patient with known MS*: If the lesion was judged to possibly be an acute MS lesion, then high-dose corticosteroids can be used; if they fail to resolve the lesion, then biopsy is needed. Patients with MS can get brain tumors as an independent primary or metastatic process.

Myelitis can be from multiple reasons: immune, infectious, neoplastic, vascular. Paraparesis can be the reason for ED presentation of a patient ultimately diagnosed with demyelinating disease. There are some differentiating features that help with diagnosis:

- *Myelitis due to MS*: Usually develops over days and tends to be found in younger patients. Other lesions are revealed from history or exam or on studies such as MRI or evoked potentials.
- *Myelitis due to NMO*: Usually affects a broader range of spinal segments on MRI, best seen on sagittal studies. MRI brain should not show plaque burden. Blood may show NMO-IgG.
- *Myelopathy from infarction*: Usually develops in an older patient with vascular disease, often after surgery affecting aortic flow. Acute onset of symptoms suggests infarct, much more acute than demyelinating disease. MRI may show subtle findings such as regional signal change in the cord but often the lesion is not identifiable unless the scan is of excellent quality.
- *Transverse myelitis*: A rapidly developing myelopathy with inflammatory change seen in the CSF and often on imaging. Causes are diverse, so some of these patients are likely to have MS, some have NMO, and some have an infectious or other immune etiology.

Exacerbation of MS

In those with known MS, patients with *acute exacerbations* are usually treated as outpatients, but occasionally they must be treated as inpatients because of comorbid conditions (e.g., brittle diabetes) or because the severity of the deficit necessitates inpatient rehabilitation.

DIAGNOSIS usually consists of MRI to ensure no other pathology is present and to assess acute and chronic disease burden. Patients with MS can develop tumors, CNS infections, and strokes related or unrelated to the MS (e.g., progressive multifocal leukoencephalopathy [PML]).

MANAGEMENT of the acute exacerbation consists of one of the corticosteroid options discussed earlier. We tend to use IV corticosteroids for patients with severe deficits; however, it is not clear that IV administration is superior.[3] Plasma exchange may be helpful for patients with acute attacks who cannot take corticosteroids.

Complication of MS

Complications of MS include effects of the disease process, including progressive deficits. Complications of MS therapy are discussed in the next section.

Dementia can occur late in the course of MS, but there are reports of dementia developing early. Certainly, there can be early psychiatric manifestations. As the disease progresses, cognitive changes are noticed in about half of patients. However, rapidly progressive or profound dementia should raise concern for other pathology, especially PML in susceptible individuals. There is no evidence that cholinesterase inhibitors have a consistent significant impact on dementia associated with MS.

Spasticity is treated with standard medications, as discussed in Chapter 41. Most commonly used is baclofen. Recently, cannabinoids have shown some potential benefit.[4]

Diplopia or *nystagmus* may be an indication for corticosteroid treatment if it is felt to be an acute attack. However, often this is encountered long after onset. There are no medications that are effective for chronic ocular motor deficits. Initially, patching one eye and reassurance that diplopia often improves is sufficient. If there is no resolution, then prism lenses may be needed.

Depression is common in patients with MS, affecting about 50% of patients at some time in their disease process.[5] Suicide ideation and attempts are significantly increased in patients with MS. Depression should be queried, and, if identified, standard multimodal therapy should be offered.

Ataxia and *tremor* are common and affect at least 80% of patients with MS. No medications have proved to be beneficial, although several are occasionally tried especially for tremor—including primidone, clonazepam, buspirone, and propranolol. Cannabis is consumed by at least 20% of patients with MS, and there is at least some evidence that it may be beneficial.[6]

Pain in MS can be of a variety of origins. Some include trigeminal neuralgia, the Lhermitte phenomenon, painful spasticity, and dysesthesias. But the most common is headache,[7] which is relatively nonspecific and not of certain origin.

- *Trigeminal neuralgia* is treated with standard medications for the disorder in unaffected patients, including anticonvulsants. Microvascular decompression has been tried with conflicting results, including a negative experience at Mayo clinic.[8]
- *Spasticity pain* is treated as elsewhere, including therapy and medications (Chapter 41).
- *Lhermitte sign* is shooting neuropathic pain typically from the cervical spinal cord and associated with cord involvement. Movement of the neck tends to precipitate the pain. This unpleasant sensation usually abates without specific treatment, but if there is active spinal cord inflammation this should be treated as above.
- *Headache* appears to be more common in patients with MS than in the general population. Tension-type headache and migraine predominate. Treatment is similar to that discussed in Chapter 20.
- *Neuropathic pain* and *dysesthesias* are common and can be treated with anticonvulsants as used for other neurologic disorders, especially oxcarbazepine, carbamazepine, gabapentin, and pregabalin. Cannabis may be helpful.[9]

Seizures are uncommon with MS but can occur.[10] Seizures can be generalized, simple partial, or complex partial. Partial seizures often have secondary generalization. Surprisingly, there does not appear to be a correlation between disease duration, severity of MS, and seizures. Medications should be used which would be appropriate for the seizure type while trying to avoid medications that might exacerbate cognitive or motor function.

Complication of MS Therapy

Medication-Specific Complications

Natalizumab (Tysabri): Progressive multifocal leukoencephalopathy (PML) and associated immune reconstitution inflammatory syndrome (IRIS) are the most worrisome complications of MS therapy and are discussed later. Relatively common reported adverse effects included urinary tract infection, pneumonia, and hypersensitivity reactions. PML is also discussed in Chapter 17.

Interferons (Avonex, Betaseron, Rebif): These agents can all produce injection-site reaction, exacerbation of depression, headache, and flu-like symptoms. Serious complications such as hepatotoxicity and seizures are rare and often not clearly related to medication.

Glatiramer (Copaxone): An episode can occur after injection characterized by any of flushing, chest pain, palpitations, anxiety, dyspnea, constriction of the throat, and urticaria. Symptoms are usually self-limited and do not come to the attention of the hospital neurologist.

Immune Reconstitution Inflammatory Syndrome

IRIS is a destructive inflammatory response seen by neurologists mainly due to abrupt withdrawal of MS therapy in response to development of PML.[11]

PRESENTATION is with new and recurrent neurologic deficits. Fever and seizures can develop. This has been described after discontinuation of natalizumab for PML. IRIS is seen especially after plasma exchange has been performed to remove residual natalizumab.

DIAGNOSIS is clinical and supported by MRI, which shows enhancement in the regions of PML lesions.

MANAGEMENT is most commonly with corticosteroids, often high-dose IV to begin with followed by oral corticosteroids; however, at the time of this writing, there is no consensus guideline.

NEUROMYELITIS OPTICA

NMO is a demyelinating disease of unknown etiology. Historically called Devic disease, the hallmark is ON and myelitis without other signs of demyelination.

PRESENTATION is classically with the combination of bilateral ON and myelopathy. The ON may precede the myelopathy; at this point, NMO might not be considered. However, bilateral ON, especially severe, raises this concern. MS usually does not affect both eyes simultaneously.

DIAGNOSIS is suspected by the two locations of neurologic deficits. An MRI brain scan is unlikely to show lesions. MRI of the affected spinal region usually shows inflammatory change spanning several segments, as opposed to MS, which would have a more restricted region of involvement.

MANAGEMENT is with corticosteroids for acute attacks followed by plasma exchange if there is not a good response. Suppression of disease is often tried with rituximab.

ACUTE DISSEMINATED ENCEPHALOMYELITIS

ADEM is an inflammatory disorder that affects mainly myelinated regions but can affect some gray matter as well. Some cases are postinfectious, but for many there is no identified preceding illness.

PRESENTATION is with a variety of neurologic deficits representing multifocal involvement. Spinal cord and cerebral involvement can occur. In addition, cognitive changes are common early, unusual for MS. Patients may progress to lethargy and coma.

DIAGNOSIS is suspected when a young individual presents with neurologic deficits and MRI suggests demyelinating disease. However, the extent of lesions and the absence of variably aged lesions argues against MS. Also, a recent history of fever or other signs of infectious illness raises this concern. Involvement of subcortical gray matter suggests ADEM and would be unusual for MS. CSF is not specific and may show mild CSF pleocytosis and elevated protein. If a patient does not respond to treatment, brain biopsy should be considered, with the chief conditions of concern being neoplastic (e.g., lymphoma, glioma), infectious (e.g., PML), vascular (e.g., vasculitis), or posterior reversible encephalopathy syndrome (PRES). Definite differentiation from MS might not be possible initially.

MANAGEMENT is with high-dose corticosteroids as would be used for MS (we use IV administration). A prolonged steroid taper is used—weeks—longer than commonly used for MS. IVIg might be considered as an alternative.[12]

OPTIC NEURITIS

ON can occur with MS, with NMO, or as an isolated entity. Inflammatory change can occur in the optic nerve near insertion into the eye or behind the globe.

PRESENTATION is usually with loss of vision in one eye. Some eye pain is often present. The visual loss may start in central vision and then progress. Exam shows an afferent pupil defect if there has been severe involvement. Fundus exam may show papilledema, but, in the majority of patients, the inflammatory change is posterior to the eye so there is no funduscopic manifestation.

DIAGNOSIS is considered when a patient presents with unilateral visual difficulty. Ophthalmoscopic exam must be done to rule out other structural causes. An MRI brain scan is performed to look for cerebral lesions that could indicate MS. CSF is usually unremarkable, but oligoclonal bands and an elevated IgG index favor subsequent development of MS. Positive NMO-IgG supports the diagnosis of NMO.

MANAGEMENT is with high-dose corticosteroids—usually similar to that used in the Optic Neuritis Treatment Trial: Solu-Medrol 1,000 mg/day IV × 3 days, followed by an oral steroid taper. If the MRI showed white matter lesions suggestive of MS, then immunomodulating treatment should be considered.

TRANSVERSE MYELITIS

Transverse myelitis (TM) can be an isolated entity or a component of MS or NMO. Most cases are immune-related. Direct infection can also occur. General information is presented here. MS, NMO, and ADEM were discussed earlier in this chapter, and infectious myelitis is discussed in Chapter 17.

PRESENTATION is with a progressive myelopathy, developing over days but with worsening often noted within a single day. Motor, sensory, and sphincter abnormalities are common. As with other early myelopathies, the paralysis is initially flaccid then becomes spastic. Spinal level can be from upper cervical to conus.

DIAGNOSIS is suspected when a patient has acute to subacute onset of myelopathy. The rapidity of acute onset is not as abrupt as with spinal cord infarct. MRI is performed to rule out tumor or hematoma, and with TM typically shows various findings depending on the etiology of the TM. Most common is increased T2 signal with enlargement of the cord, with the rostrocaudal extent usually being at least one verte-bral segment. In contrast, patients with NMO usually have a lesion that extends over multiple segments. CSF in TM may be normal or may show a mild mononuclear pleo-cytosis. Differentiation of TM from many other causes of myelopathy must rest on the clinical presentation plus CSF or MRI evidence of an inflammatory process.

MANAGEMENT depends on the etiology. Autoimmune causes are usually treated with immune suppressants, which can include high-dose corticosteroids, plasma exchange, or IVIG. Infectious causes may be treated, but, for many causes, there is no specific treatment. If the cause is unknown and the risk is relatively low, then a trial of high-dose methylprednisolone or similar should be considered if there are no contraindications.

23 Movement Disorders

John Y. Fang, MD and
David A. Isaacs, MD

CHAPTER CONTENTS

- Overview
- Syndromes
  - Tremor
  - Myoclonus
  - Rigidity and Stiffness
  - Athetosis, Chorea, Dystonia, Dyskinesia, Hemiballismus, and Tics
  - Ataxia
- Movement Disorders
  - Parkinsonis
  - Tremor
  - Myoclonus
  - Hemiballismus
  - Restless Leg Syndrome and Periodic Limb Movement Disorder
  - Other Hyperkinetic Disorders
  - Ataxias

OVERVIEW

Abnormal movements are a common reason for hospital neurology consultation. Tremor and myoclonus are the most common abnormal movements seen in the inpatient setting. Medications and metabolic disturbances are the most common identified etiologies. Abnormal movements may occur in association with encephalopathy or as an isolated entity. As with encephalopathy, it is more common to identify multiple contributing factors rather than a single cause. Occasionally, a single medication can precipitate tremor or myoclonus, either directly or via a drug–drug interaction. Equally important, drug withdrawal can result in abnormal movements. When abnormal movements occur concurrently with encephalopathy, seizures should be considered and an electroencephalogram (EEG) may be needed for diagnosis. Some abnormal movements commonly seen in the hospital setting include:

- *Tremor*: Rhythmic involuntary movement, described by the frequency and by its presence at rest, in posture, or with action.
- *Myoclonus*: Abrupt, lightning-like muscle contractions, which may also occur in trains and be confused with tremor, described by its distribution (generalized, segmental or focal). Negative myoclonus (or asterixis) is abrupt muscle relaxation.

- *Asterixis*: Abrupt loss of muscle tone resulting in a negative twitch, such as in the arm if the arm is being held up against gravity; it is also known as negative myoclonus.
- *Chorea*: Dancelike, irregular involuntary movements described as generalized, hemi-, segmental or focal.
- *Dystonia*: Irregular movements with abnormal posture of the affected body part, often twisting the neck, limbs, or trunk; it may also be seen with tremor and other types of movements.
- *Athetosis*: Slow, writhing involuntary movements, generally in the upper extremities.
- *Hemiballismus*: Unilateral, high-amplitude movements resembling more severe chorea.
- *Dyskinesia*: Term generally used to describe drug-induced chorea, though literally any abnormal movement; specific syndromes involving chorea or dystonia are also often grouped under dyskinesia.
- *Tics*: Sudden, stereotyped, purposeless movements that are suppressible; they are described as *simple* if brief and limited to one muscle group (such as a grimace) or *complex* if of longer duration and affecting multiple muscle groups (such as touching or grabbing, or grunting after grimacing).
- *Rigidity*: Increased muscle tone that is independent of velocity or position, primarily seen in parkinsonism. Parkinsonian rigidity increases when the contralateral limb is activated, and stiffness is increased resistance to passive movement that is not necessarily from muscle.
- *Spasticity*: Increased muscle tone that changes with velocity on passive movement, primarily seen with lesions in the motor tracks in the brain and spinal cord.
- *Seizure*: Episodic motor or sensory disturbance due to synchronous cortical discharges; seizures are not considered a movement disorder, although they can sometimes appear stereotyped like a tic, tremorlike, or even dystonic. Seizures are generally distinguished from movement disorders by a discrete start and stop and a consistent pattern from episode to episode. Consciousness is also often affected, and the impairment may persist after termination of the movements (the postictal period). Focal status epilepticus or epilepsia partialis continua can mimic tremor.

Movement disorders may overlap; a firm distinction is not always possible. Writhing movements may have features of both athetosis and chorea. Twisting movements can be seen in both chorea and dystonia. Tremor and rhythmic myoclonus appear similar.

SYNDROMES
Tremor

Tremor has a broad differential diagnosis, and physical examination cannot always make a clear etiologic diagnosis. Tremors exacerbated by medications and metabolic disturbance can all have similar appearance. Tremor is broadly classified by its occurrence in action versus rest or kinetic versus postural. Features include:

- *Resting*: Present when at rest, with the body part relaxed; attenuated by posture or voluntary movement; most commonly seen with parkinsonism

- *Postural*: Tremor seen while holding a sustained posture, such as hands outstretched; essential tremor and enhanced physiologic tremor are postural.
- *Kinetic (or action)*: Present with voluntary movement and attenuated by rest or posture

Differential diagnosis of tremor in hospitalized patients includes:

- *Essential tremor*: Predominantly postural tremor involving hands or arms, onset in youth to young adult age, often hereditary. Head and voice, or lower extremities, can sometimes be affected as well. Usually no other neurologic deficit, occasional ataxia may appear later in course.
- *Renal failure*: Tremor and multifocal myoclonus can develop from renal insufficiency, especially with acute exacerbation of renal insufficiency. In metabolic disturbances, abnormal movements are usually multifocal.
- *Hepatic failure*: Tremor, myoclonus, and asterixis are common.
- *Parkinsonian tremor*: Resting tremor may be due to Parkinson disease, although drug-induced and other secondary parkinsonisms are also common. Very symmetric tremor is supportive of secondary parkinsonism.
- *Medication-induced tremor*: Multiple drugs can cause tremor, but some of the most important are corticosteroids, neuroleptics, valproate, lithium, amiodarone, theophylline/adenosine analogs, amphetamines. Withdrawal from medications can also cause tremor. Serotonin syndrome is another important consideration in hospitalized patients with unexplained tremor.
- *Psychogenic tremor*: Almost any type of tremor. Clues to etiology are abrupt onset, changing direction, marked variability/inconsistency on examination.

Myoclonus

A variety of conditions can appear as phasic motor activities or jerking of a body part. Other conditions that can resemble myoclonus include tics, tremor, and occasionally seizure. Common causes of myoclonus are:

- *Hepatic failure*: Myoclonus and asterixis are common and are often accompanied by other stigmata of hepatic encephalopathy.
- *Renal insufficiency*: Myoclonus can occur with renal insufficiency, usually when fairly advanced. Note that medication-induced myoclonus is also more common with renal insufficiency.
- *Medications*: Multiple medications can cause myoclonus, and it is more prominent with coexistent renal or hepatic impairment (e.g., gabapentin toxicity developing in a patient with chronic, but stable, renal insufficiency).
- *Epilepsy*: Epileptic myoclonus is most commonly seen with juvenile myoclonic epilepsy but also with severe epilepsies such as progressive myoclonus epilepsy and Lennox-Gastaut syndrome.
- *Essential myoclonus*: Myoclonus without seizures or other neurologic conditions; it is nonprogressive; it may be sporadic or familial.
- *Post-hypoxic myoclonus*: Can develop after hypoxic cardiopulmonary arrest, both early while still encephalopathic, and delayed, after intellectual recovery.

- *Palatal myoclonus*: Fast, rhythmic oscillation of the soft palate and sometimes surrounding muscles, often associated with a clicking sound in the ear. Also known as palatal tremor.
- *Juvenile myoclonic epilepsy*: Common idiopathic generalized epilepsy with myoclonus (often in the morning), frequently co-existing with generalized tonic-clonic seizures and absence seizures
- *Progressive myoclonus epilepsy (PME)*: Family of disorders with myoclonus, epilepsy, and degenerative changes in neurons
- *Cortical reflex myoclonus*: Myoclonic movements with cortical discharge; often evoked by an intention to move or a stimulus

Rigidity and Stiffness

Rigidity and stiffness are features of many disorders. The list shows some of the conditions that produce sustained stiffness or rigidity. These two terms have subtly different meanings but are considered together for our discussion.

- *Spasticity*: Rigidity with increased tendon reflexes, velocity- and direction-dependent resistance to passive movement, and corticospinal tract signs
- *Dystonia*: Increased tone without corticospinal tract signs. Associated with abnormal posture, often with some slow superimposed tremor or chorea
- *Stiff-person syndrome*: Increased tone of mainly proximal and paraspinal muscles. Slow and stiff movements and gait
- *Tetanus*: Rigidity and spasms starting in facial muscles, extending to body and limb muscles
- *Parkinsonism*: Rigidity and bradykinesia as components of the syndrome; resting tremor may also be present.
- *Neuromyotonia*: A neuromuscular condition with excessive muscle contraction that may occur with fasciculations, myokymia, muscle rigidity, or muscle cramps
- *Myokymia*: A neuromuscular condition with involuntary spontaneous firing of muscle fibers that is visible but insufficient to move a joint, often described as rippling, quivering, or "bag of worms" appearance
- *Neuroleptic malignant syndrome*: Rigidity with fever and mental status changes, usually after initiation or change in dose of neuroleptics. Sometimes called Parkinsonism-hyperpyrexia syndrome, such as when it occurs in patient with pre-existing parkinsonism.
- *Malignant hyperthermia*: Rigidity and hyperthermia, usually precipitated by medications, especially inhaled anesthetics along with succinylcholine or other paralytic drugs

Athetosis, Chorea, Dystonia, Dyskinesia, Hemiballismus, and Tics

Athetosis and *chorea* classically have distinct features, but clinical discrimination can be blurred.

- *Athetosis* is characterized by slow, involuntary, writhing movements, often associated with an abnormal posture, which can have a dystonic appearance. Important causes are Huntington disease (HD), neuroleptics, and metabolic disorders, especially hepatic insufficiency.

- *Chorea* is characterized by more rapid involuntary movements. Some movements can have features of athetosis and chorea. Athetosis can blur the distinction from dystonia, since the slow movement of some dystonias can resemble athetosis. Causes of chorea are numerous but include HD, other hereditary choreas, Fahr disease, Wilson disease, and some paraneoplastic disorders.[1]
- *Dystonia* is abnormal posture that often has superimposed movement that can have the appearance of athetosis. The spontaneous movement is slow and can be temporarily suppressed. Important causes include dystonia musculorum deformans, metabolic disorders such as kernicterus, and degenerative disease including HD. However, the most common cause is medication, often neuroleptics or dopamine-blocking antiemetics.
- *Dyskinesia* is repetitive movements that have features of chorea with dystonia and have a fairly stereotyped appearance. Common causes are medications, especially dopaminergic agents for Parkinson disease.
- *Hemiballismus* is a special form of unilateral choreiform movements with often violent involvement of proximal muscles that risk injury. This is among the most violent disorders seen in neurology and often requires hospitalization. The most common cause is infarction of the subthalamic nucleus.
- *Tics* are brief movements that are stereotyped but differentiated from chorea by their brief character, suppressibility, and the frequent presence of an urge preceding the movement. Tourette syndrome is characterized by a mixture of different tics developing in the first or second decade. (However, the history may be unreliable in some cases so there may be an apparent older age of onset.)
- *Hemifacial spasm* consists of episodes of clonic movements of the face, typically unilateral, although occasional movements on the opposite side can occur. Symptoms are initially brief clonic movements but evolve to more sustained hemifacial contractions. Cause is typically vascular impingement on the facial nerve.
- *Spasmodic dysphonia* is a focal dystonia affecting the laryngeal muscles and it comes with a varied presentation. More than 90% of patients have *adductor spasm*, causing a strained voice, sometimes to the point of making speech almost incomprehensible. The remainder of patients have *abductor spasm*, which presents with a breathy, whispering voice.[2] Both conditions are worse with stress.

Ataxia

Ataxia can have several origins. Localization of the ataxia is the first step to diagnosis:

- *Cerebellar ataxia*: Ataxia of the limbs and/or gait. Repetitive movements are unequal, irregular, and off-target. Often associated with decreased tone, nystagmus. Abnormal saccades may be present.
- *Sensory ataxia*: Deficits in balance with proprioceptive difficulty and without vertigo. Worse with eyes closed. Associated with other signs of peripheral neuropathy: sensory deficit, reduced reflexes

- *Vestibular ataxia*: Prominent vertigo. No other cranial nerve deficits such as diplopia or speech change

With localization of the ataxia, a differential diagnosis can be established:

- *Cerebellar infarction*: Acute onset of cerebellar ataxia, usually unilateral
- *Miller Fisher syndrome*: Variant of acute inflammatory demyelinating neuropathy with subacute onset of ataxia, areflexia, and ocular motor deficits
- *Multiple sclerosis*: Stepwise progression of ataxia with cerebellar and corticospinal features
- *Wernicke encephalopathy*: Associated with ethanol toxicity or malnutrition, prominent nystagmus, plus ataxia
- *Ethanol toxicity*: Predominately gait ataxia, often without other deficits
- *Paraneoplastic cerebellar degeneration*: Subacute development of vertigo and nystagmus, often with nausea, progressing to cerebellar ataxia, dysarthria; usually precedes diagnosis of cancer, often ovarian or small-cell lung cancer
- *Spinocerebellar ataxias*: Family of hereditary cerebellar ataxias usually with corticospinal, brainstem, motor neuron, or cognitive deficits
- *Wilson disease*: Familial disorder with mainly hepatic presentation but can have cerebellar and/or corticospinal deficits
- *Friedreich ataxia*: Hereditary cerebellar ataxia with corticospinal deficits, peripheral neuropathy, and cardiac disease; cardiomyopathy is commonly associated.
- *Multiple system atrophy*: Neurodegenerative condition with a combination of ataxia, dysautonomia, and parkinsonism, although not all findings are present at onset
- *Peripheral vestibulopathy*: Vertigo, sometimes with gait ataxia. No speech or other findings to suggest brainstem involvement

Specific entities are discussed in the following sections or in respective chapters on vascular, demyelinating, genetic, developmental, toxic, and nutritional disorders.

MOVEMENT DISORDERS

Clinical features and differential diagnoses of individual abnormal movements were discussed earlier. Here, we will discuss specific disorders, with a focus on hospital neurology implications. Comprehensive discussion of movement disorders is not provided here, and the reader is referred to excellent comprehensive sources.[3]

Parkinsonism

Parkinson Disease

Parkinson disease (PD) is usually idiopathic, although genetic forms have been identified. Drug-induced parkinsonism is discussed later. PD onset is usually between 50 and 70 years, although older and younger cases do occur. Most cases are sporadic, although up to 25% of cases may be familial.

PRESENTATION is usually with resting tremor of one hand. Occasionally decreased arm swing or leg-dragging occur without tremor. At early stages, other motor deficits might not be noticed. However, eventually, patients or clinicians notice slowed and stiff gait with decreased arm swing, stooped posture, and shortened stride. Exam classically shows resting tremor, bradykinesia, rigidity, and postural instability. Cognitive difficulties, particular word-finding trouble, occur late in the disease.

DIAGNOSIS is suspected on the basis of tremor with other motor signs representing a parkinsonian appearance. Diagnosis of PD is clinical; there are no specific diagnostic tests. However, a robust response to levodopa is typical. Due to individual variation in absorption and metabolism, levodopa doses must be pushed above 1,000 mg per day in order to determine responsiveness. Differential diagnosis includes other parkinsonian syndromes, parkinson-plus syndrome, dementia with Lewy bodies, normal pressure hydrocephalus (NPH), essential tremor (in combination with other conditions), multiple system atrophy (MSA), progressive supranuclear palsy (PSP), corticobasal syndrome (CBS), and vascular parkinsonism, among others. Magnetic resonance imaging (MRI) and computed tomography (CT) show no specific findings in patients with PD, and imaging is mainly to rule out structural lesions such as NPH or vascular disease. Routine labs are also negative. Lumbar puncture (LP) is rarely helpful and should only be done if NPH or chronic CNS infection is considered.

MANAGEMENT is generally symptomatic. There are no proven agents that slow the progression of the disease. The approaches to treatment fall into the following categories:

- Levodopa/carbidopa (available in multiple formulations)
- Dopamine agonists
- Anticholinergics
- Amantadine
- Monoamine oxidase inhibitors (MAOI)
- Catechol-O-methyl transferase (COMT) inhibitors
- Surgery

Levodopa is converted to dopamine in the brain. Peripheral conversion of levodopa to dopamine can cause severe nausea and hypotension; carbidopa is added to reduce this peripheral conversion. A variety of preparations, both short-acting and varying degrees of longer-acting, are available, such as Sinemet, Sinemet CR, Parcopa, Rytary, and Duopa. Doses are not equivalent from formulation to formulation, and time of administration is critically important for many patients. Levodopa is often used first-line and is mainly effective for rigidity and bradykinesia, but it can also be helpful for tremor. Long-term use and high doses predispose to dyskinesias, fluctuations, GI distress, and psychosis. Dopamine agonists are associated with less severe dyskinesias but a higher risk of sleepiness and impulsivity.

Anticholinergics are used mainly for tremor. When symptoms are early and mild and tremor is predominant, anticholinergics may be sufficient to control symptoms. However, more commonly, these are combined with dopaminergic agents. Most commonly used agents are trihexyphenidyl (Artane) and benztropine (Cogentin). Tricyclic antidepressants such as amitriptyline (Elavil) have significant anticholinergic effects and have also been used. Potential anticholinergic side effects, including cognitive impairment, can limit use.

Amantadine is a weak N-methyl-D-aspartate (NMDA) receptor antagonist with dopaminergic activity. It is most often used to reduce dyskinesias associated with levodopa therapy. It can also be effective for tremor when levodopa or anticholinergics cannot be used or are not tolerated.

Dopamine agonists are broadly used for PD. They can be helpful as monotherapy or in combination with levodopa preparations. They are less likely to produce dyskinesia but are generally less effective than levodopa at typical doses. They are often used when patients are developing fluctuations and dyskinesias, although they can be effective at all stages of the disease. Commonly used dopamine agonists include ropinirole (Requip) and pramipexole (Mirapex). Rotigotine (Neupro) is available as a once-daily skin patch. Apomorphine (Apokyn) is an injectable dopamine agonist used for sudden off-episodes.

MAO-B inhibitors inhibit the metabolism of dopamine. They can be used as monotherapy but are fairly weak alone and are more commonly used as adjunctive therapy to levodopa. Commonly used agents are selegiline (Deprenyl or Eldepryl) and rasagiline (Azilect).

COMT inhibitors reduce the metabolism of levodopa, and dopamine to a lesser extent, so they are used as an adjunct to levodopa therapy, especially in patients with wearing-off effects. The most common drug used in this class is entacapone (Comtan).

Surgery for PD is beyond our scope of discussion and is not done on an emergent basis. However, lesioning surgery and deep brain stimulation (DBS) can be helpful for select patients who have complications of medical management, mainly fluctuations with an otherwise very good response. Lesional therapies are mainly used for tremor, but can cause dysarthria or even hemiparesis. DBS can be helpful for motor fluctuations, dyskinesia, and tremor. In hospitalized patients, DBS can pose a problem due to special restrictions on MRI scanning and also artifacts on head and upper torso CT scans or plain x-rays. Diathermy is contraindicated in patients with DBS, and cardioversion or cardiac defibrillation must avoid contact with the DBS system. Trauma to the head or neck can also result in damage to the DBS system. Lead fractures can sometimes be detected on plain x-ray, although interrogation of the device may be necessary.

Drug-Induced Parkinsonism

Drug-induced parkinsonism (DIP) is a common cause of parkinsonism and may be even more common in hospitalized patients. Common causative agents include both typical and most atypical antipsychotics, metoclopramide, and antiemetics. Prominent parkinsonism may develop both in patients previously normal and in patients with pre-existing parkinsonism.

PRESENTATION is typically limited to bilateral rigidity and bradykinesia, but tremor also occurs commonly. There are no specific findings with DIP. Dopamine replacement therapy may exacerbate underlying psychosis and often fails to relieve DIP if the offending agent is not discontinued.

DIAGNOSIS rests on a parkinsonian presentation plus history of exposure to an exacerbating agent. Brain imaging with CT or MRI can be helpful if a structural lesion is suspected or if encephalopathy is present. Dopamine transporter imaging (DaTscan) may be useful to distinguish from PD, although discontinuation of the offending drug is probably a more useful diagnostic and therapeutic intervention.

MANAGEMENT consists of withdrawal of the offending agent. More than 80% of patients showed improvement following discontinuation of the offending drug in one large study.[4] Symptomatic improvement can take several weeks to occur, depending on the culprit drug and the duration of use by the patient.

Multiple System Atrophy

Multiple system atrophy (MSA) is a family of related degenerative conditions that likely exist on a pathophysiological continuum. They affect mainly extrapyramidal, cerebellar, and autonomic functions. The parent term, MSA proper, incorporates the former Shy-Drager syndrome with earlier onset of dysautonomia. The subtypes of MSA-P and MSA-C are divided as follows:

- MSA-P: For patients with mainly parkinsonism, mainly bradykinesia and rigidity, less commonly tremor
- MSA-C: For patients with prominent cerebellar findings, mainly gait over appendicular ataxia, nystagmus and abnormal saccades, and scanning dysarthria

MSA-P includes the historical entity of striatonigral degeneration (SND), whereas MSA-C includes olivopontocerebellar degeneration (OPCA). These distinctions are not felt to be exclusive because almost any combination of parkinsonism, cerebellar ataxia, and autonomic deficit can occur.

Autonomic findings in MSA include orthostatic hypotension, urinary incontinence, and reduced sweating and salivation.

DIAGNOSIS of these disorders is clinical. However, MRI brain scans may show a characteristic cross-shaped T2 intensity— the *hot cross bun sign*—in the pons.

MANAGEMENT is supportive. Interestingly, oral water therapy is generally more effective than intravenous fluids for orthostatic hypotension, and care must be exercised to avoid excessive heat causing peripheral vasodilation or bladder distension. Supine hypertension is very common, and shorter acting anti-hypertensives administered at bedtime can be very effective at addressing this without exacerbating daytime orthostatic hypotension.

Dementia with Lewy Bodies and Parkinson Disease with Dementia

Dementia with Lewy bodies (DLB) and *Parkinson disease with dementia (PDD)* are both degenerative disorders with parkinsonism plus dementia. PDD is characterized by dementia developing at least 1 year after the onset of the motor symptoms of PD. DLB is characterized by dementia-onset within 1 year (or earlier) of motor symptoms. Pathologically, both PDD and DLB have Lewy bodies, so these may not be distinct disorders. Hallucinations early in the disease course are suggestive of DLB.

PRESENTATION is typical parkinsonism, with dementia either near contemporaneously (DLB) or separated by substantial time (PDD). The dementia differs from Alzheimer's disease (AD) by affecting attention and concentration more prominently than memory, but overlap is common. Hallucinations can occur in DLB, PDD, and AD, but they are characteristically an early symptom of DLB. In the hospital setting,

DLB is suspected when a patient with dementia has marked exacerbation of parkinsonism following neuroleptic administration for sedation or psychosis.

DIAGNOSIS is clinical, with dementia and parkinsonism. Brain imaging may be performed to rule out hydrocephalus, tumor, multiple infarctions, or other structural conditions.

MANAGEMENT of parkinsonism is as described for PD. Management of dementia is supportive. Rivastigmine is US Food and Drug Administration (FDA)-approved for dementia with parkinsonism. In patients with severe hallucinations, neuroleptics are sometimes necessary to control severe behavioral disturbances; one must exercise caution in using these agents in DLB because many patients are hypersensitive to this class of medication. Rivastigmine may help with behavior, but quetiapine in low doses (less than 100 mg/day) and clozapine are frequently needed in more severe cases.

Progressive Supranuclear Palsy

PSP is a progressive neurodegenerative condition with cognitive and motor manifestations and a characteristic impairment of downgaze. Onset is usually age 50 years and older.

PRESENTATION is with slow and stiff movements, gait difficulty, and supranuclear vertical gaze palsy. Patients often tilt their heads back in order to activate the vestibulo-ocular reflex. In neutral head position, patients cannot voluntarily look down. Other manifestations include dementia, dysphagia, dystonia, and abnormal facial expression with lid retraction and forehead muscle contraction, giving the appearance of being surprised. The gait is often broad-based; early falls are a hallmark of the disease.

DIAGNOSIS is clinical. PSP is differentiated from PD by the paucity or absence of tremor, the very abnormal facial expression, and broad-based gait, as well as the head position and supranuclear gaze palsy. Brain imaging shows no specific findings, but midbrain atrophy can suggest the diagnosis. CSF can be useful to rule out infectious etiologies. CNS Whipple disease can appear like PSP.

MANAGEMENT is generally supportive. The motor symptoms do not respond well to dopaminergic medications, but a trial of levodopa is often offered. Very limited data are available, but there is no evidence for benefit of cholinesterase inhibitors in PSP.[5]

Corticobasal Syndrome (and Degeneration)

Corticobasal syndrome (CBS) is the diagnosis applied to a combination of cognitive and motor deficits. *Corticobasal degeneration*, also known as *corticobasal-ganglionic degeneration*, is another term applied to some cases as described herein, with CBS being a broader diagnostic entity. CBS can include some cases of PSP.

PRESENTATION is a combination of cognitive deficits and extrapyramidal symptoms. Neglect and apraxias are common cognitive findings. Ideomotor apraxia, the inability to generate hand gestures, is often prominent. Alien limb can also occur. In this unusual condition, one hand contradicts the activity of the contralateral limb, such as removing eyeglasses placed on the head by the other hand. Rigidity and unilateral dystonic posturing are common extrapyramidal signs. Upgoing toes and other corticospinal tract signs may also be present.

DIAGNOSIS is clinical. There are no specific diagnostic findings on MRI or routine laboratory tests. Testing can be done to rule out other diseases. Tests for tau protein have been suggested but are not routinely done.

MANAGEMENT can include a trial of dopaminergic agents, but these are often ineffective. Botulinum toxin injections can temporarily improve hand dystonia, but dosing can be difficult to determine. There are no FDA-approved therapies.

Hospital Implications of Parkinsonism

Hospital consultation of patients with PD most often occurs because of comorbid conditions rather than the disease itself. Neurologic consultation on patients with PD can include:

- First diagnosis of the disease.
- Exacerbation of PD symptoms
- Disturbance of PD medication schedule
- Inability to take PD medications
- Hospital delirium and psychosis
- Medical complications of reduced mobility
  - Decubitus ulcer
  - Pneumonia
  - UTI
  - DVT

First diagnosis of PD is uncommon in hospitalized patient and seldom a cause of an ED visit. However, patients may be admitted with a small stroke or other deficit requiring therapy and be identified as having tremor, rigidity, or balance difficulty. History is key to determine if the deficits are related to the present illness or if deficits developed prior to the admission.

Misdiagnosis of PD is more common than a first diagnosis of the disorder. Our non-neurologist colleagues often consider PD when a patient has tremor, imbalance, or gait difficulty, leading to the provisional diagnosis of PD. More common diagnoses for tremor are essential tremor (ET), enhanced physiologic tremor, and medication-induced tremor. More common diagnoses for gait and coordination difficulty are stroke, medications, metabolic derangements, and neuropathies.

Exacerbation of PD symptoms during hospitalization occurs when concurrent illness causes PD symptoms to become decompensated. Corticosteroids may produce superimposed tremor as well as sleep disturbance. Deconditioning and nutritional deficiency can impair motor function and balance. Nutritional and specifically protein deficiency can increase levodopa bioavailability, effectively increasing the dose and resulting in increased adverse effects (e.g., dyskinesias, psychosis, or nausea).

Disturbance of PD med schedule is a common reason for worsening symptoms. Physicians, patients, and their families have often established a careful timing of meds to balance benefits on mobility and to reduce adverse effects, but in the hospital, medications are often given erratically and at different times than home administration. Formulary restrictions can create additional problems. Our solution is usually to ask the caregivers to administer the PD meds on their own effective schedule. PD meds should generally be given no longer than fifteen minutes from the targeted time.

Inability to take PD medications is common, especially around the time of surgery or when bowel rest is required. None of the dopaminergic agents is routinely available for IV use. Subcutaneous apomorphine (Apokyn) injection might be appropriate for some patients. However, NG or other alternative enteral administration can suffice when the inability to take oral medication lasts longer than one or two doses. The rotigotine (Neupro) patch may be an option for some patients. Patients with PD who endure prolonged periods without their dopaminergic medications are at risk for a neuroleptic-malignant syndrome-like condition (*parkinsonism hyperpyrexia syndrome*) with hyperthermia, rigidity, and altered mental status. This condition can be fatal.[6,7]

Acute akinesia is a marked exacerbation in parkinsonism, often precipitated by concurrent illness including infection, injury, and sometimes by medication change such as sudden reduction in levodopa or adding a dopamine blocker. Management focuses on the underlying cause.

Hospital delirium and *psychosis* are more common in patients with PD, especially if they have pre-existing cognitive changes. Cognitive deficits are common with PD even in the absence of dementia.[8]

Medical complications of PD are multiple. Some of the most common include dysphagia, pneumonia, UTI, and decubitus ulcer. Deep vein thrombosis (DVT) is associated with immobility as well. Neurologist input can be helpful if dosage adjustments are necessitated by new side effects or if comorbidities develop during hospitalization.

Tremor

Hospital neurologists are commonly consulted for tremor, either as an exacerbation of a pre-existing tremor or development of a new tremor.

Enhanced Physiologic Tremor

Enhanced physiologic tremor is a common diagnosis among hospitalized patients. Some of these are exacerbated by medications, which are discussed in an upcoming section.

Hypoglycemia produces restlessness, anxiety, sweating, and tremor. The tremor can begin with an internal shakiness not visible externally that worsens to a visible fine finger tremor, which occurs mainly with action. If untreated, encephalopathy, coma, and seizures can result. Diagnosis is by measurement of blood glucose. Management is to treat the hypoglycemia emergently because delay or failure can result in permanent neurologic deficit. Intravenous thiamine is often given as well to prevent Wernicke encephalopathy.

Metabolic disorders can enhance physiologic tremor. Among the metabolic causes are renal failure, hepatic failure, and hypercarbia. The tremor appears more coarse and can resemble myoclonus and asterixis if severe. Diagnosis depends on identification of the metabolic disturbance. Often reviewing the chart shows new renal insufficiency, increased LFTs, CO_2 retention, or some other derangement that can be responsible. Brain imaging is usually unrevealing but should be done if there are mental status changes or focal neurologic deficits.

Alcohol withdrawal can cause mild tremulousness in the early stages, with subsequent evolution into more severe tremor. More severe withdrawal can cause delirium with hallucinations and marked tremors. The most extreme manifestation is *delirium tremens* (DTs), consisting of worsening tremor, encephalopathy, autonomic hyperactivity, and possibly seizures. DTs have a significant mortality rate: between 5% and 25%. At least 5% of patients are reported to have seizures. Diagnosis is clinical. Vigilance should be maintained for possible sepsis since it can have a similar appearance to DTs. In the face of cognitive changes, brain imaging is usually needed to look for subdural hematoma or other structural lesions. LP may be needed to exclude meningitis or encephalitis. Management of alcohol withdrawal consists of benzodiazepines to reduce the agitation and to prevent or treat withdrawal seizures; most conventional antiepileptic drugs are relatively ineffective for alcohol withdrawal seizures.

Essential Tremor

ET is the most common tremor and the most common movement disorder seen in routine practice. Evaluation and management of ET is uncommon for hospital neurology practice, but neurologists can be called to evaluate patients with unexplained tremor. Often, these patients carry the errant diagnosis of Parkinson disease. ET is often exacerbated by illness and medications in hospitalized patients.

PRESENTATION is with a mainly postural tremor—present with the arms extended. The tremor with movement can interfere with functions. Most patients have bilateral tremor, but one arm may be more severely affected. Tremor tends to abate with walking. Head tremor can occur. The tremor is usually mild but can be disabling. Notably, chin tremor is more typical of parkinsonism, whereas head tremor is more typical of ET.

DIAGNOSIS is clinical, with the postural nature being the most specific finding. Brain imaging is unrevealing, and, in a patient with typical tremor without other findings, imaging is likely not needed, especially if there is a family history.

MANAGEMENT is conservative for most patients. If the tremor interferes with important activities, then primidone or propranolol can be effective. Side effects can limit utility, and titration should be done over several days to weeks. Gabapentin, pregabalin, zonisamide, and topiramate can be effective alternatives in many patients.

Medication

A host of medications can cause or exacerbate tremor. The list is extensive, but some include valproate, amiodarone, caffeine, lithium, metoclopramide, theophylline, mexiletine, procainamide, prednisone, and sometimes selective serotonin reuptake inhibitors (SSRIs). Select agents include:

- *Valproate* can cause tremor, and there are rare reports of it causing parkinsonism. The tremor does not appear to depend on hepatic insufficiency.
- *Amiodarone* has been reported to cause multiple tremor types, including postural tremor suggestive of ET, cerebellar tremor, and even parkinsonism. Associated thyroid abnormalities can confuse the clinical picture. Discontinuing amiodarone is recommended in tremor patients if other antiarrhythmic drugs are available.

- *Metoclopramide* can produce parkinsonism, as well as tardive dyskinesia (TD). The incidence of these is difficult to establish. Litigation has resulted in a marked increase in reporting of TD.[9]

Psychogenic Tremor

Psychogenic movement disorders are usually hyperkinetic disorders resembling tremor or myoclonus, although other patterns can develop.[10] Differentiation from organic tremor rests on details of the presentation and inconsistency in exam and observation.

Myoclonus

Myoclonus is a common trigger for neurologic consultation. Myoclonus is more often positive than negative.

Drug-Induced Myoclonus

Drug-induced myoclonus is usually caused by doses of medications higher than normally used in practice. Among some of the most important are:

- *Opiates*: At high doses although also with withdrawal
- *Anticonvulsants*: Carbamazepine, valproate, phenytoin
- *Antibiotics*: Penicillins and cephalosporins
- *Antidepressants*: SSRIs and tricyclic antidepressants (TCAs)
- *Benzodiazepines*: Which can also improve myoclonus at lower doses

Offending meds should be reduced and do not necessarily need to be replaced. Diagnosis can be difficult since often patients are on multiple potential causative meds; high-dose meds are more likely to be implicated.

A host of metabolic derangements can cause myoclonus. Among these are:

- Hepatic failure
- Renal failure
- Hypercarbia
- Hyponatremia

Best management of these is to correct the metabolic derangement, but if that is not possible or effective, then the alternative is medical treatment. Depending on cause, treatment options include clonazepam, levetiracetam, valproate, or primidone. Sedatives should be avoided in patients with CO_2 retention. Levetiracetam might be preferable for a patient with hepatic dysfunction. Valproate can be a potent hepatic enzyme inhibitor and may increase levels of other drugs. Primidone can be a potent hepatic enzyme inducer and may reduce levels of other drugs.

Hemiballismus

Hemiballismus is due to dysfunction in the subthalamic nucleus. The most common cause is infarction, generally in a small branch of the posterior cerebral artery. Patients with nonketotic hyperglycemia may also develop hemiballismus. Younger patients may display hemiballismus due to inflammatory and infectious disorders causing focal basal ganglia dysfunction.

MANAGEMENT is among one of the more difficult tasks of hospital neurologists. First-line are generally dopamine receptor blockers, especially haloperidol.[11] Atypical neuroleptics, such as clozapine and risperidone, are potential alternatives. For sustained treatment, tetrabenazine is preferred, but the response may require weeks to achieve efficacy. Reserpine was occasionally used before tetrabenazine became available. The movements often subside over time.

Restless Leg Syndrome and Periodic Limb Movement Disorder

Restless legs syndrome (RLS) has multiple causes but can be idiopathic. Among common causes are renal failure, hepatic insufficiency, iron-deficiency anemia, and pregnancy. Periodic limb movement disorder (PLMD) is often seen in these patients and in patients with narcolepsy.

PRESENTATION of RLS is with an uncomfortable sensation that improves with motor activation and movement. It occurs mainly in the evening.

PRESENTATION of PLMD is with episodic limb jerking during sleep that may cause arousals.

DIAGNOSIS is suspected from the symptoms. PLMD may require polysomnography (PSG) for diagnosis. Screening for inciting medical disorders is key.

MANAGEMENT begins with identification and correction of inciting causes, if possible. Dopamine agonists such as ropinirole or pramipexole are used. Gabapentin may be of some benefit.

Other Hyperkinetic Disorders

Tardive Dyskinesia

TD is an occasional cause for hospital neurology consultation. TD is due to a precipitating drug, but there are some cases where the offending agent cannot be identified. Neuroleptics and metoclopramide are the most common agents implicated in TD. The atypical antipsychotics are less likely to produce TD, but they are not without risk. Note that the drug exposure may have occurred in the past.

PRESENTATION is with continuous choreoathetoid movements of the oro-facial muscles or limbs. The movements may be coupled with elements of tremor or dystonia. The clinical appearance is not unique from other disorders that cause dyskinesia, like Huntington disease (HD), so accurate diagnosis depends on documentation of med use.

DIAGNOSIS is clinical, with the movement disorder generally developing weeks after exposure to the neuroleptic. In the absence of a history of drug exposure, one should search for etiologies other than TD, such as HD. Edentulous patients may also display frequent mouth movements, but these typically resolve once dentures are inserted.

MANAGEMENT begins with withdrawal of the offending medication if possible. Acutely lowering the dose of medication often results in transient worsening of the movement disorder. For severe worsening with medication tapering, tetrabenazine is commonly used. Psychotic patients on older neuroleptics may be transitioned to newer atypical neuroleptics, which pose a lower risk of TD. Clozapine and quetiapine are generally preferred in this situation. Other therapies that might be helpful include clonazepam, branched chain amino acids and ginkgo biloba,[12] although data are limited.

Huntington Disease

HD is a rare cause for hospital neurology consultation and, when requested, is usually for management of the movements or a medical complication in an affected patient. Making a first diagnosis in the hospital is uncommon for this autosomal dominant, degenerative condition.

PRESENTATION is initially with chorea and later development of dystonia and parkinsonism with rigidity, bradykinesia, and ataxia. Cognitive changes begin with behavioral and psychiatric symptoms, usually irritability and depression, but psychotic features may manifest early. Late in the disease, parkinsonism and dementia predominate.

DIAGNOSIS is established prior to hospitalization for most patients. The diagnosis is suspected when there are choreiform movements in the absence of other identified causes, especially if there is a family history. The development of cognitive symptoms early in the disease is supportive. Brain imaging with MRI or CT shows abnormal configuration of the caudate. Confirmation by genetic testing is available. The main differential diagnoses are drug-induced dyskinesia, Wilson disease, and a familial chorea that is not associated with the remaining neurodegenerative manifestations.

MANAGEMENT is of the movement disorder, the cognitive disturbance, and related complications. Chorea can be treated with tetrabenazine or haloperidol, but other potentially effective medications include reserpine, valproate, and clonazepam. Dementia seldom responds to acetylcholinesterase inhibitors, but the associated depression can be treated with SSRIs. Psychosis requiring treatment may also respond to neuroleptics.

Dystonias

Dystonias seldom require hospital admission in adults, but can be problematic in children. Generally, the diagnosis has already been established or suspected prior to hospitalization.

PRESENTATION depends on the type. Some of the most important types include:

- *Torsion dystonia* affects any body region(s), though it typically affects limbs and trunk. A wide variety of genotypes produce an array of phenotypic presentations, generally starting in childhood years.
- *Cervical dystonia* or *spasmodic torticollis* is twisting of the neck, often with an anterior or posterior tilt.
- *Tardive dystonia* is a prominent dystonic component of tardive dyskinesia.
- *Cranial dystonia* includes a variety of presentations of orofacial dystonias. One manifestation is craniocervical dystonia or *Meige syndrome*: one example of Meige syndrome is blepharospasm plus oromandibular dystonia. *Spasmodic dysphonia* is a laryngeal dystonia.

DIAGNOSIS is clinical. Other causes of dystonia must be considered, including Wilson disease. In middle-aged adults, degenerative dystonias are very uncommon. MRI with gradient echo sequences can be helpful to detect the basal ganglia iron accumulation associated with several hereditary younger onset dystonias, termed neurodegeneration with brain iron accumulation (NBIA).

MANAGEMENT is often multimodal. Physical therapy is recommended for most patients, especially since medications produce modest improvement at best.

- *Anticholinergics*: Trihexyphenidyl (Artane) is often used first-line, with the alternative of benztropine (Cogentin).
- *Anti-spasmodics*: Baclofen (Lioresal) is commonly used, with an alternative being Tizanidine (Zanaflex).
- *Benzodiazepines*: Clonazepam (Klonopin) or Lorazepam (Ativan)
- *Dopaminergics*: Levodopa/Carbidopa (Sinemet, and others). If there is going to be response, it is typically early and robust. Effective doses are often lower than in PD.
- *Botulinum toxin*: Injections can very helpful for focal dystonias.

Hemifacial Spasm

Hemifacial spasm can be disabling and trigger neurologic consultation. Onset is usually late in life, and there may be no trigger.

PRESENTATION is with paroxysms of usually unilateral facial muscle contraction. Initially, the symptoms may be limited to periorbital muscles. Contractions occur spontaneously but can be triggered by movement or eye closure. Rare patients may have bilateral involvement.

DIAGNOSIS is clinical. A MRI brain scan is performed to look for focal structural lesions affecting the facial nerve. Special sequences with thin cuts are recommended. Electromyogram (EMG) is supportive. MR/CT angiography (e.g., MRA/CTA) is performed before considering decompressive surgery.

MANAGEMENT can include carbamazepine and other select antiepileptic drugs, baclofen, or benzodiazepines. Oxcarbazepine is often used in place of carbamazepine because of the improved side-effect profile. Botox injections are often the most effective treatment.

Ataxias

Differential diagnosis of ataxia was discussed earlier in this chapter. Here, we discuss some of the most important disorders not found elsewhere. The following ataxic disorders are discussed elsewhere:

- Stroke: Chapter 16
- Demyelinating diseases: Chapter 22
- Spinal cord disorders: Chapter 24
- Ethanol: Chapter 30
- Nutritional deficiency: Chapter 29
- Paraneoplastic cerebellar degeneration: Chapter 25

Hereditary ataxias rarely present in an acute setting other than when hospital evaluation is needed for medical complication or comorbid condition.

Major hereditary ataxias possibly encountered in a hospital practice are the multiple types of spinocerebellar ataxia (SCA), Friedreich ataxia (FA), and Wilson disease.

Spinocerebellar Ataxia

SCA is a family of disorders with various genetic and clinical manifestations. Most cases are autosomal dominant, but with incomplete penetrance. Onset is usually in early adult years but can be much later.

PRESENTATION is with progressive cerebellar ataxia, often affecting gait initially. Appendicular ataxia and tremor can occur. If they are to occur, cognitive, corticospinal, and noncerebellar motor involvement usually develop later. An exception is SCA3, where parkinsonism or dystonia may be the initial findings.

DIAGNOSIS is clinical with progressive cerebellar ataxia, a positive family history, and genetic testing. Brain imaging is usually done to exclude other causes of cerebellar ataxia.

MANAGEMENT is supportive. No medications have been proved to improve cerebellar ataxia or alter the course of the degeneration. There is some experimental evidence to support trialing amantadine.

Friedreich Ataxia

FA is an autosomal recessive, degenerative ataxia with associated non-neurologic manifestations. Neuronal degeneration extends beyond the cerebellum with involvement of corticospinal tracts, spinal neurons, and peripheral nerves.

PRESENTATION is with ataxia, mainly affecting gait but appendicular ataxia can occur early also. Ataxia has ultimately both cerebellar and spinal deficits, including sensory ataxia.

DIAGNOSIS is suspected when a patient seen for cerebellar ataxia is found to have peripheral neuropathic and corticospinal tract signs. An MRI brain scan can show the cerebellar atrophy, but, more importantly, imaging is used to exclude other etiologies of cerebellar and corticospinal dysfunction. Genetic testing is available.

MANAGEMENT is supportive. There is no approved treatment for the neurologic manifestations.

Wilson Disease

Wilson disease is an autosomal recessive disorder of copper metabolism, rarely seen in hospital neurology practice; when it is, it is usually for complications in a patient with known disease.

PRESENTATION is usually with hepatic insufficiency; neurologic manifestations occur in a smaller proportion of patients. About half of patients present with neurologic manifestations that can be extrapyramidal or cerebellar. Neurologic findings include the classic wing-beating tremor, as well as other tremor types, ataxia, parkinsonism, and chorea.[13] In the hospital setting, Wilson disease should be considered in younger (under age 40) patients with unexplained hepatic insufficiency.

DIAGNOSIS is suspected neurologically with extrapyramidal and cerebellar findings of unknown cause. Hepatic functions are often abnormal. Kayser-Fleischer rings in the eye are often evident if specifically looked for but subtle enough to be missed on casual exam. Labs include measurement of serum copper and ceruloplasmin and urinary copper excretion, in addition to assessment of liver function tests (LFTs). LFTs are generally elevated. Ceruloplasmin is usually but not invariably reduced. Copper excretion is increased, often markedly so. However, in severe disease, copper excretion can be so severely impaired that urine copper levels are normal. Slit-lamp exam can be done for accurate identification of the Kayser-Fleischer rings. Liver biopsy can be diagnostic.

MANAGEMENT consists of administration of a copper-chelating agent, such as penicillamine (Cuprimune) or trientine (Syprine). Patients are also instructed to restrict daily copper intake. Zinc supplementation is commonly used to block dietary absorption of copper. Transient worsening of neurologic symptoms can occur when a chelating agent is initiated.

Psychogenic Gait

Psychogenic gait is sometimes called *hysterical gait.* This is usually a conversion disorder and often associated with symptoms other than gait.

PRESENTATION can be with a wide variety of findings. Some of the gait syndromes can be dancing or bouncing, knees bent persistently, dragging one or both legs across the floor without lifting the foot, or use of cane in an unconventional or inconsistent manner.

DIAGNOSIS is clinical with observation of the character of gait. Also, patients with psychogenic gait usually have other signs of nonorganic neurologic deficit, such as nonanatomic sensory loss or inconsistent weakness.

MANAGEMENT is difficult, and direct confrontation is seldom effective. Chapter 38 discusses the approach to psychogenic deficits in detail.

24 Spinal Cord Disorders

Karl E. Misulis, MD, PhD and
E. Lee Murray, MD

CHAPTER CONTENTS

- Overview
- Differential Diagnosis
- Clinical Diagnosis
- Disorders
  - Degenerative Spine Disease
  - Cervical Radiculopathy
  - Lumbosacral Radiculopathy
  - Thoracic Radiculopathy
  - Spondylotic Myelopathy
  - Cauda Equina Syndrome and Conus Medullaris Syndrome
  - Traumatic Spinal Cord Injury

OVERVIEW

Differential diagnosis of myelopathy is broad and can include almost any of the cardinal mechanisms of disease. The following list presents common and important conditions that can cause myelopathy. Additional details are subsequently presented in this chapter for disorders not discussed elsewhere.

DIFFERENTIAL DIAGNOSIS

The differential diagnosis of myelopathy includes:

- *Inflammatory disorders*
  - *Transverse myelitis*: Rapidly progressive inflammatory myelopathy. Thoracic spine is most common site.
  - *Neuromyelitis optica (NMO)*: Rapidly progressive inflammatory myelopathy associated with optic neuritis
  - *Multiple sclerosis*: Episode of myelopathy but usually incomplete, less severe than NMO; also history or magnetic resonance imaging (MRI) evidence of brain lesions
  - *Acute disseminated encephalomyelitis (AEDM)*: Rapidly progressive myelopathy with other deficits including confusion, headache, neck pain, cranial nerve deficits

- o *Paraneoplastic myelitis/Necrotizing myelopathy*: Rapidly progressive myelopathy with inflammatory and hemorrhagic findings on MRI.
- *Structural disorders*
  - o *Cauda equina syndrome*: Compression of the cauda equina with progressive asymmetric leg weakness, sensory disturbance, and sphincter disturbance, with back and radicular pain
  - o *Conus medullaris syndrome*: Compression, infiltration, or inflammation of the conus produces rapidly progressive symmetric motor, sensory, and sphincter deficits
  - o *Syringomyelia*: Fluid-filled cavity in the spinal cord, often associated with Chiari malformation; often produces central cord syndrome
  - o *Compressive myelopathy from vertebral disease*: Compression from bony or disc elements
  - o *Spinal cord tumor*: Primary or metastatic lesion at any level of the cord initially produces mainly local pain then progressive myelopathy
  - o *Spinal hematoma*: Back pain followed rapidly by myelopathy or cauda equina syndrome
  - o *Epidural abscess*: Rapidly progressive myelopathy, back pain, often with headache and malaise
- *Degenerative disorders*
  - o *Hereditary spastic paraparesis*: Family of disorders of various inheritance with progressive myelopathy, but also can produce nonspinal neurologic manifestations—cerebral, brainstem, cerebellar
  - o *Primary lateral sclerosis*: Progressive spastic paraparesis without sensory loss or lower motoneuron involvement
- *Vascular disorders*
  - o *Spinal cord infarction*: Acute onset of paralysis, usually at the level of the lower thoracic spine
  - o *Spinal arteriovenous malformation* (AVM): Widely variable but generally stepwise-progressive asymmetric myelopathy; usually but not invariably painless
- *Metabolic/nutritional disorders*
  - o B_{12} *deficiency*: Spinal manifestations are spastic paraparesis, sensory disturbance affecting especially vibration and position sense
  - o *Copper deficiency*: Can present with weakness from myelopathy of neuropathy; can resemble and be combined with B_{12} deficiency
- *Cancer-related disorders (nonstructural)*
  - o *Radiation myelopathy*:
    - *Acute myelopathy*: Quadriplegia or paraplegia with acute onset. There is a transient form.
    - *Chronic progressive radiation myelopathy*: Progressive ascending deficit with sensory, motor, and sphincter disturbance. Spasticity is prominent.
  - o *Upper motor neuron degeneration*: Spasticity as a component of encephalomyelitis, usually with small-cell lung cancer
  - o *Lower motor neuron degeneration*: Progressive paralysis, often upper extremities, especially with lymphoma

CLINICAL DIAGNOSIS

Clues from clinical presentation can suggest a shorter list of differential diagnoses.

Acute myelopathy following fall:

- Intraspinal extra-medullary hematoma
- Intramedullary spinal hematoma
- Spinal cord contusion
- Acute herniated disc with compressive myelopathy
- Vertebral fracture with bony compression of the spinal cord

Subacute myelopathy:

- Transverse myelitis: infectious or autoimmune (MS, NMO, etc.)
- Epidural abscess
- Paraneoplastic myelitis.

Chronic progressive painless myelopathy:

- Primary lateral sclerosis
- Hereditary spastic paraparesis
- Disc disease with progressive cord compression
- Intrinsic tumor of the cord.

Progressive myelopathy with regional spine pain:

- Spinal epidural abscess
- Intraspinal tumor
- Degenerative disc disease or spondylosis with cord compression

Acute painless paraparesis:

- Spinal cord infarction
- Transverse myelitis (relatively acute, but not as acute as infarction)

Paraparesis with lumbar region pain:

- Cauda equina syndrome, from compression
- Conus medullaris syndrome, from compression, inflammation, or infiltration

Quadriparesis with upper neck pain:

- Chiari malformation
- Syringomyelia
- Cervical spondylotic myelopathy

Myelopathy with spine pain and fever:

- Spinal epidural abscess

DISORDERS

Specific myelopathies not covered elsewhere are discussed here. The locations of discussion of some specific disorders include:

- Multiple sclerosis: Chapter 22
- Neuromyelitis optica: Chapter 22
- Neoplastic cord compression: Chapter 25
- B_{12} deficiency: Chapter 29
- Hereditary spastic paraparesis: Chapter 37
- Infectious myelopathies: Chapter 17
- Syringomyelia: Chapter 37
- Transverse myelitis: Chapter 22
- Spinal cord infarction: Chapter 16
- Radiation myelopathy: Chapter 25

Degenerative Spine Disease

Degenerative spine disease usually does not produce myelopathy but can do so with significant spinal stenosis. Cervical and lumbar spine involvement is much more common than thoracic spine involvement largely due to biomechanical factors.

PRESENTATION to the hospital service usually occurs when neurologic deficits develop. Radiculopathy is more common with sensory and motor symptoms. Myelopathy is less common but an emergent condition. The vast majority of patients with degenerative spine disease have spine pain without neurologic deficit.

DIAGNOSIS is suspected with spine pain and, in the hospital setting, usually with weakness and sensory disturbance including paresthesias. With involvement of the cervical spine a central cord syndrome is most common, with weakness especially affecting the hands and arms with relative preservation of leg function due to integrity of the descending tracts. Imaging with computed tomography (CT) or MRI shows the cord compression. If MRI cannot be done, CT myelography is an alternative.

MANAGEMENT for patients developing neurologic deficit is usually surgery. This is especially the case for patients with myelopathy, although severe radiculopathy may also necessitate surgery. Symptomatic treatment with therapy and medications suffice for many patients not needing surgery.

Cervical Radiculopathy

Cervical radiculopathy is nerve compression due to osteophytes or disc material. Disc disease is more common with younger patients, osteophytes are more common with older patients.

PRESENTATION is usually with neck pain associated with pain radiating into the arm in a distribution that aids anatomic localization. Motor deficit may appear although often radicular pain is present prior to weakness.

- C5: Motor deficit in the deltoid or biceps; sensory deficit on the lateral upper arm
- C6: Motor deficit in the biceps and brachioradialis; sensory deficit on the radial forearm and first and second digits; reduced biceps and brachioradialis reflexes

- C7: Motor deficit in the triceps, wrist extensors; sensory deficit on the third and fourth digits; reduced triceps reflex
- C8: Motor deficit in the intrinsic hand muscles; sensory deficit on fifth digit and ulnar forearm
- T1: Motor deficit in the intrinsic muscles of the hand, especially abductor pollicis brevis; sensory deficit in the axilla

DIAGNOSIS is by MRI of the cervical spine. CT may show the lesion, but intrathecal contrast might be needed if MRI cannot be done. An electromyogram (EMG) is often done to determine if there is nerve root damage.

MANAGEMENT is conservative for most patients.

- *Medications* can include anti-inflammatories, muscle relaxants, and/or meds for neuropathic pain.
- *Therapy* is recommended especially for patients with reduced function due to pain or weakness.
- *Select nerve root blocks* can be helpful for refractory pain.
- *Surgery* is typically offered to patients with persistent weakness or pain.

Lumbosacral Radiculopathy

Lumbosacral radiculopathy is nerve compression due to osteophytes or disc material. As with cervical radiculopathy, disc material is more common in younger patients, osteophytes are more common in older patients.

PRESENTATION is commonly with back pain plus pain radiating into the leg in a distribution that depends on the nerve root. Weakness may be present. Dermatomal symptoms are as follows:

- L2: Motor deficit in the psoas and quadriceps; sensory deficit on the lateral and anterior thigh
- L3: Motor deficit in the psoas and quadriceps; sensory deficit of the lower medial thigh; may have reduced patellar reflex
- L4: Motor deficit of the tibialis anterior and quadriceps; sensory deficit in the medial lower leg; may have reduced patellar reflex
- L5: Motor deficit in the peroneus longus, gluteus medius, tibialis anterior, extensor hallucis longus; sensory deficit of the lateral lower leg
- S1: Motor deficit of the gastrocnemius and gluteus maximus; sensory loss on the lateral foot and fourth and fifth digits; may have reduced Achilles reflex

DIAGNOSIS is made by MRI of the lumbar spine. If MRI cannot be done, then CT may show the lesion, but intrathecal contrast may be needed. EMG can be done to evaluate for pattern of denervation.[1] Nerve conduction studies (NCS) are usually normal although F-waves and H-reflex can be abnormal. Sensory studies are normal.

MANAGEMENT is medical for most patients, as with cervical radiculopathy.

- *Medications* are commonly anti-inflammatories, muscle relaxants for patients with muscle tightness or spasm, and/or meds for neuropathic pain.

- *Therapy* is recommended, especially for patients with limited function due to pain or weakness.
- *Select nerve root blocks* can be helpful for refractory cases.
- *Surgery* is often offered to patients with refractory pain or persistent weakness.

Thoracic Radiculopathy

Thoracic radiculopathy can be from a variety of causes including disc disease, osteophytes, tumor, diabetes, or herpes zoster.

PRESENTATION is with pain and often sensory loss in one nerve root distribution. Weakness is not expected unless there is associated spinal cord compression with myelopathy below the lesion.

DIAGNOSIS is usually by MRI of the thoracic spine. CT with intrathecal contrast can show the lesion if MRI cannot be performed.

MANAGEMENT depends on the etiology. Surgical decompression is considered mainly if there is incipient myelopathy.

Spondylotic Myelopathy

Spondylotic myelopathy is compression of the spinal cord from degenerative disease. Most commonly this is in the cervical region.

PRESENTATION is with progressive myelopathy, usually with pain at about the level of the lesion.

DIAGNOSIS is by MRI of the spine in the appropriate region. CT is performed if MRI cannot be done and is most sensitive with intrathecal contrast.

MANAGEMENT is generally surgical, with decompression.

Cauda Equina Syndrome and Conus Medullaris Syndrome

Cauda equina syndrome is due to compression below the conus medullaris. Potential causes are multiple, including spinal stenosis, lumbar disc disease, neoplastic compression, meningioma, trauma, or other intrinsic lesion.

Conus medullaris syndrome is due to a lesion of the conus, and potential causes include all of those mentioned for cauda equina syndrome. In addition, inflammatory conditions such as multiple sclerosis can occasionally involve the conus.

PRESENTATION is similar, but there are important differences. Both produce motor, sensory, and sphincter abnormalities. Differences depend on etiology and localization.

- *Cauda equina* is associated with more severe pain in the spine and nerve root distributions, and the level of the lesion is lower. Tone is reduced and reflexes are usually absent.
- *Conus medullaris* is usually less painful both in regional and radicular distributions. Tone acutely will be reduced but can become spastic with increased tone and hyperreflexia.

DIAGNOSIS is suspected with paraparesis associated with back and limb pain. Imaging of the lumbosacral region with CT or MRI shows the lesion. If none is seen, then contrast-enhanced MRI should be considered to look for inflammatory lesion. Depending on imaging, if no compression is seen, then CSF analysis may show signs of inflammatory, infectious, or neoplastic disease.

MANAGEMENT depends on etiology.

- *Compressive lesions that are not neoplastic* depend on surgery for most clinical scenarios.
- *Compression due to tumor* may respond to urgent radiation therapy and chemotherapy.
- *Inflammatory causes* are treated with high-dose corticosteroids.
- *Infectious causes* are treated with appropriate anti-infective agents and surgery if compressive.

Prognosis depends on the severity of the lesion and the time from onset to definitive treatment. Patients with complete paralysis have a very low chance of restoring ambulation. Patients with incomplete and especially mild weakness have a much better prognosis.

Traumatic Spinal Cord Injury

Spinal cord injury is usually the province of neurosurgery and/or trauma surgeons, so this discussion is brief and covers mainly areas of interest for hospital neurologists.

PRESENTATION is with neurologic deficit after an injury that is appropriate to the level of the lesion. Note that in patients with dementia, encephalopathy from another reason, or transient loss of consciousness (e.g., syncope, seizure), the actual trauma may not have been witnessed or immediately appreciated.

DIAGNOSIS begins with standard x-rays. With neurologic deficit, spine and often cerebral imaging with CT is performed. MRI spine is performed if the etiology of the deficit is not identified.

MANAGEMENT begins with the basics, including spine stabilization. Corticosteroids had been standard of care, but recent data review has cast doubt on the risk versus benefits of treatment.[2] Still, many neurosurgeons advocate high-dose corticosteroids if they can be given within 8 hours of injury. Neurosurgery should be urgently consulted with traumatic myelopathy.

Prognosis depends on a variety of factors including the timing of the injury and treatment, severity of the trauma, and mechanism of trauma. The American Spinal Injury Association (ASIA) has developed a grading scheme that can be used to classify injuries and guide prognosis; it is publicly available.[3]

25 Neuro-Oncology

Mark D. Anderson, MD and
Karl E. Misulis, MD, PhD

CHAPTER CONTENTS

- Overview
- Primary Brain Tumors
- Metastatic Brain Tumors
- Spinal and Leptomeningeal Tumors
- Tumor Mimics
- Remote Manifestations of Cancer
  - Paraneoplastic Encephalitis
  - Lambert-Eaton Myasthenic Syndrome
  - Paraneoplastic Cerebellar Degeneration
- Neurologic Effects of Cancer Treatment
  - Chemotherapy Neuropathy
  - Radiation Injury to the Brain
  - Radiation Plexopathy
  - Radiation Myelopathy
  - Radiation Effects on the Brain
- Stroke in the Cancer Patient

OVERVIEW

Cancer and other tumors can affect the nervous system by local effect of a primary or metastatic lesion; by remote effect due to metabolic, vascular, or autoimmune effects of the cancer; or by side effects from the cancer therapy. Most common is the local effect of the tumor, whether primary or metastatic.

PRIMARY BRAIN TUMORS

Primary brain tumors are not as common as metastatic tumors to the brain but they are an occasional reason for neurology consultation in the hospital. Half of primary brain tumors are gliomas. Many are meningioma and are benign. Causes of primary brain tumors are unknown, and although there is an increased incidence in relation to radiation exposure, associations with cell phones are unsubstantiated.

PRESENTATION is with headache in 80% of patients, and many will have seizures, cognitive changes, weakness, numbness, or speech changes.

Diagnosis is best with magnetic resonance imaging (MRI) with and without contrast because computed tomography (CT) imaging is not very sensitive or specific. Biopsy is needed to make a diagnosis.

The World Health Organization (WHO) has a comprehensive classification scheme for tumors in general and brain tumors specifically. This was summarized best in the article by Louis,[1] the full text of which is freely available from PMC. In general, primary brain tumors are described by grades, with grade I representing well-differentiated, generally benign tumors and grade IV representing the most malignant tumors.

Primary brain tumor types are summarized here:

- *Glioblastoma (GBM)*
  - WHO Grade IV
  - Highly malignant glial tumor; most common of the glial tumors
  - Presents with focal deficit or seizures appropriate to the location of the tumor or headache; on MRI, a thick, ringlike enhancement with surrounding edema
- *Anaplastic astrocytoma/Anaplastic oligodendroglioma*
  - WHO Grade III
  - Common glial tumors that are less aggressive than GBM, with distinct histopathology and molecular markers. Presents with focal deficit or seizures appropriate to the location. Anaplastic astrocytoma may progress to GBM; may not enhance on MRI.
  - Anaplastic oligodendroglioma has the better prognosis.
- *Astrocytoma/Oligodendroglioma*
  - WHO grade II
  - Common low-grade glial tumors, with distinct histopathology and molecular markers; often progress to a higher grade. These lesions rarely enhance on MRI; usually present due to seizure.
  - Oligodendroglioma has the better prognosis.
- *Meningioma*
  - WHO grade I–III
  - Tumors arising from the meninges, from the arachnoid layer. In the brain, they are typically over the convexity, midline interhemispheric, or skull-based.
  - Produces focal symptoms depending on location from dysfunction of the adjacent parenchyma
  - More than 90% are grade I with an excellent prognosis.
- *Sellar masses*
  - Includes craniopharyngioma, pituitary adenoma, usually histologically benign but invasive. Common symptoms are headache, visual disturbance, and endocrine dysfunction. Visual disturbance is due to compression of the optic chiasm resulting in bitemporal hemianopia. Occasionally, rare glial tumors or brain metastasis can develop here.
- *Medulloblastoma*
  - WHO grade IV
  - Tumor of embryonal origin located in the cerebellum and 4th ventricle; commonly seeds CSF
  - Presents with headache, diplopia, ataxia, mental status changes, nausea, vomiting
- *Ependymoma*
  - WHO I–III

- o Less common glial tumor of ependymal origin; can be intraventricular or spinal arising in the central canal.
- o Presents with symptoms depending on location. Intracranial tumor usually produces lethargy, nausea, headache, brainstem, and/or cerebellar dysfunction. Spinal tumor produces regional pain with myelopathy appropriate to the location.
- *Primary CNS lymphoma*
  - o Lymphoma that is isolated to the brain or spinal cord. Secondary involvement of the CNS is necessary to rule out by looking for systemic lymphoma. Typically, a B-cell lymphoma with a distinct appearance on MRI.

Initial management in the ED involves stabilization. If there is symptomatic edema or mass effect, high-dose corticosteroids may be necessary, using a one-time IV dose of 10 mg of dexamethasone followed by 4 mg three to four times a day. Antiepileptic medication is indicated only if a seizure has occurred.

Further management depends on grade, stage, and host factors such as age and comorbid conditions.

METASTATIC BRAIN TUMORS

Metastatic brain tumors are the most common CNS tumors. Increased survival from systemic cancers has resulted in increased prevalence of brain metastases.[2] The most common sources are lung, breast, melanoma, renal cell, and colon cancers. Metastatic tumors with the highest propensity to cause intracerebral hemorrhage include melanoma, renal cell carcinoma, thyroid cancer, and choriocarcinoma

PRESENTATION is similar to primary brain tumors with headache, focal symptoms, seizure, and/or mental status changes.

DIAGNOSIS begins with imaging in any patient with symptoms of brain tumor whether there is known cancer or not. Diagnosis is generally confirmed by MRI brain with and without contrast, which is the most sensitive. Positron emission tomography (PET) with CT is less sensitive, but preferable to PET alone.[3] Patients without a history of cancer will need body imaging because brain metastasis can be the initial presentation of systemic cancer. A small percentage of patients diagnosed with brain metastases have no identified systemic cancer. Occasionally, biopsy is necessary to confirm diagnosis or help guide therapy.

MANAGEMENT of metastatic tumors depends on the primary site, number of metastases, and prior treatment. Corticosteroids are indicated for symptomatic edema. A solitary or single brain metastasis can be treated by resection if systemic cancer is controlled. Additionally, a brain metastasis that is large and symptomatic can be resected. With a few small brain metastases, stereotactic radiosurgery is commonly used, while whole brain radiation therapy is used for numerous or large brain metastasis. Systemic chemotherapy is generally not effective for brain metastases of most cancers but may be indicated in select patients.

SPINAL AND LEPTOMENINGEAL TUMORS

Spinal tumors are most commonly metastatic but can be primary. Metastases from remote tumors are most common; however, tumors affecting the brain and upper spine can seed the spinal fluid and produce drop metastases.

PRESENTATION of spinal tumors is with back pain and focal symptoms in the extremities, with weakness, numbness, or radiating pain. Evaluation with MRI of the spine is recommended. Urgent consultation with neurosurgery or radiation oncology is recommended.

PRESENTATION of leptomeningeal metastases may be with a myriad of symptoms but should be suspected with multifocal involvement (e.g., radiculopathies, cranial neuropathies).

DIAGNOSIS: MRI spine with contrast often shows meningeal disease. Lumbar puncture (LP) with at least 10 mL of spinal fluid should be sent for cytology. Opening pressure is usually elevated. Protein is increased. Glucose may be reduced. Leptomeningeal metastasis represents an end-stage involvement of cancer and portends a poor prognosis, with most patients living just weeks after diagnosis. However, young, healthy patients can do well with aggressive treatment.

Spinal cord tumors, their locations, and common etiologies include:

- Intramedullary
  - Astrocytoma
  - Ependymoma
- Intradural extramedullary
  - Meningioma
  - Neurofibroma
  - Schwannoma
- Extradural
  - Systemic cancers including lung, breast, lymphoma, renal, sarcoma, chordoma
- Leptomeningeal
  - Systemic cancers can be many, but common sources are lung, breast, lymphoma

TUMOR MIMICS

Even with the appearance of a brain tumor on imaging, care should be taken to exclude entities that can mimic a brain tumor, including demyelinating disease (tumefactive multiple sclerosis), infarction, vasculitis, infection (abscess, encephalitis, progressive multifocal leukoencephalopathy [PML]), textiloma (with a history of prior neurosurgery), and neurosarcoidosis.[4]

REMOTE MANIFESTATIONS OF CANCER

Remote effects of tumors are uncommon but should be considered with neurologic deficits of uncertain etiology. Many times, the paraneoplastic condition precedes the diagnosis of cancer.

Paraneoplastic Encephalitis

Paraneoplastic encephalitis is a diffuse or multifocal inflammatory disorder most commonly seen in patients with small-cell lung cancer. Common panels will test for more than a dozen different identified antibodies. *Limbic encephalitis* is a form of this. Another is paraneoplastic anti-N-methyl-D-aspartate receptor encephalitis

(*Anti-NMDA-R encephalitis*); this is classically related to ovarian teratoma, but not invariably so and can occur in men.

PRESENTATION can be with any combination of cerebral, brainstem, or peripheral nerve involvement.

- *Cerebral involvement*: Confusion, psychosis. seizures
- *Brainstem involvement*: Diplopia, dysarthria, dysphagia
- *Sensory, motor, or autonomic neuropathy*

DIAGNOSIS is suspected with a constellation of confusion, headache, psychiatric disturbance, seizures, and/or brainstem deficits, which could not all be explained by a single lesion. Patients may also demonstrate motor neuron degeneration, Lambert Eaton Myasthenic Syndrome (LEMS), or subacute neuropathy. In new-onset epilepsy without a structural lesion on MRI, consider autoimmune or paraneoplastic epilepsy. Especially in young women without known cancer, consider anti-NMDA-R encephalitis.[5]

- *CSF*: Often shows signs of inflammation, moderate pleocytosis with positive cytology. Repeat high-volume CSF analysis is sometimes needed.
- *MRI*: May show temporal lobe or brainstem increased signal on fluid attenuated inversion recovery (FLAIR) and T2, usually bilateral
- *EEG*: Usually slow or epileptiform activity
- A broad paraneoplastic panel is recommended in serum or CSF.

MANAGEMENT is usually treatment of the primary tumor. Occasionally, immune therapy with IV immunoglobulin (IVIg) or plasma exchange can be used.

Lambert-Eaton Myasthenic Syndrome

Lambert-Eaton Myasthenic Syndrome (LEMS) is weakness and fatigue due to antibodies to the voltage-gated calcium channel.[6] Most patients have malignancy, although at least 30% do not have a demonstrated cancer. The most common associated cancer is small-cell lung cancer.

PRESENTATION is usually with proximal weakness, legs more than arms. Dry mouth is common. Ocular muscle involvement can occur but is usually not seen at onset and not as severe as systemic weakness.

DIAGNOSIS is suspected when a patient presents with weakness and often has dysautonomia. Labs are done to look for myasthenia as well as LEMS. Electromyographic (EMG) distinction between LEMS and myasthenia gravis (MG) requires specific testing that should be requested.

- *EMG* shows incremental response in post-exercise compound motor action potential (CMAP) amplitude on high-frequency repetitive stimulation. Motor units show instability on routine and single-fiber studies.
- *Antibodies to VGCC* are present in most patients with cancer and in the majority of those without cancer who have LEMS.[7]

Differentiation from MG can be difficult, but MG typically has earlier and more prominent ocular muscle involvement with ptosis and diplopia.

MANAGEMENT includes immunotherapy, which is used for patients both with and without identified malignancy. Treatment of the underlying cancer can produce clinical improvement. Treatment can include:

- Prednisone or other corticosteroids
- IVIg
- Plasma exchange
- Azathioprine and other immunosuppressants
- Guanidine hydrochloride helps many patients but toxicity limits use.
- 3,4-diaminopyridine is not approved by the US Food and Drug Administration (FDA) at the time of this writing but has been studied and has had expanded access.
- Pyridostigmine or other cholinesterase inhibitors are often ineffective but do help some patients, so these may be considered.

Paraneoplastic Cerebellar Degeneration

Paraneoplastic cerebellar degeneration (PCD) is a progressive cerebellar ataxia due to the remote effect of cancers, especially breast, ovarian, lymphoma, and small-cell lung cancer.[8]

PRESENTATION can be with vertigo and nystagmus, and progress to cerebellar ataxia with both axial and appendicular involvement. Early symptoms might suggest vestibulopathy. Symptoms might be so acute as to suggest stroke.

DIAGNOSIS is suspected in cerebellar syndromes of subacute onset with negative MRI and lab studies. Some patients will have cerebellar atrophy. It may be mistaken for vestibulopathy before development of appendicular ataxia.

- *MRI brain*: Performed to rule out other etiologies and to evaluate for cerebellar atrophy
- *Blood work*—Paraneoplastic panel is recommended on serum or CSF; Anti-Tr and Anti-Yo are the most common causes. Check labs for B_{12} deficiency, neurosyphilis.
- *CSF*: To look for neoplastic, infectious, demyelinating, or inflammatory disorders. CSF pleocytosis or elevated protein is common.

Differential diagnosis includes vestibulopathy early in the course. With more severe symptoms, consider demyelinating disease, stroke, local cerebellar tumor, or central pontine myelinolysis (CPM).

MANAGEMENT begins with completing the search for occult malignancy, particularly ovarian. Treatment of the underlying cancer can improve symptoms. Medical treatment with IVIg, corticosteroids, or cyclophosphamide can be tried, but there is no treatment that has been proved effective.

NEUROLOGICAL EFFECTS OF CANCER TREATMENT

Among the most important neurologic complications of cancer treatment are:

- Chemotherapy neuropathy
- Radiation injury to the brain

- Radiation myelopathy
- Radiation plexopathy
- Chemotherapy-related posterior reversible encephalopathy syndrome (PRES)
- Nutritional deficiency syndrome.

PRES is discussed in Chapter 13. Management does not differ from that in patients without cancer, except that the offending medication would be discontinued.

Chemotherapy Neuropathy

Peripheral neuropathy is common with chemotherapy, especially with combinations. Certain chemotherapies are more likely to produce neuropathy than others, especially platinum-based agents (e.g., cisplatin), vinca alkaloids (e.g., vincristine), and taxanes (e.g., paclitaxel).

PRESENTATION usually begins with sensory symptoms and includes pain, dysesthesias, paresthesias, and sensory loss. The neuropathy progresses during chemotherapy and usually improves following cessation but might progress for a limited time following cessation of treatment.

DIAGNOSIS is suspected with distal pain or sensory loss in a patient undergoing chemotherapy. For many patients, this is expected and is not dose-limiting. Clinical presentation of neuropathic symptoms is usually only necessary for diagnosis. EMG/ nerve conduction studies (NCS) can document the neuropathy but is seldom necessary. Additional labs to look for contributing factors such as metabolic or nutritional causes for neuropathy should be done.

MANAGEMENT is symptomatic. Rarely will a change in chemotherapy regimen have to be made because of neuropathy. However, for some patients, neuropathy may limit duration of therapy, especially when used for tumor recurrence. Pain is managed by a variety of medications; gabapentin and similar agents are commonly used. Symptoms can improve with cessation of therapy.

Radiation Injury to the Brain

Radiation injury to the brain can be acute or delayed; the delayed state is divided into early delayed and late delayed. At both acute and delayed stages it is often difficult to differentiate this from tumor growth.

PRESENTATION is usually with worsening focal neurologic deficit, confusion, or signs of increased intracranial pressure.

DIAGNOSIS is suspected with symptomatic worsening. MRI is performed and may show no change, edema, or increased signal change near the region of tumor, which can be difficult to differentiate from progressive tumor. Enhancement has been described as having different patterns in tumor versus radiation injury, but this is not consistent. PET can show hypometabolism with radiation injury in contrast to high metabolism in regions of active tumor growth. Biopsy may be needed for definitive diagnosis.

MANAGEMENT begins with corticosteroids for most patients. Anticoagulation can be used because late radiation necrosis is felt to be a vascular occlusive process; however, there are limited data on this use. Bevacizumab (Avastin) may be effective since it inhibits angiogenesis, although it is not FDA-approved for this indication.[9]

Radiation Plexopathy

Radiation plexopathy can involve the brachial or lumbosacral plexus, depending on the focus of radiation.

PRESENTATION *of brachial plexopathy* is with arm weakness, especially involving muscles innervated by the upper plexus (e.g., deltoid). Sensory symptoms are common, including paresthesias and decreased sensation, but there is usually little pain. *Lumbosacral plexopathy* presents with leg weakness. Sensory loss is common but a less reported symptoms than motor deficit.

DIAGNOSIS is suspected with weakness in a single limb, which is appropriate to previous radiation therapy. The main differential diagnosis is tumor infiltration, which is often quite painful.

- *MRI with and without contrast* is most sensitive for identifying tumor infiltration of nerves or nerve roots. Lack of enhancement favors radiation plexopathy.
- *EMG* may show myokymia, but this is not a dependable finding. Denervation can be seen with neuronal damage from radiation or tumor, so this is not a reliable differentiating feature.
- *CSF* may be needed to look for neoplastic meningitis.

Differentiation of radiation plexopathy from tumor infiltration can be difficult. In general, tumor infiltration is quite painful, whereas radiation plexopathy is relatively painless. For the brachial plexus, radiation plexopathy generally involves the upper plexus, whereas tumor infiltration usually involves the lower plexus because of the lesser tissue attenuation for radiation in the former and proximity to involved tissues in the latter.

MANAGEMENT is supportive. There is no specific treatment to improve neural function. Pain may be managed by typical meds for neuropathic pain.

Radiation Myelopathy

Radiation myelopathy can be early or late. Early-onset radiation myelopathy generally has a better prognosis for improvement than does late-onset radiation myelopathy.

PRESENTATION *of early radiation myelopathy* is with transient leg weakness and sensory loss. This usually starts at least 2 and up to 6 months after the treatments. Lhermitte sign is common. There is gradual spontaneous improvement over months.

PRESENTATION *of late radiation myelopathy* is with a progressive myelopathy between 6 and 12 months following treatment. Weakness and sensory loss develop without the electrical sensation of early myelopathy. Findings are often asymmetric, especially initially. Progression is expected; only rare patients have late improvement in the chronic myelopathy.

DIAGNOSIS is suspected with myelopathy starting months after radiation. If deficit occurs at the time of radiation, alternative diagnoses including tumor and infarction should be considered. MRI shows increased signal on T2 and FLAIR at the level of the lesion. Contrasted MRI may show cord enhancement with radiation myelopathy, but this would also suggest tumor.

MANAGEMENT is supportive. Early myelopathy remits spontaneously. Late myelopathy usually continues to progress. There is no proven treatment to alter the course of either condition.

Radiation toxicity in the brain in most cases results in a leukoencephalopathy, usually asymptomatic, but it can result in cognitive impairment. Acutely, patients can present with encephalopathy or seizures after initiation of radiation therapy and may need antiepileptic treatment or corticosteroids during the remainder of cranial radiation.

About 20% of patient will have persistent or delayed development of enhancement and vasogenic edema from the radiation within the first 6 months of treatment, often termed *pseudo-progression* and responsive to corticosteroids. Around 5% of patient can develop a more severe local tissue reaction with signs of a disrupted blood–brain barrier, edema, and mass effect for up to several years after completion of radiation, termed *radiation necrosis*. Often, on standard MRI, these changes look identical to recurrent tumor and require advanced imaging with MRI, PET, or biopsy to establish the diagnosis.

STROKE IN THE CANCER PATIENT

Strokes may be a complication from a hypercoagulable state, from vessel compression and/or infiltration by a tumor, or as a side effect from chemotherapy or radiation therapy. The survival rate of patients hospitalized with cerebral infarction is worse in patients with cancer.[10]

The typical pattern of stroke from a hypercoagulable state is embolic. MRI will reveal strokes involving multiple arterial territories. The workup of a stroke in a cancer patient should always seek to rule out nonbacterial thrombotic endocarditis (NBTE) with a transesophageal echocardiogram if possible.[11] Additionally, a stroke from a tumor embolus can result in an aneurysm, so CT angiography should also be performed. Occasionally the stroke will be from a cerebral venous thrombosis (CVT). If suspected, check with MR or CT venography (MRV or CTV). If CVT or NBTE is suspected, treatment with heparin is usually begun.

26 CSF Circulation Disorders

Karl E. Misulis, MD, PhD and
E. Lee Murray, MD

CHAPTER CONTENTS

- Overview
- Increased CSF Pressure
  - Nonobstructive Hydrocephalus from Increased CSF Production
  - Nonobstructive Hydrocephalus from Reduced CSF Resorption
- Obstruction of CSF Flow
  - Colloid Cyst
  - Aqueductal Stenosis
  - Fourth Ventricular Outflow Lesions
  - Chiari Malformation
  - Syringomyelia
- Low CSF Pressure
  - Low-Pressure Headache
  - Persistent CSF Leak
- Normal Pressure Hydrocephalus

OVERVIEW

Cerebrospinal fluid (CSF) is formed by the choroid plexus and ependyma and absorption is by the arachnoid granulations that protrude into the venous sinuses, as well as by CNS lymphatics. CSF circulation can be disordered by a mismatch in formation and resorption or occlusion of CSF conduits. Some of the potential defects affecting CSF circulation include:

- *Increased CSF pressure* from increased CSF production, decreased CSF resorption, or, in the case of pseudotumor cerebri, from unknown causes
- *Decreased CSF pressure*, especially CSF leak
- *Occlusion of CSF flow* at various levels producing obstructive hydrocephalus
- *Normal-pressure hydrocephalus*, a specific condition possibly related to impaired absorption

INCREASED CSF PRESSURE

Increased CSF pressure can be from:

- Nonobstructive hydrocephalus from increased CSF production
- Nonobstructive hydrocephalus from reduced CSF resorption
- Increased CSF pressure without hydrocephalus, e.g., pseudotumor cerebri

Pseudotumor cerebri is discussed in detail in Chapter 20. This is differentiated from the other disorders by the absence of increased ventricular size.

Nonobstructive Hydrocephalus from Increased CSF Production

Nonobstructive hydrocephalus from increased CSF production is usually a disorder of children but can occur in adults. A *choroid plexus papilloma* produces more CSF than is usually resorbed. The lesion is usually benign but can be malignant. Location is most commonly in the lateral ventricle.

PRESENTATION is with symptoms of increased intracranial pressure (ICP), which can include headache, nausea, and vomiting. With markedly increased ICP, patients can become drowsy. Exam often shows papilledema unless the onset is fairly acute. Visual loss can be insidious but detectable on exam. Cranial nerve palsies are most commonly of CN 3 and CN 6.

DIAGNOSIS is suspected when a patient presents with headache and papilledema and there is concern for increased ICP. Brain imaging with computed tomography (CT) or magnetic resonance imaging (MRI) shows increased ventricular size and can visualize choroid plexus lesions.

MANAGEMENT is usually surgical. Some patients need urgent shunting to relieve pressure, followed later by surgical excision of the lesion. Depending on pathology, location, and success of surgery, other treatments including radiation therapy and/or chemotherapy may be considered.

Nonobstructive Hydrocephalus from Reduced CSF Resorption

Nonobstructive hydrocephalus from reduced CSF resorption is usually due to one of the following:

- *Meningitis*, can be early or late
- *Subarachnoid hemorrhage* can be early or late even months after the event
- *Congenital defect* in children; this will not be discussed further here

PRESENTATION is usually with typical symptoms of increased ICP including head-ache, nausea, vomiting, and, ultimately, mental status changes with drowsiness or confusion.

DIAGNOSIS is suspected in the presence of symptoms of increased ICP with brain imaging showing increased ventricular size but no occlusion and no lesion which would be suspected of evoking increased CSF production.

MANAGEMENT is usually with shunt placement. Medications to reduce CSF production, such as acetazolamide, can be helpful especially as a prelude to surgery, but long-term medical treatment is ineffective. Serial lumbar punctures (LP) also are used to produce an immediate reduction in ICP but are usually not long-term solutions.

OBSTRUCTION OF CSF FLOW

CSF flows from the lateral ventricles to the third ventricle, through the cerebral aqueduct to the fourth ventricle, where it exits to the subarachnoid space.

Occlusion at any level can produce increased CSF pressure, specifics of which are dependent on location. Here, we discuss structural occlusion of flow rather than defective resorption.

Colloid Cyst

Colloid cysts usually develop in the third ventricle but can develop in the fourth ventricle. Other locations are much more rare.

PRESENTATION is usually with headache, which is positional and especially worse in the morning. Change in head position can produce marked exacerbation of the pain, often when bending forward. Signs of increased ICP can include papilledema, nausea, vomiting, and, with more severe obstruction, confusion, drowsiness, and gait ataxia.

DIAGNOSIS is suspected with symptoms and signs of increased ICP. Brain imaging with CT or MRI shows the cyst. These are occasionally incidental, but are more likely to be symptomatic when there is increased ventricular size.

MANAGEMENT is usually surgical. Urgent ventricular drain placement may be needed prior to definitive surgery if hydrocephalus is critical.

Aqueductal Stenosis

Aqueductal stenosis is typically congenital but usually is not symptomatic until adult life.

PRESENTATION is with symptoms and signs of increased ICP with headache, nausea, vomiting, ataxia, and confusion, ultimately progressing to lethargy. Diplopia may develop.

DIAGNOSIS is suspected when a patient with presentation of increased ICP has enlargement of the lateral and third ventricles without enlargement of the fourth ventricle and without a visible mass occluding CSF flow. Contrast can help to rule out tumor. A high-quality MRI can often show the aqueduct anatomy.

MANAGEMENT is usually surgical, with a variety of techniques used. Shunting is historically most common. Third ventriculostomy is effective for many patients.

Fourth Ventricular Outflow Lesions

Fourth ventricular outflow obstruction is usually due to tumors or other lesions in the region of the fourth ventricle and can produce hydrocephalus. These are less common than aqueductal occlusive conditions.

PRESENTATION of the resultant hydrocephalus is with all of the symptoms and signs of increased ICP already discussed plus diplopia, nystagmus, and prominent ataxia, which provide a clue to the posterior fossa location.

DIAGNOSIS is suspected by presentation of increased ICP with brainstem signs. Brain imaging is best with MRI and contrast is recommended.

MANAGEMENT depends on the etiology. Some tumors of the posterior fossa can be debulked or resected, others are treated with radiation therapy and/or chemotherapy. Ventricular drain is sometimes used when normal CSF flow cannot be restored.

Chiari Malformation

Chiari malformation can be sufficiently severe to extend the cerebellar tonsils and caudal brainstem tissue through the foramen magnum, thereby producing obstructive hydrocephalus.

PRESENTATION is often with symptoms and signs of increased ICP, including headache, nausea, and vomiting, but also signs of brainstem dysfunction including dysphagia, vertigo, and appendicular as well as gait ataxia, often worse with changes in position or Valsalva maneuver. Pain in the craniocervical junction can develop.

DIAGNOSIS is suspected with symptoms of increased ICP with headache, nausea, and vomiting. MRI shows descent of the cerebellar tonsils through the foramen magnum and often visible compression of the brainstem, best seen on sagittal images. Cervical spine imaging should also be done to look for syrinx.

MANAGEMENT is surgical if the Chiari malformation is not an asymptomatic incidental finding. We often see patients who attribute severe symptoms to a Chiari malformation that would be expected to be asymptomatic.

Syringomyelia

Syringomyelia is a fluid-filled cavity in the spinal cord. Most cases are due to an associated Chiari malformation with obstruction to CSF flow. Other causes include spinal cord injury, CSF hemorrhage, infection, or tumor.

PRESENTATION is usually with local back or neck pain and weakness of the arms and legs. Associated symptoms can be incontinence of bowel and bladder and sensory disturbance of the extremities, often with prominent muscle stiffness and pain. The correlation of the location of the pain and level of the neurologic deficit is a clue to the diagnosis.

DIAGNOSIS is suspected with spine pain and findings of myelopathy. At the time of presentation, the differential diagnosis is large but the principal concern is cord compression from disc or tumor. The syrinx is seen best on MRI of the spine with sagittal images.

MANAGEMENT of patients with neurologic deficits from syringomyelia is usually surgical. If a syrinx is thought to be due to a clinically significant Chiari malformation, then decompression of this is usually tried.

LOW CSF PRESSURE
Low-Pressure Headache

Low-pressure headache is often due to CSF leak. Most patients will have some identifiable cause, including recent LP, spinal or cranial surgery, or other recent spinal procedure, such as epidural block, where the dura might have been punctured. However, low-pressure headache can develop with cough, sneeze, Valsalva maneuver, sinus surgery or erosion, or nonsurgical injury to the head or spine. LP is the most common cause encountered in hospital neurology practice.

PRESENTATION is usually with holocephalic headache that is relieved by recumbency. The positional nature is a useful diagnostic clue. Neck pain and stiffness is often associated with this presentation.

DIAGNOSIS is considered mostly in a patient who has had recent LP or other spinal instrumentation. Brain imaging may need to be performed to rule out serious intracranial structural lesion, but it is usually normal. Repeat LP for infection may be needed if there is fever or increased WBC but is usually not needed.

MANAGEMENT includes blood patch for many patients. LP is the most common cause and thus a self-limited etiology. This produces prompt and lasting relief for many patients. High-volume fluids and caffeine have been advocated, and these plus bedrest may result in some patients not requiring a blood patch. Corticosteroids may be considered for some refractory cases.

Persistent CSF Leak

Persistent CSF leak produces low-pressure headache but does not abate because the leak continues. Persistent CSF leak predisposes to meningitis.

DIAGNOSIS is suspected with positional headache. Brain imaging is performed, preferably with MRI. If contrast is administered, MRI may show dural enhancement from venous distention. If the leak is in the region of the sinuses, demonstration may require radionucleotide study. CSF is under low pressure, usually 6 cm H_2O or less. There are special procedures for examination for possible CSF leak and use of these should involve consultation with neurosurgery. Severe cases can result in subdural hematoma.

MANAGEMENT begins with fluids, caffeine, bedrest, and if needed and appropriate, blood patch. Surgery for dural repair is often needed for persistent leak.

NORMAL PRESSURE HYDROCEPHALUS

Normal pressure hydrocephalus (NPH) is usually considered in the differential diagnosis of dementia. The etiology is likely an abnormality in CSF flow, but the exact cause is not known. Ventricles are increased in size, out of proportion to cortical atrophy yet CSF pressure is not increased at the time of diagnosis.

PRESENTATION is classically described as a triad of:

- Dementia
- Gait ataxia
- Incontinence

Most patients do not have all three at the time of presentation. Gait ataxia is often the principal finding in patients with NPH. Gait is broad-based and shuffling, having features of a frontal lobe ataxia. Dementia also has a prominent frontal lobe appearance, with slowness of cognition and response in addition to memory loss.

DIAGNOSIS is usually suspected when a patient has gait ataxia and signs of increased ventricular size on brain imaging. Often there is significant cortical atrophy accompanying the increased ventricular size, so, for NPH to be felt likely, a significant discrepancy between ventricular size and cortical atrophy should be present.

Clinical findings include:

- Gait difficulty is the predominant clinical finding—a "magnetic gait."
- Removal of at least 30 mL of CSF produces clinical improvement especially in gait. This can be done by removal of a specified amount or placement of an external lumbar drain

MRI imaging findings can include:

- Increased ventricular size is out of proportion to sulcal atrophy.
- Frontal horns of the lateral ventricles are rounded.
- Flow void may be seen in the aqueduct as dark on T2-weighted imaging when the rest of the CSF is bright, however this is not specific or diagnostic.
- Temporal horns of the lateral ventricles are large.
- Periventricular signal is increased on fluid attenuated inversion recovery (FLAIR) and T2 imaging suggests transependymal fluid, which suggests NPH and other causes of hydrocephalus rather than the ex vacuo effect of cerebral atrophy.

We recommend that testing mental status and gait before and after CSF removal be performed to look for interval improvement.

MANAGEMENT of NPH is surgical, with ventriculoperitoneal shunt being the most common. This is offered especially to patients who showed a good response to CSF drainage since this has a fairly high predictive value for response to shunting. However, select patients with negative clinical response to CSF drainage may be considered for shunting because some of these patients respond.

27 Pregnancy and Neurology

Georgia Montouris, MD and
Maria Stefanidou, MD, MSc

CHAPTER CONTENTS

- Spectrum of Neurologic Problems in Pregnancy
  - Headache
  - Seizures
  - Encephalopathy
  - Focal Neurologic Deficit
- Neurologic Disorders in Pregnancy
  - Eclampsia and Pre-Eclampsia
  - Cerebral Venous Thrombosis
  - Migraine
  - Epilepsy
  - Myasthenia Gravis
  - Peripheral Nerve Injuries
  - Multiple Sclerosis

SPECTRUM OF NEUROLOGIC PROBLEMS IN PREGNANCY

The most common problems for which neurologists see pregnant patients in the ED and hospital are:

- Headache
- Seizure
- Confusion/encephalopathy
- Focal neurologic deficit

Most obstetricians do not consult neurology for eclampsia unless seizures are refractory or focal neurologic symptoms develop.

Headache

Headache has a broad differential diagnosis, almost all of which can potentially occur during pregnancy. Chapter 20 discusses headache in depth. However, there are some etiologies of particular note during pregnancy. Features of some of these, as well as their differential diagnoses, include:

- *Migraine*: Recurrent, episodic unilateral or bilateral headache lasting 4–72 hours and associated with nausea, vomiting, and/or photophobia. Migraines improve during pregnancy in 60–70% of women with pre-existing migraine, but may occasionally worsen or appear for the first time.
- *Pre-eclampsia*: Headache often with nausea; visual obscurations are common. Non-neurologic findings are key, including hypertension, proteinuria, and edema.
- *Cerebral venous thrombosis*: Headache often with encephalopathy or focal deficits. May develop seizure or signs of increased intracranial pressure.
- *Intracerebral hemorrhage*: Headache, focal deficit, and often encephalopathy related to intraparenchymal hemorrhage.
- *Subarachnoid hemorrhage*: Acute onset of headache often associated with neck stiffness. Aneurysmal bleed has an increased incidence during pregnancy, which peaks at 30–34 weeks gestational age and among older mothers (>35 years).
- *Postpartum cerebral angiopathy*: Severe headache developing in the 6 weeks postpartum and associated with reversible segmental narrowing and dilation of large and medium-sized cerebral arteries. Often complicated by seizures, reversible brain edema, intracerebral or nonaneurysmal subarachnoid hemorrhage.
- *Arterial dissection*: Acute onset of focal deficits, often with headache. In a woman of childbearing age, dissection must always be considered, but pregnancy may increase the risk.
- *Pituitary apoplexy*: Acute onset of headache and visual disturbance including visual loss and/or diplopia due to acute hemorrhage into the pituitary. Clinical signs of pituitary insufficiency follow.
- *Meningitis*: Headache associated with fever, stiff neck, nausea, and vomiting, often with encephalopathy.
- *Pseudotumor cerebri*: Headache and visual change with papilledema on exam. Must look for venous thrombosis if this diagnosis is considered.

MANAGEMENT of most of these does not markedly differ from that in the nonpregnant population (Chapter 20), but there are some differences that deserve note and these are discussed in the following sections.

Seizures

Seizure in pregnancy can have a variety of causes. Among some of the most important are:

- Idiopathic seizure
- Eclampsia
- Cerebral venous thrombosis
- Tumor
- Cerebral infarction
- Cerebral hemorrhage
- CNS infection
- Psychogenic nonepileptic seizures

PRESENTATION is with any of the seizure manifestations discussed in Chapter 19. Associated symptoms will not be expected unless there is a new causative neurologic problem, such as stroke, tumor, or infection. Seizures can be focal-onset or primarily generalized.

DIAGNOSIS is established by the clinical seizure activity. Approach to diagnosis depends on the clinical scenario.

- *Recurrent seizure with known epilepsy*: Further study is often not needed unless change in seizure semiology or breakthrough in well-controlled epilepsy occurs.
- *New seizure without neurologic deficit*: Electroencephalogram (EEG) is performed. Brain imaging with computed tomography (CT) or magnetic resonance imaging (MRI) is recommended. LP is recommended if CNS infection is suggested by clinical parameters or imaging (e.g., temporal signal change suggesting HSV encephalitis).
- *New seizure with new neurologic deficit*: Brain imaging with CT or MRI is recommended. EEG is performed. Eclampsia is considered in patients with pregnancy-induced hypertension, edema, proteinuria, or evidence of hemolysis, elevated liver enzymes and low platelet count (HELLP) syndrome. LP is recommended if clinical findings suggest infection (fever, increased WBC) or subarachnoid hemorrhage (CSF signal change on CT or MRI)
- *Suspected nonepileptic seizure*: Recommend continuous video EEG if possible to document whether the paroxysmal activity is nonepileptic. Routine EEG may not capture a spell.

MANAGEMENT: Anticonvulsants used during pregnancy are similar to those used in nonpregnant patients (Chapter 19), but agents with increased incidence of developmental defects and cognitive effects, such as valproate, are to be avoided if possible.

Encephalopathy

Encephalopathy in pregnancy is usually pre-eclampsia or eclampsia, but there are a host of other potential causes. Some of the important causes of encephalopathy during pregnancy include:

- *Pre-eclampsia*: Severe pre-eclampsia can produce cognitive change in addition to hypertension, proteinuria. Visual obscuration can also occur.
- *Eclampsia*: Presents with symptoms of severe pre-eclampsia, progressing to seizure or coma.
- *Cerebral venous thrombosis*: Confusion with headache often occurs. Patients may have focal deficits.
- *Intracranial hemorrhage*: Acute onset of headache and confusion is common, often with focal signs if the hemorrhage is intraparenchymal, less so if subarachnoid.
- *Seizure*: Presents as acute onset of encephalopathy that usually has an observed clinical seizure. May present as encephalopathy if the motor component was subtle or unobserved.

- *CNS infection*: Presents with headache, encephalopathy, sometimes with fever. Meningeal signs, including neck stiffness, may develop.
- *Metabolic encephalopathies and drug toxicity*: Presents with altered mental status, marked sedation. Seizures may occur.

DIAGNOSIS of patients with encephalopathy in pregnancy usually begins with urgent CT brain. MRI is felt by many to be safer for the baby but is often not available urgently. LP may be indicated in some cases. EEG can be helpful to rule out nonconvulsive status in patients who are unresponsive.

Focal Neurologic Deficit

Focal neurologic deficit during pregnancy is always an indicator for urgent evaluation. The differential diagnoses of focal deficit during pregnancy include:

- *Cerebral venous thrombosis*: Focal deficits are combined with headache, confusion. Seizures may develop.
- *Acute ischemic stroke (AIS)*: Acute onset of focal deficit.
- *Arterial dissection*: One cause for AIS. Acute onset of focal deficit. Note that the dissection can be carotid or vertebral.
- *Intracranial hemorrhage*: Acute onset of focal deficit often with headache, nausea, vomiting, and/or encephalopathy.
- *Brain tumor*: Subacute or chronic progressive focal deficit and/or headache. Seizures may develop.

Tumors can be identified during pregnancy and may complicate evaluation and management. Primary tumors are more common than metastatic at this age.

DIAGNOSIS usually begins with brain imaging. CT is relatively safe because of the low radiation exposure. MRI is believed to be of even less risk to the fetus.[1]

- *Tumor?* If the etiology of the focal deficit is possibly tumor, MRI with contrast is preferable to CT with contrast.[1]
- *Infarction?* Vascular studies are better performed with MR angiography (MRA) than CT angiography (CTA) because of the lack of need for contrast, but CTA does show better anatomy and may be preferable emergently if endovascular therapy is considered.
- *Hemorrhage?* Hemorrhage is identified on CT brain or MRI. MRA is able to show many aneurysms and vascular malformation, but not all, and CTA may be needed.

NEUROLOGIC DISORDERS IN PREGNANCY

Disorders occurring during pregnancy are discussed here unless they are discussed elsewhere in more detail:

- Pseudotumor cerebri: Chapter 20

In cases of pseudotumor cerebri presenting or being exacerbated during pregnancy avoid acetazolamide because of the potential for adverse effects on the developing fetus. Lumbar punctures (LPs) and most other treatments can usually be done safely. Surgical treatments can also be considered.

- Pituitary apoplexy: Chapter 28
- Cerebral infarction or hemorrhage: Chapter 16

Regarding acute ischemic stroke in pregnancy, IV tissue plasminogen activator (tPA) and endovascular therapy have, historically, been withheld from pregnant patients, but this is being revisited and should not be dismissed as a possibility[2] for potentially disabling strokes, as both these reperfusion therapies have been used successfully in patients at different stages of pregnancy. Evaluation with genetic testing for thrombophilia and hypercoagulable state may have to wait at least 6 weeks after childbirth for the accurate evaluation of protein C and S activity and antithrombin III deficiency. Study for sickle-cell disease and lupus antiphospholipid antibody may be indicated on a case-by-case basis, in addition to standard stroke workup.

Eclampsia and Pre-Eclampsia

Pre-eclampsia is hypertension and proteinuria associated with pregnancy after 20 weeks gestation. *Eclampsia* is seizure and/or encephalopathy or coma in a patient with pre-eclampsia. Onset can be postpartum typically, within 48 hours of childbirth, but sometimes up to 6 weeks after childbirth. Pre-eclampsia is more common with a personal history of hypertension, diabetes including gestational diabetes, or other vascular disease.

PRESENTATION of eclampsia is with seizures and/or coma in a pregnant patient with pre-eclampsia. The seizures are typically generalized, although they may be of focal onset. Encephalopathy or coma can be present before or after seizure activity. Associated findings are hypertension and proteinuria.

DIAGNOSIS is suspected when a pregnant patient develops seizures or unexplained encephalopathy. Since idiopathic seizures can occur during pregnancy, not all seizures during pregnancy are due to eclampsia. Brain imaging is often not needed if the patient has recurrence of a known seizure disorder with typical seizure semiology. CT or MRI brain is performed if the patient has new-onset seizures, there are atypical features, or the seizures are prolonged or refractory. Other diagnoses to consider are arterial or venous infarction, cerebral hemorrhage, or CNS infection. Imaging may show findings typical of posterior reversible encephalopathy syndrome (PRES).

MANAGEMENT is usually with magnesium sulfate. Most obstetricians do not consult neurology for eclampsia unless seizures are refractory or focal neurologic symptoms develop. If seizures are refractory, benzodiazepines should be considered. BP management is addressed.

Cerebral Venous Thrombosis

Cerebral venous thrombosis (CVT) risk peaks in the early postpartum period and can occur in a variety of locations including cortical veins, sagittal sinus, lateral sinus, or cavernous sinus. A full-text review by Sasidharan is available at PMC.[3]

PRESENTATION is most commonly with headache. Nausea and vomiting are a common accompaniment. Neurologic symptoms depend on the location of the thrombosis and can include seizures, altered mental status, focal motor or sensory deficit, visual deficits, papilledema, or cranial nerve deficits.

DIAGNOSIS is suspected with headache that is more severe and of a different character than previous headaches. Seizures or focal deficits should raise particular concern over possible CVT. Brain imaging with CT may show no abnormalities acutely, but may show hemorrhagic change and, with time, may show signs of focal infarction. CT venogram (CTV) can show the thrombosis. MRI brain can show infarction that does not fall within an expected arterial distribution. MRA and MRV can be done together and can often show the venous occlusive disease.

MANAGEMENT has traditionally been with anticoagulation. This is discussed in detail in Chapter 16. Antibiotics are given if the thrombosis was induced by infection, particularly sinus.

Migraine

Migraine is common in women of childbearing age and can become worse or better during pregnancy. Occasionally, the first clinical manifestations of migraine may occur during pregnancy.

PRESENTATION is with typical migrainous headache as outlined in Chapter 20. Common symptoms are throbbing pain that is unilateral or bilateral, lasting 4–72 hours, often with nausea, vomiting, and photophobia. A visual or other aura may occur.

DIAGNOSIS is suspected with a migraine-type headache. Usually no imaging is needed and should be avoided in pregnancy if possible. But if the headache is prolonged, very severe, or if there are neurologic deficits, imaging with MRI is preferable to CT, especially since vascular visualization with MRA and MRV can be performed without contrast. Infarction and venous thrombosis are two differential diagnoses of particular concern, although they usually are much more prolonged than typical migraines and associated with neurologic deficits. New onset or prolonged (>1 hour) visual or other auras may warrant further workup.

MANAGEMENT:[4] Nonpharmacologic management of headaches during pregnancy is of utmost importance, and pregnant women should be encouraged to stay well hydrated, keep a regular sleep schedule, avoid skipping meals, and exercise regularly.

Some key points include:

- Acetaminophen is first-line therapy. Aspirin and nonsteroidal anti-inflammatory drugs (NSAIDs) should be avoided in the third trimester because they are associated with postpartum bleeding, neonatal bleeding, and premature closure of the fetal ductus arteriosus.
- Antiemetics (e.g., metoclopramide) are effective and safe during pregnancy.
- Triptans are avoided, but may be used for severe attacks when first-line drugs have failed; sumatriptan may also be used during lactation. Triptans do not seem to increase the risk of major congenital malformations, but there may be an increase in spontaneous abortions.
- Ergots are contraindicated.
- Many patients on preventative meds for migraine can discontinue them during pregnancy and ideally should discontinue them before a planned pregnancy. Medications with potential adverse effects on the fetus should be avoided, including especially valproate, but also topiramate.

- For women whose migraines improved during pregnancy, breast-feeding is encouraged because it helps maintain headache control during the postpartum period.

Epilepsy

Epilepsy can be exacerbated or improved during pregnancy. Concerns during pregnancy include:

- Effects of seizures on the mother
- Effects of seizures on the child
- Effects of the antiepileptic drugs (AEDs) on the child

Effects of seizures on the mother: Pregnancy can lower drug levels, thereby increasing the risk of seizure.[5] Seizures during pregnancy can lead to bodily injury to the mother, miscarriage, and ischemic changes to the fetus. Serum concentrations drop during pregnancy, varying from drug to drug, and these also vary depending on which trimester(s) are associated with the greatest drug level alterations. Close, often monthly, monitoring of serum concentrations is strongly recommended, with adjustments in dosing when appropriate.[6] Lower drug levels increase the risk of having a seizure while driving, placing the mother and others at a risk that is at least somewhat predictable.

Effects of seizures on the child: Seizures in the mother may have a deleterious effect on the child through the possibility of traumatic injury or hypoxia. If the seizure is not severe and limited in duration, then the risk of fetal injury is low.

Effects of AEDs on the child: The risk of congenital malformations in women without epilepsy who are on no AEDs is about 2–4%; women with epilepsy on first-generation AEDs carry a 4–8% risk, and women with epilepsy on second-generation AEDs appear to carry about a 3–4% risk as currently reported. More than 90% of women with epilepsy have normal, healthy outcomes. Particular drugs appear to have a higher risk of defects than others (e.g., valproate). Also, the risk is likely increased with multiple AEDs and high doses of AEDs.

MANAGEMENT *of epilepsy prior to pregnancy* begins with selecting those AEDs in women of childbearing potential that have the lowest risk of congenital malformations. Also, reducing the number of drugs can reduce the risk of malformations. Vitamin supplementation including folate before pregnancy is recommended. AEDs should be used at the lowest effective dose.

MANAGEMENT *of epilepsy during pregnancy* includes all the recommendations just mentioned. If a patient was on a regimen with significant risk much of the damage may have already been done.[7] However, there is still merit to improving the AED regimen. No medication is absolutely free from risk, but among the currently most commonly used AEDs during pregnancy are lamotrigine, levetiracetam, and oxcarbazepine. Doses often have to be increased during pregnancy and reduced following delivery, so clinical and laboratory monitoring are indicated. Seizure precautions are emphasized to patients.

Postpartum issues need to be addressed as well, including:

- Breastfeeding is not contraindicated in women with epilepsy.

- Barbiturates and benzodiazepines often cause sedation in the infant and can cause issues such as poor suck.
- Patients need to avoid sleep deprivation by having assistance with nighttime feeding to avoid risk of seizure due to sleep deprivation.

Myasthenia Gravis

Myasthenia gravis (MG) can worsen during pregnancy, especially in the first trimester, although at least half of patients have no change in disease severity or an actual improvement.

PRESENTATION of an exacerbation during pregnancy is worsening of fatigue, diplopia, ptosis, swallowing, or other deficit. An exacerbation of pre-existing deficit is more common than a new deficit heralding a new diagnosis of MG. Respiratory muscle involvement may progress to myasthenic crisis.

DIAGNOSIS is usually known, with documented electrophysiological and laboratory tests as described in Chapter 21. If the patient does not already carry the diagnosis, MG is suspected especially with ocular motor abnormalities, diplopia, and ptosis; diffuse weakness might be passed off as an effect of the pregnancy.

MANAGEMENT is similar to that for patients who are not pregnant.

- Acetylcholinesterase inhibitors (e.g., pyridostigmine) may have to be increased with pregnancy, but overuse should be avoided because they may induce uterine contractions or premature labor.
- Corticosteroids may be used for acute exacerbation, being cognizant of the transient worsening that is common with institution of therapy and an increased risk for cleft palate when given during the first trimester, as well as an increased risk of premature rupture of membranes with prednisone.
- Plasma exchange and IV immunoglobulin (IVIg) may also be used during pregnancy for exacerbations, but should be given only for severe MG symptoms or myasthenic crisis, and the patients need to be closely monitored for hypotension, hyperviscosity, and volume overload. Induced abortions are a potential risk.
- Other immunosuppressants should be avoided during pregnancy.
- Magnesium should be avoided because it can block neuromuscular transmission and precipitate an exacerbation of MG.

If the patient is unable to deliver vaginally for any reason including systemic weakness, the anesthesiologists needs to be aware of the MG diagnosis for medication selection. Close attention is paid to respiratory function since this can acutely deteriorate. These patients benefit most from a multidisciplinary team that includes obstetricians, perinatologists, and neurologists who follow the patient closely throughout the pregnancy.

Peripheral Nerve Injuries

Peripheral nerve injuries can develop from direct compression in the pelvis or of vulnerable peripheral nerves or from indirect effects of pregnancy with edema and weight gain. Common syndromes are neuropathies affecting the lower extremities (lateral femoral cutaneous nerve-meralgia paresthetica, lumbosacral radiculopathy), carpal tunnel syndrome, and Bell palsy.[8]

Most of these syndromes spontaneously improve. We try to avoid use of corticosteroids for Bell palsy in pregnancy.[9]

Multiple Sclerosis

Multiple sclerosis (MS) attacks are usually lessened in patients during pregnancy. At the time of this writing, none of the disease-modifying agents has been approved for use in pregnancy. Recommendations are that patients discontinue these meds prior to becoming pregnant. If a patient becomes pregnant on disease-modifying medications, it is generally recommended that she stop the med. The risk seems to be higher for interferons and chemotherapy agents than for glatiramer. Corticosteroids are sometimes used during pregnancy, but these also have the potential for complications. Consult the most current literature and recommendations when discussing this crucial issue with patients.

28 Endocrine Disorders

Karl E. Misulis, MD, PhD and
E. Lee Murray, MD

CHAPTER CONTENTS

- Overview
- Diabetes Mellitus
  - Diabetic Neuropathy
- Thyroid Disorders
  - Hyperthyroidism
  - Hypothyroidism
  - Hashimoto Encephalopathy
  - Thyroid Ophthalmopathy
- Adrenal Disorders
  - Cushing Syndrome
  - Addison Disease
  - Pheochromocytoma
- Pituitary Disorders
  - Pituitary Tumor
  - Pituitary Apoplexy
  - Diabetes Insipidus
  - SIADH

OVERVIEW

Some of the most important endocrine disorders with neurologic manifestations are listed here, and details of most of these disorders are included in the following sections. Disorders discussed elsewhere are so indicated.

- *Diabetic neuropathy*: Can be polyneuropathy with mainly sensory symptoms, mononeuropathy, mononeuropathy multiplex, ocular motor palsy, or diabetic amyotrophy
- *Thyroid ophthalmopathy*: Proptosis and diplopia, typically bilateral
- *Thyrotoxicosis*: Fatigue, weakness, tremor, associated with tachycardia, weight loss
- *Hashimoto encephalopathy*: Memory difficulty, personality change, symptoms of hypothyroidism, with possibly seizures and/or neurologic deficits.
- *Pheochromocytoma*: Episodic headache with hypertension, tachycardia, diaphoresis, orthostatic hypotension

- *Cushing syndrome*: Neurologic presentation of proximal muscle weakness with central obesity, moon facies
- *Addison disease*: Neurologic symptoms include progressive muscle weakness, occasionally acute, with hyperkalemia, depression, orthostatic hypotension; systemic symptoms of hyperpigmentation, weight loss, nausea, vomiting
- *Pituitary tumor*: Headache, visual field disturbance, ocular motor deficit, sometimes associated with hormonal derangements
- *Pituitary apoplexy*: Abrupt onset of headache, visual deficit, ocular motor deficit from pituitary infarction or hemorrhage
- *Diabetes insipidus (DI)*: Polyuria and polydipsia due to loss of antidiuretic hormone (ADH; also known as arginine vasopressin, AVP). Commonly in the setting of cerebral trauma or surgery but can be due to brain tumors
- *Syndrome of inappropriate antidiuretic hormone (SIADH)*: Weakness, depression, confusion, lethargy due to profound hyponatremia; usually caused by acute cerebral lesion (e.g., trauma, infection)

DIABETES MELLITUS

Hospital neurology consultation in patients with diabetes is usually for the following indications:

- Diabetic neuropathy
- Hypoglycemic encephalopathy (Chapter 11)
- Ocular motor palsy (Chapter 33)
- Stroke in a patient with diabetes (Chapters 11 and 16)
- Neurologic symptoms with hyperglycemic state (Chapter 11)
- Seizures with hyper- or hypoglycemic state (Chapters 11 and 19)

Some important disorders in diabetics who come to neurology consultation are discussed here; others are discussed in their respective chapters as indicated.

Diabetic Neuropathy

Diabetes mellitus neuropathic complications:

- *Peripheral neuropathy*: Mixed polyneuropathy with sensory symptoms predominating but also motor and autonomic manifestations.
- *Mononeuropathy*: Acute symptomatic neuropathy with involvement of almost any of the arm, leg, or cranial nerves.
- *Mononeuropathy multiplex*: Almost any nerve can be affected, but most common are ulnar, median, radial, peroneal.
- *Ocular motor palsy*: Painful CN 3 palsy, pupil-sparing, is the most common. CN-6 palsy can be seen less commonly. Usually unilateral.
- *Autonomic neuropathy*: Broad range of symptoms including orthostatic hypotension, decreased pupil response, impaired sweating, bladder distention with incomplete emptying, and gastroparesis with abdominal pain, nausea/vomiting, and constipation.

- *Lumbar radiculoplexopathy (diabetic amyotrophy)*: Proximal plexopathy and/or radiculopathy with lumbar involvement producing unilateral weakness in an L2–L4 distribution. Associated with pain in the back extending to the thigh.

Details of the evaluation of neuropathy are found in Chapter 21. *Electromyogram (EMG)* and *nerve conduction studies (NCS)* are indicated for most patients with peripheral neuropathy. Some patients have mononeuropathies superimposed on polyneuropathy.

CSF analysis is not needed unless there is concern for an infectious or inflammatory cause.

MANAGEMENT begins with best diabetes care. Note that many of the medications used for diabetic neuropathic pain are not approved by the US Food and Drug Administration (FDA) for that indication.

- *Polyneuropathy*
  - Anticonvulsants, antidepressants; especially amitriptyline, gabapentin, pregabalin, and duloxetine
  - Others include nortriptyline, paroxetine, citalopram, carbamazepine; NSAIDs are sometimes tried.
- *Mononeuropathy and mononeuropathy multiplex*
  - Occasional patients may benefit from decompression when entrapment is believed to be a significant contributing factor.
  - Pain is managed as for polyneuropathy.
  - Mononeuropathy can be exacerbated by compression, so protection and avoidance can be helpful, especially in patients who have had significant weight loss.
- *Lumbar radiculoplexopathy*
  - Best diabetes management and physical therapy
  - Pain can be managed as for polyneuropathy.
- *Autonomic neuropathy*
  - Orthostatic hypotension can be managed by elastic hose to thigh or higher, increasing Na intake, midodrine, fludrocortisone; use caution in those with supine hypertension.
  - Pyridostigmine can be used in those with supine hypertension.
  - Droxidopa is another option for orthostatic hypotension.[1]

THYROID DISORDERS
Hyperthyroidism

Hyperthyroidism has many potential causes, including Graves disease, thyroid adenoma, pituitary adenoma producing thyroid stimulating hormone (TSH), and thyroiditis. Most common is Graves disease, an autoimmune disorder.

PRESENTATION is with both neurologic and systemic symptoms:

- *Neurologic symptoms* include weakness especially proximal, fatigue, tremor, proptosis, eyelid retraction, and lid lag, Tendon reflexes may be enhanced.
- *Systemic symptoms* can include thyroid enlargement (esp. with Graves disease), weight loss, tachycardia.

DIAGNOSIS is suspected when patients present with weakness and weight loss and is supported by tachycardia. TSH is low with Graves disease and thyroiditis, and thyroid antibodies are demonstrated in many patients with Graves disease and thyroiditis. Radioactive iodine imaging of the thyroid may have to be performed to look for cancer. Thyroid ultrasound and sometimes biopsy may be needed.

MANAGEMENT of Graves disease can be by radioactive iodine, antithyroid meds, or thyroidectomy:

- Medical management of the hyperthyroid state includes beta-blockers especially for cardiovascular symptoms and tremor, and antithyroid drugs. Some patients will need thyroid replacement after treatment.
- Surgery may be needed for severe or refractory cases or in patients with adenoma or multinodular goiter.

Hypothyroidism

Hypothyroidism is a low thyroid hormone level due to a variety of causes that localize to the hypothalamus, pituitary, or thyroid. Autoimmune thyroiditis is common, with other important possibilities being post-thyroid treatment for hyperthyroidism or goiter, radiation treatment of the neck for other reason, iodine deficiency, some medications including lithium, some anticonvulsants[2] (phenytoin, valproate, phenobarbital, carbamazepine, and oxcarbazepine), or reduced pituitary TSH production.

PRESENTATION depends on severity: symptoms can be from mild to marked encephalopathy. Systemic features can be weight gain, dry skin, constipation, cold intolerance.

DIAGNOSIS is suspected with cognitive deficits or depression with weight gain or unexplained encephalopathy precipitating thyroid function tests.

- TSH and free T4 are the usual first steps in lab evaluation.
- Antithyroid antibodies may be elevated, especially in Hashimoto thyroiditis.
- Thyroid ultrasound may be needed. Fine-needle aspiration may be needed for thyroid nodules.

MANAGEMENT begins with thyroid hormone replacement for most patients. TSH or T4 levels are monitored depending on the location of the defect (thyroid or pituitary, respectively).

Hashimoto Encephalopathy

Hashimoto encephalopathy is associated with *Hashimoto thyroiditis*. It is sometimes called *steroid-responsive encephalopathy with autoimmune thyroiditis (STREAT)*.

PRESENTATION is classically with encephalopathy that can be accompanied by multifocal myoclonus, focal deficits, tremor, psychosis, or seizures. Presentation may suggest a host of metabolic disorders. Other symptoms of hypothyroidism are common (e.g., weight gain, constipation, cold intolerance).

DIAGNOSIS is suspected with encephalopathy plus myoclonus, yet metabolic parameters are insufficient to explain the findings. Anti-thyroperoxidase and anti-thyroglobulin antibodies are typically elevated, but might be normal. TSH is often elevated in symptomatic patients but might be normal. Electroencephalogram (EEG) usually shows slowing, but epileptiform discharges can be seen. Magnetic resonance imaging (MRI) does not show any specific abnormalities.

MANAGEMENT begins with corticosteroids that often produces improvement within just a few days. Associated seizures and/or thyroid status must also be addressed.

Thyroid Ophthalmopathy

Thyroid ophthalmopathy is a restrictive disorder of extraocular muscles caused by an antibody-mediated effect that causes a lymphocytic inflammatory response.

PRESENTATION is usually with proptosis. Neurologic presentation can be with diplopia. Lid retraction is seen. Findings can include especially median and inferior rectus restriction even to passive movement. Esotropia or visual loss can occur.

DIAGNOSIS suspected with proptosis and ocular motor deficits. Labs show a hyperthyroid state, which is diagnostic with a typical clinical presentation.

MANAGEMENT of the hyperthyroid state is standard, and corticosteroids are used for patients with optic neuropathy or a significant symptomatic inflammatory component.

ADRENAL DISORDERS

Adrenal disorders of principal importance to the hospital neurologist include:

- Cushing syndrome
- Addison disease
- Pheochromocytoma

Cushing Syndrome

Cushing syndrome produces excess glucocorticoids. This is most commonly due to systemic administration of corticosteroids, but may be due to overstimulation by adrenocorticotropic hormone (ACTH) from the pituitary, stimulation from occult malignancy (e.g., small-cell lung cancer), or a primary adrenal-secreting tumor.

PRESENTATION is with neurologic and medical manifestations:

- *Neurologic*: Weakness from proximal myopathy. Neuropsychiatric abnormalities can include depression, confusion, occasional psychotic features.
- *Medical*: Obesity, diabetes, hypertension, striae, bruising, moon facies, buffalo hump. Many of these are only seen with long-term effect.

DIAGNOSIS is mainly suspected when a history of glucocorticoid use suggests an iatrogenic cause. Otherwise, diagnosis is suspected from body changes and weakness and then documentation of excess cortisol production with failure of dexamethasone suppression. Additional imaging for pituitary or other tumor location may be indicated depending on the study results.

MANAGEMENT begins with cessation of any exogenous corticosteroids. If tumor is found, treatment depends on location, type, and stage. After treatment, it is essential to watch for glucocorticoid deficiency. In case of an inability to remove the cause of ACTH excess, medical treatment may be helpful with ketoconazole, metyrapone, or mitotane.

Addison Disease

Addison disease is hypoadrenalism usually due to destruction of the adrenal; it has many potential causes, including autoimmune disorders, tumors, infection, hemorrhage, or from adrenal surgery.

PRESENTATION has neurologic and medical manifestations:

- *Neurologic*: Progressive muscle weakness; sometimes acute weakness due to hyperkalemia. Some patients have myalgias, depression.
- *Medical*: Hyperpigmentation, nausea, vomiting, orthostatic hypotension, salt-craving

DIAGNOSIS is suspected especially in patients with progressive weakness with hyperpigmentation. Rapid ACTH stimulation test shows low aldosterone level and failure of an adequate increase with stimulation.

MANAGEMENT begins with replacement with hydrocortisone or prednisone plus fludrocortisone. Doses often must be increased during illness. Management is more complex in diabetics due to difficulty with glucose control.

Pheochromocytoma

Pheochromocytoma is a tumor that releases catecholamines, usually from the adrenal medulla. Neurologic manifestations are due to severe hypertension. The tumors are usually benign but can be malignant. Most common occurrence is in middle-aged or younger patients.

PRESENTATION has neurologic and medical manifestations:

- *Neurologic*: Episodes of headache, palpitations, associated with marked hypertension. Can present with hypertensive intracranial hemorrhage with a history suggestive of episodic hypertension.
- *Medical*: Often associated with diaphoresis, nausea, with acute episodes. Chronic symptoms may include weight loss, orthostatic hypotension.

DIAGNOSIS is suspected with episodes of headache, palpitations, and hypertension, or in a patients with intracranial hemorrhage who has a history of similar symptoms. Catecholamine levels support the diagnosis. Imaging of the adrenal is warranted if tumor is suspected.

MANAGEMENT is best with removal of the tumor if possible. Preoperative treatment is given to reduce the risk of crisis during surgery. This can be by combined alpha- and beta-adrenergic blockade. Metyrosine reduces catecholamine synthesis and is prescribed specifically for pheochromocytoma.

PITUITARY DISORDERS
Pituitary Tumor

Pituitary tumors are usually benign and may be functional or nonfunctional. Hormonal change can be from increased or decreased production. Pituitary tumors are generally not susceptible to hypothalamic control. Neurologic symptoms can be from changes in hormonal release due to the tumor or due to mass effect.

PRESENTATION depends on size, whether they are functional or nonfunctional, and on which hormones are affected:

- *Common findings independent of alteration in hormone levels*: Headache, visual field disturbance, diplopia, ptosis. Visual field defect is typically bitemporal hemianopia. More extensive mass effect can produce diabetes DI, encephalopathy, and even seizures, but this is uncommon.
- *Prolactin-secreting adenomas*:
  o Males: Hypogonadism, rarely galactorrhea
  o Females: Galactorrhea, amenorrhea, infertility
- *Growth hormone-producing*: Acromegaly, often with headache; patients may develop diabetes mellitus.
- *ACTH-producing adenomas*: Cushing syndrome

DIAGNOSIS is suspected by core symptoms of headache, visual field defect, and ocular motor abnormalities or by hormonal abnormalities as described:

  o *Hormonal assay* is directed by symptoms, measurement for prolactin, growth hormone, ACTH.
  o *MRI with special attention to pituitary* is the best imaging study.

MANAGEMENT depends on the size and function of the tumor:

- Prolactin-producing adenomas are usually treated with bromocriptine.
- Growth hormone-producing adenomas are often treated with octreotide.
- ACTH-producing adenomas involve surgical treatment or medical management (Chapter 28).

Endocrinology consultation is recommended for assistance in evaluation and management of these disorders.

Pituitary Apoplexy

Pituitary apoplexy is infarction or hemorrhage into the pituitary, usually occurring postpartum or due to a pituitary adenoma. Symptoms are due to involvement of optic nerves and chiasm and ocular motor nerves in the cavernous sinus. Headache is likely from dural stress from the lesion.

PRESENTATION is classically with abrupt onset of headache, visual deficit, ocular motor deficit with diplopia, and often ptosis. Headache is present in almost all cases. Nausea and vomiting are common. Incipient visual field deficit might not be noted until acute presentation. Non-neurologic complications can include profound hypotension and syncope.

DIAGNOSIS is suspected with acute onset of headache with visual field and/or ocular motor deficits. A bitemporal superior quadrant defect is classic:

- Emergent computed tomography (CT) of the brain often shows pituitary enlargement, sometimes with evidence of hemorrhage.
- MRI brain and pituitary shows ischemic or hemorrhagic pituitary changes that can be characteristic.
- CSF usually shows increased WBC, increased RBC, and increased opening pressure.

MANAGEMENT is a combination of medical and surgical treatment:

- Emergent hemodynamic stabilization is provided as needed.
- Electrolyte management
- Corticosteroids are given, typically at high dose.
- Surgical decompression might be needed for ongoing mass effect with neurologic symptoms.

Diabetes Insipidus

DI is a fluid-electrolyte disorder producing polyuria and polydipsia due to loss of ADH/AVP. Neurologic causes are usually head injury, cranial surgery, or tumor.

PRESENTATION is with polyuria, polydipsia, and nocturia in the setting of a recent neurologic event. No specific neurologic signs are present other than of the precipitating event unless the patient develops encephalopathy and/or seizures.

DIAGNOSIS is usually suspected with polyuria. Diagnosis is confirmed with electrolyte and osmolarity determination of urine and blood. ADH can be measured but is not required for diagnosis.

MANAGEMENT begins with oral or IV replacement of fluids. Monitoring of electrolytes and tailoring fluids to electrolyte levels are essential. Desmopressin (DDAVP) is used to reduce renal losses.

SIADH

Syndrome of inappropriate anti-diuretic hormone (SIADH) is the inappropriate secretion of ADH/AVP with regard to serum osmolality. SIADH is usually due to an acute cerebral lesion such as trauma or surgery. It can also be due to ectopic production by tumor.

PRESENTATION is commonly with weakness, depression, confusion, and lethargy, with profound hyponatremia. Early symptoms may be minimal and may be only nausea. Severe cases may show encephalopathy, tremor, myoclonus, seizures, and coma.

DIAGNOSIS is suspected usually when a patient has unexplained hyponatremia, especially with an implicated neurologic event. Labs show continued renal release of sodium despite the hyponatremia and hypo-osmolality.

MANAGEMENT begins with water restriction. Demeclocycline is seldom used because of its potential toxicity and the effectiveness of other therapies. NaCl infusions may be needed for severe symptomatic hyponatremia.

29 Nutritional Deficiencies and Toxicities

Karl E. Misulis, MD, PhD and
E. Lee Murray, MD

CHAPTER CONTENTS

- Overview
- B_{12} Deficiency
- B_1 Deficiency
- Protein-Energy Malnutrition
- Folate Deficiency
- B_6 Deficiency
- B_6 Toxicity
- Copper Deficiency
- Vitamin D Deficiency

OVERVIEW

The most common nutritional disorders seen in hospital neurology practice are:

- B_{12} deficiency
- B_1 deficiency
- Malnutrition

These and some other important disorders are discussed here. Links to related disorders discussed in other chapters are also shown.

B_{12} DEFICIENCY

B_{12} deficiency is usually from impaired absorption especially with advanced age. Dietary deficiency is uncommon.

PRESENTATION is neurologic and systemic:

- *Neurologic:* Symptoms of neuropathy, myelopathy, or cognitive impairment may occur. Signs can include confusion and tendon reflexes reduced (neuropathy) or increased (myelopathy).
- *Systemic:* Common symptoms are fatigue and weakness from anemia. Glossitis occurs uncommonly.

DIAGNOSIS is considered in patients with a broad range of neurologic dysfunction, and is usually part of routine testing for neurologists.

- B_{12} *level* is usually reduced; methylmalonic acid (MMA) level testing is performed if B_{12} deficiency is suspected; high MMA suggests B_{12} deficiency.
- *Folate level* testing is also performed. Note that folate supplementation can prevent hematologic manifestations of B_{12} deficiency but not the neurologic events.
- *Schilling test* is performed for pernicious anemia, especially in younger patients but is seldom needed in older patients.

MANAGEMENT with B_{12} replacement is usually IM initially followed by oral replacement. Intra-oral absorption is better than gastric absorption for many patients so dissolvable or liquid preparations may be used.[1]

B₁ DEFICIENCY

B_1 deficiency usually occurs in the setting of starvation (cancer, anorexia nervosa, situational), alcoholism, or gastric bypass. Increased thiamine demand can occur with a variety of stresses including renal failure on dialysis, sepsis, pregnancy, or intractable diarrhea.

PRESENTATION classically has two related presentations: *Wernicke encephalopathy* and *Korsakoff syndrome.*

- *Wernicke encephalopathy* may present with a classic triad of confusion, ataxia, and ophthalmoplegia. The diagnosis is suspected especially when at least two of the triad are present. Ocular findings are incomplete, with nystagmus most common; pupil involvement is less likely. Ataxia is mainly of gait.
- *Korsakoff syndrome* follows episodes of Wernicke encephalopathy. Patients develop confusion and memory loss, usually with residual nystagmus or other ocular motor abnormality, plus gait ataxia. Peripheral neuropathy is often present.

DIAGNOSIS is considered in any patient presenting with confusion and/or ophthalmoplegia. Clinical suspicion is sufficient to start treatment. Unexplained confusion even in the absence of ocular motor abnormalities or ataxia should trigger consideration, especially if there is a possibility of alcohol abuse or malnutrition.

- *Lab*: Erythrocyte transketolase activity can be measured but is not needed for most cases and should not delay treatment. CSF analysis is often needed for unexplained encephalopathy but would show no specific findings for Wernicke encephalopathy.
- *Imaging*: Cerebral imaging is usually needed because at-risk populations may develop subdural hematoma, abscess, infarction, or other structural abnormalities. Magnetic resonance imaging (MRI) may show signal change in the mammillary bodies and periaqueductal gray.

MANAGEMENT with thiamine replacement improves Wernicke encephalopathy and reduces the chance of development of Korsakoff syndrome. We usually give parenteral thiamine and administer it before other IV fluids; symptoms may worsen with glucose-containing fluids.

PROTEIN-ENERGY MALNUTRITION

Protein-energy malnutrition is often undiagnosed in hospitalized patients. This is a deficiency of multiple nutrients, energy-containing materials, and protein.

PRESENTATION begins with weight loss, although edema may mask this initially. Complications of malnutrition can occur before the patient becomes underweight. Fatigue and weakness are common. Exam may reveal nonhealing wounds, decubitus ulcers, dystrophic nail changes, and other findings that are dependent on specific vitamin deficiencies.

DIAGNOSIS is considered in any patient with prolonged decrease in oral intake, prolonged hospitalization, alcoholism, cancer, or other significant risk factor. Labs show low albumin and protein and often low glucose. Other findings can include elevated cortisol level, low cholesterol, and often iron-deficiency anemia.

MANAGEMENT begins with fluids and electrolyte management to correct deficits. Nutritional supplementation with multivitamins is given.

Refeeding syndrome is an underdiagnosed condition with edema, electrolyte abnormalities, and hyperglycemia. Risk of this can be reduced by a gradual institution of full refeeding.

FOLATE DEFICIENCY

Folate deficiency is usually due to decreased intake, especially with alcoholism and other causes of malnutrition, in which case folate deficiency is combined with other deficiencies. Other important causes include pregnancy or the use of some meds, including methotrexate, metformin, and trimethoprim, as well as enzyme-inducing anticonvulsants. Folate deficiency can resemble B_{12} deficiency and is often coexistent with it and megaloblastic anemia.

PRESENTATION can be neurologic or systemic:

- *Neurologic*: Confusion, mood change with depression, weakness
- *Systemic*: Glossitis, often with diarrhea
- *Pregnancy*: Mothers who do not receive sufficient folate have a higher risk of neural tube defects in their children.

DIAGNOSIS is considered in patients with confusion, especially with glossitis and/or identified with megaloblastic anemia. Folate levels are low. B_{12} levels should be checked also. Since many patients at risk for folate deficiency are also at risk for other deficiencies, these should be considered, especially B_{12} and thiamine.

MANAGEMENT begins with folate supplementation combined with other vitamins and nutrients as indicated by studies. Folate supplementation during pregnancy is at a higher dose than for other patients.

B_6 DEFICIENCY

B_6 is a complex of chemicals of which pyridoxine is just one. Deficiency is uncommon but can occur especially with malnutrition due to starvation or alcoholism and with certain medications that inactivate pyridoxine, including isoniazid. Manifestations can be peripheral neuropathy, encephalopathy, and/or seizures. Associated findings can be glossitis, dermatitis, and anemia. Seizures are more of an issue in young children.

B₆ TOXICITY

B_6 toxicity is not expected with dietary intake but rather from aggressive supplementation. Peripheral neuropathy is most prominent, initially with sensory symptoms including pain and dysesthesias of the extremities and loss of vibration and proprioception.

PRESENTATION may be with a sensory ataxia. Motor neuropathy can develop with weakness affecting ambulation.

DIAGNOSIS is considered when a patient with progressive neuropathic symptoms, perhaps considered to have acute inflammatory demyelinating polyneuropathy (AIDP), is identified as taking supplements. Nerve conduction studies do not differentiate well between these disorders because in both AIDP and B6 toxicity nerve conduction velocities can be slowed with increased F-wave latency.

COPPER DEFICIENCY

Acquired cooper deficiency is uncommon in adults but is looked for especially in patients with unexplained weakness. Causes in adults can include gastric bypass surgery. Weakness can be from myelopathy or neuropathy. The diagnosis is suspected especially when progressive weakness is accompanied by anemia or myelodysplasia. Copper deficiency in adults is often combined with B_{12} deficiency.

VITAMIN D DEFICIENCY

Neurologic presentation of vitamin D deficiency is not expected other than muscle pains associated with the skeletal manifestations. However, vitamin D deficiency may increase the risk of multiple sclerosis (MS). Also, vitamin D supplementation in patients who already have MS may reduce the frequency and severity of acute attacks. Therefore, many clinicians check vitamin D levels in patients with confirmed or suspected MS.

30 Neurotoxicology

Karl E. Misulis, MD, PhD and
E. Lee Murray, MD

CHAPTER CONTENTS

- Overview
- Prescription Medications
- Ethanol and Other Alcohols
  - Ethanol
  - Alcoholic Neuropathy
  - Alcoholic Myopathy
  - Isopropanol
  - Methanol
  - Ethylene Glycol
- Heavy Metals
  - Lead Poisoning
  - Mercury Poisoning
  - Arsenic Poisoning
- Cholinesterase Inhibitors

OVERVIEW

Toxin exposure is a common reason for a ED visit, and although most of these are managed by emergency physicians and internists, neurologists are sometimes called on to assist with selected toxin exposures. Prescription medications and household chemicals are common causes of toxic neurologic symptoms, some acute, some insidious. Here, we focus on some of the most important toxic exposures, selected by virtue of frequency or severity.

PRESCRIPTION MEDICATIONS

A list of medications with potential neurologic toxicity is far beyond the scope of this book, but a brief synopsis of some of the most important is discussed. It is sometimes difficult to distinguish between idiosyncratic effect, hypersensitivity, allergy, and dose-dependent toxicity, so some of these are blended in this discussion. The neurologic toxicity of some common medications includes:

- Anticonvulsants
  - *Sedation*: Many

- o *Exacerbation of seizures*: Several, especially carbamazepine.[1]
- o *Hyponatremia*: especially carbamazepine and oxcarbazepine.
- Neuroleptics
  - o *Acute dystonic reaction*: Many
  - o *Tardive dyskinesia*: Many, less for atypical neuroleptics
  - o *Neuroleptic malignant syndrome*: Many
  - o *Parkinsonism*: Especially typical neuroleptics
- Antidepressants
  - o *Seizures*
  - o *Headaches*
  - o *Orthostatic hypotension*
  - o *Confusion*
- Amiodarone
  - o *Tremor*: Most common neurological complication, postural and intention[2]
  - o *Parkinsonism*: Uncommon[3]
- Baclofen
  - o *Encephalopathy*: Can be profound

Antidepressants are associated with a variety of neurologic complications; however, they are overrepresented even in patients who are not treated.[4]

ETHANOL AND OTHER ALCOHOLS

Alcohol intoxication is usually presumed to be ethanol, but this term includes others, especially isopropanol, methanol, and ethylene glycol. This section will focus on ethanol with subsequent brief discussions of the other alcohols.

Ethanol

Hospital neurologists see the spectrum of ethanol effects from acute intoxication to chronic neuronal degeneration to neurologic manifestations of liver failure. The list presents some of the important syndromes resulting in neurologic consultation:

- Acute intoxication
- Hepatic failure: Chapter 11
- Wernicke-Korsakoff syndrome: Chapter 29
- Ethanol withdrawal
- Cerebellar degeneration
- Optic neuropathy
- Central pontine myelinolysis (CPM): Chapter 13
- Optic neuropathy
- Neuropathy
- Myopathy

Ethanol Intoxication

Ethanol intoxication manifests a range of symptoms that depend on individual susceptibilities and metabolism. Levels that are well-tolerated by some may produce severe intoxication in others. Chronic ethanol use can produce neuronal degeneration directly and/or manifest neurologic symptoms through coexistent nutritional deficiency.

PRESENTATION may be excitatory or depressive. Patients may have agitation, excitement, and enhanced loquaciousness. Alternatively, they may be lethargic or somnolent. There may be cognitive dysfunction with disinhibition progressing to confusion, stupor, and even coma. Motor manifestations are most commonly dysarthria and gait ataxia. Rare complications are acute psychosis and "blackouts"—epochs for which the patient is amnestic.

DIAGNOSIS is suspected with the clinical presentation of cognitive and behavioral deficits with ataxia and dysarthria. Clinicians usually notice the typical breath of ethanol intoxication. Confirmation is by documentation of elevated ethanol levels. Note that identification of ethanol intoxication does not rule out coexistent disorder so computed tomography (CT) should be performed if the symptoms are out of proportion to the ethanol level or if there are clinical signs of head injury, mental status changes, focal deficits, or seizures.

MANAGEMENT begins with supportive care for most patients. Hemodialysis is considered for refractory patients and those with extremely high ethanol levels.

Ethanol Withdrawal

Ethanol withdrawal can cause an array of neurologic manifestations. Timing of onset depends on the manifestation. Persistent intake and abrupt withdrawal can begin to produce symptoms within 6 hours, whereas delirium tremens (DTs) has an onset 48–72 hours later.

PRESENTATION begins in about 6 hours with mild tremor, the "morning shakes." With progressive time and severity, progression through delirium to DTs can occur. Symptoms of ethanol withdrawal are summarized here:

- Mild: Tremulous, sweating, headache, and often GI symptoms
- Moderate: Restlessness, agitation; may be hyper-alert
- Severe: Delirium tremens with confusion, agitation, hallucinations, often with associated fever, tachycardia, and diaphoresis

Seizures are common during the withdrawal period, usually around 12 hours from last intake. They are usually single; repetitive seizures are less likely.

DIAGNOSIS is suspected with the development of agitated delirium especially with seizure in the absence of another obvious cause. Studies include CT brain for structural lesion, electroencephalogram (EEG) for seizure activity, and sometimes lumbar puncture (LP) for infection. Fever and encephalopathy should prompt consideration of LP even if the patient is a known alcoholic since meningitis and encephalitis still would be in the differential diagnosis.

MANAGEMENT begins with supportive care including fluid and electrolyte management. Patients commonly are dehydrated, malnourished, and are predisposed to hyponatremia, hypokalemia, and hypomagnesemia.

- Thiamine supplementation is given if ethanol abuse is suspected, even if the diagnosis is not confirmed.
- Sedation with chlordiazepoxide, diazepam, or lorazepam is often helpful. Phenobarbital is sometimes used for refractory cases.

- *Seizure* recurrence can be reduced by lorazepam (often 2 mg IV) after the first seizure. Long-term antiepileptic drugs are usually not needed.

Alcoholic Cerebellar Degeneration

Alcoholic cerebellar degeneration is progressive gait ataxia due to neuronal degeneration. Although this is most commonly seen in alcoholics, it is also seen in patients with nutritional deficiency for other reasons.

PRESENTATION is with gait ataxia, consisting of a wide-based stance. Gait often has a shuffling appearance. Ocular findings are uncommon but can include nystagmus and saccadic pursuit. The presentation of unexplained gait ataxia should prompt questioning and investigation of possible ethanol use.

DIAGNOSIS is suspected with progressive gait ataxia without another evident cause. Ethanol toxicity is suspected especially with ocular motor findings. Limb ataxia or dysarthria as part of a cerebellar syndrome suggests other diagnoses.

Brain imaging shows no strokes or other structural lesion, but there is prominent atrophy of the superior cerebellar vermis on sagittal magnetic resonance imaging (MRI); this finding may not be noted by some radiologists—yet another reason for neurologists to view images themselves.

MANAGEMENT is supportive. There is no specific treatment for the ataxia. Cessation of ethanol intake is key. Nutritional supplementation is given, including thiamine as well as other vitamins and nutrients. The ataxia often persists despite abstinence.

Optic Neuropathy with Alcohol Abuse

Optic neuropathy can develop in patients with ethanol abuse. This is likely multifactorial, a direct effect of ethanol plus other agents. Tobacco-alcohol amblyopia is a manifestation of this. Effects may be indirect, including nutritional deficiency, B_1 and B_{12} deficiency, or mediated by accumulation of formic acid with resultant mitochondrial dysfunction.

PRESENTATION is with subacute development of blurred or dim vision. Visual difficulty develops over weeks and is painless. Exam shows centrocecal scotoma. Optic nerves may show pallor, especially on the temporal aspect of the discs.[5] Visual loss may progress to blindness.

DIAGNOSIS is suggested by the presentation of bilateral painless visual loss in a patient with a history of significant ethanol use, especially if there is also a smoking history. Coexistent cerebellar ataxia or neuropathy supports the diagnosis. MRI brain and even LP often have to be performed to look for other causes. However, optic neuritis is usually not painless and also can be associated with very different funduscopic findings.

MANAGEMENT begins with cessation of ethanol consumption. Nutritional supplementation is given to ensure adequate protein-calorie intake and specifically sufficient B_1 and B_{12}. Improvement in vision is expected with optimal treatment and ethanol abstinence.

Alcoholic Neuropathy

Alcoholic neuropathy is a common complication of chronic ethanol use. It is seldom found in isolation; it usually is seen in combination with other complications of alcoholism.

PRESENTATION is with sensory more than motor symptoms, although both develop. Pain and paresthesias can develop.

DIAGNOSIS is suspected with symptoms and signs of neuropathy and a confirmed or suspected history of ethanol abuse. Nerve conduction studies and electromyogram (NCS/EMG) can confirm the neuropathy. Additional labs for hepatic and other associated abnormalities are helpful.

MANAGEMENT is with cessation of ethanol intake and adequate nutrition. Medications for neuropathic pain may be needed; non-narcotic meds are preferred.

Alcoholic Myopathy

Alcoholic myopathy can be acute or chronic. It can lead to rhabdomyolysis (Chapter 21).

PRESENTATION is with muscle weakness, usually proximal, with pain, and this is usually contemporaneous with an increase in alcohol consumption.

DIAGNOSIS is suspected when a patient presents with rhabdomyolysis (acutely) or weakness with a myopathic character (chronically) and has a known or suspected history of ethanol abuse.

MANAGEMENT is by cessation of ethanol use and adequate nutrition. There are no other specific treatments.

Isopropanol

Isopropanol (isopropyl alcohol) is most commonly encountered as the principal ingredient of some brands of rubbing alcohol. Isopropanol is sometimes consumed by accident or intentionally as an ethanol substitute.[6]

PRESENTATION can be mild or severe. Mild symptoms include nausea and vomiting. Severe symptoms include CNS and respiratory depression and progressive deterioration. Cardiovascular collapse can develop.

DIAGNOSIS is most likely to be suspected with a history of ingestion. In the absence of this history, it is suspected when the patient is noted to have a breath with a sweet smell and is found to have ketosis without acidosis. Isopropanol levels are elevated.

MANAGEMENT is supportive for most patients. For patients with severe poisoning, hemodialysis should be considered.

Methanol

Methanol is a commonly used solvent and is also found in some home-distilled drinks. Methanol is suspected especially when a patient presents with visual difficulty after an episode of intoxication, but this is unfortunately late in the process. Formic acid is produced in the retina. Exposure may be as an ethanol substitute or in a suicide attempt.

PRESENTATION early is with clinical intoxication similar to that of ethanol. After 1–2 days, visual difficulty may develop with blurring and flashes of light. Subsequently, headache then cognitive changes can develop with confusion, possibly progressing to lethargy and coma.

DIAGNOSIS is considered with unexplained encephalopathy and increased osmolar gap. Amylase is often increased. Hemorrhagic pancreatitis can develop. Methanol level is elevated.

MANAGEMENT is supportive. Fluid and electrolytes and acid–base balance are managed. Ethanol or fomepizole are sometimes used to delay methanol metabolism until otherwise eliminated. Hemodialysis is used for selected patients with severe toxicity, especially with visual deficits, high methanol levels, or high volumes ingested.

Ethylene Glycol

Ethylene glycol is a component mainly of radiator fluids as antifreeze. Because of the sweet taste, animals and humans are susceptible to ingestion.

PRESENTATION is initially with clinical intoxication similar to that of ethanol. Mental status changes predominate. Delayed effects start after about 12 hours with tachycardia, hypertension, tachypnea, acute respiratory distress syndrome (ARDS), and or cardiac arrhythmias.

DIAGNOSIS is usually suspected by either a history of ingestion or an early osmolar gap that develops into a high anion gap metabolic acidosis. Ethylene glycol levels can be measured in some labs. Otherwise, UV light examination of urine may reveal fluorescein fluorescence because this compound is added to radiator fluid to facilitate identification of leaks.

MANAGEMENT begins with supportive care with fluid and electrolyte management. Cardiac and respiratory monitoring and management are required. Antidotes include fomepizole and ethanol, the former preferred. Thiamine and pyridoxine supplementation is occasionally used to enhance metabolism, but this is not routine.

HEAVY METALS

The most important heavy metals producing human toxicity are:

- Lead
- Mercury
- Arsenic

Although there is overlap in presentation and management, they are discussed individually. Suspicion is the key to diagnosis of heavy metal intoxication. Hypochromic microcytic anemia can occur in any of these.

Lead Poisoning

Lead intoxication is most likely to be from occupational exposure, water contamination, or household contamination.

PRESENTATION depends on the acuteness of the exposure:

- *Acute high-dose exposure*: Encephalopathy, neuropathy, renal failure
- *Chronic exposure*: Cognitive changes, especially in children; weakness, sleep disturbance

DIAGNOSIS is suspected by hypochromic microcytic anemia, which would suggest lead or other heavy metal toxicity. Blood lead levels can be measured. Free erythrocyte protoporphyrin level is increased with chronic exposure but typically not with acute exposure.

MANAGEMENT begins with cessation of exposure. Chelation is used for patients with high lead levels, especially with organ damage including encephalopathy or renal damage.

Mercury Poisoning

Inorganic mercury is not absorbed through the GI tract but *organic mercury*, particularly methylmercury, is absorbed well.

PRESENTATION is often with prominent neurologic symptoms with central and peripheral manifestations:

- *Neuropathic deficits* can include numbness, weakness, dysesthesias.
- *Central deficits* can include cognitive disturbance visual loss, and hearing loss.
- *Inhalation of mercury vapor* can acutely cause nausea, vomiting, abdominal pain and cramps, with neurologic manifestations of headache, dizziness, and weakness.

DIAGNOSIS of mercury poisoning is suspected with a history of exposure; without this, diagnosis can be difficult.

- Neuropsychiatric manifestations with renal insufficiency may suggest the diagnosis.
- Mercury can be measured in blood and urine.
- EMG may show neuropathic findings.

MANAGEMENT starts with supportive care and cessation of exposure.

- Gastric lavage can be used for recent organic mercury ingestion. Abdominal x-ray may show mercury still in the stomach.
- Chelation can be helpful for patients with prominent symptoms.
- Hemodialysis is used especially if renal function has deteriorated.

Arsenic Poisoning

Arsenic poisoning can be intentional or from contaminated food or drink or occupational exposure. Presentation can be acute or chronic:

- *Acute*: Confusion, delirium; possible seizures; tachycardia, hypotension
- *Chronic*: Neuropathy, dermatitis; Mees lines on the fingernails. Hemolytic anemia can occur.

DIAGNOSIS may be suspected with microcytic hypochromic anemia. Urine assay is generally a 24-hour collection. If arsenic levels are elevated, the lab must differentiate between inorganic and organic arsenic because the inorganic version is responsible for most toxicity.

MANAGEMENT requires careful monitoring, especially if arrhythmia is present. Chelation is used for symptomatic patients.

CHOLINESTERASE INHIBITORS

Cholinesterase inhibitors (ChEI) are sometimes termed *acetylcholinesterase (AChE)* inhibitors, but we prefer the more generic term since there are other cholinesterases.

ChEIs are used for symptomatic treatment of Alzheimer disease and some neuromuscular transmission disorders, and as insecticides, and they are also part of a class of nerve agents used in chemical warfare. Two prominent classes of cholinesterase inhibitors are organophosphates and carbamates. They produce similar clinical presentations.

Cholinesterase-inhibitor intoxication can begin with exposure to insecticides or from overdose of ChEIs given as medications for medical reasons. A terrorist attack might also use these agents.

PRESENTATION starts with generalized muscular weakness. Fasciculations are common and suggest the diagnosis. Encephalopathy and seizures can occur with acute high-dose exposure. Cardiac arrhythmia may also occur with high-level exposure. Chronic exposure can produce progressive weakness and neuropathy.

DIAGNOSIS may be suspected with a presentation of marked weakness, respiratory difficulty, fasciculations, and miosis. RBC cholinesterase assay helps with diagnosis when available. Atropine can produce marked improvement in symptoms, which is helpful diagnostically as well as therapeutically.

MANAGEMENT is usually with a combination of the following agents:

- Atropine can improve especially the respiratory symptoms.
- Pralidoxime (2-PAM) is used for neurologic symptoms.
- Benzodiazepines (e.g., diazepam/lorazepam) is used for control of seizures.

31 Neuro-Ophthalmology

Karl E. Misulis, MD, PhD and
E. Lee Murray, MD

CHAPTER CONTENTS

- Overview
- Ocular Ischemia
  - Transient Monocular Blindness
  - Ischemic Optic Neuropathy
  - Central or Branch Retinal Arterial Occlusion
  - Central or Branch Retinal Vein Occlusion

OVERVIEW

This chapter covers disorders specific to visual deficits not described elsewhere in this text. Some important neuro-ophthalmological disorders in other chapters are as follows:

- Optic neuritis: Chapter 22
- Benign intracranial hypertension: Chapter 20
- Temporal arteritis: Chapter 20
- Stroke: Chapter 16

OCULAR ISCHEMIA
Transient Monocular Blindness

Transient monocular blindness (TMB) is usually due to retinal or optic nerve ischemia. Evaluation and treatment is as for transient ischemic attack (TIA) in a carotid distribution. TMB is associated with an increased risk for cerebrovascular accident (CVA) but less so than with a hemispheric TIA. Additional information is found in Chapter 16.

PRESENTATION is usually with abrupt onset of monocular visual loss that may be complete or partial and may have a wedge-shaped distribution. The transient nature differentiates this from central retinal artery occlusion. Fundus can be normal but can show small areas of retinal ischemia despite the clinical resolution of the symptoms.

DIAGNOSIS is suspected by transient monocular visual loss. The main differential diagnosis is migraine. Demyelination does not produce so rapid an onset and so transient a presentation. Imaging usually includes magnetic resonance imaging (MRI) of the brain to look for previous cerebral ischemia. MR angiography (MRA) or preferably computed tomography angiography (CTA) evaluates for significant carotid disease. Echo may be indicated if no carotid lesion is identified.

MANAGEMENT includes secondary prevention of TIA with antiplatelet plus statin for most patients, anticoagulation for selected patients, vascular surgery or stent for carotid disease if warranted, and best general medical management of risk factors including diabetes, hypertension, and smoking.

ISCHEMIC OPTIC NEUROPATHY

Ischemic optic neuropathy (ION) is ischemia of the optic nerve. Two forms described are nonarteritic and arteritic. Nonarteritic is more common. Differentiation is also made into anterior and posterior. Anterior ischemic optic neuropathy involves the optic disc, whereas Posterior ischemic optic neuropathy does not.

- Nonarteritic: Optic nerve infarction is usually unilateral.
- Arteritic: Most often is associated with temporal arteritis (giant cell arteritis).

PRESENTATION is with acute or subacute visual loss. Most cases are unilateral; bilateral or sequential involvement is more common with arteritic ION. Specifics of presentation depend on the pathophysiology:

- Nonarteritic: Visual loss is noted suddenly or overnight and is usually painless.
- Arteritic: Typically shows the same pattern of visual loss but with associated inflammatory symptoms including headache, especially temporal; jaw claudication; and malaise.

DIAGNOSIS is considered with acute painless visual loss. Associated headache and malaise suggests the arteritic variety.

- Differential diagnosis includes retinal artery or vein occlusion, and funduscopic exam can differentiate these. Optic neuritis should be considered especially in younger patients. Most ION patients are over 50 years of age.
- Lab: Erythrocyte sedimentation rate (ESR) is usually but not invariably elevated in arteritic ION. C-reactive protein (CRP) may be increased in patients with arteritic ION with an unremarkable ESR. CBC may show anemia with arteritic ION.
- Imaging: MRI is performed especially when demyelination is suspected or to evaluate for other regions of ischemia. CTA of carotid and orbital circulation can show occlusive disease and sometimes arteritic change.

MANAGEMENT begins with first establishing causation regarding ischemia (i.e., arteritic vs. nonarteritic). Consider a rheumatology consult if assistance with this differentiation is challenging. High-dose corticosteroids are often used if arteritic ION is suspected, even if not certain. Prednisone is usually used if there is no visual loss, but IV methylprednisolone is often used initially if there is visual disturbance.

CENTRAL OR BRANCH RETINAL ARTERY OCCLUSION

Central retinal artery or branch retinal artery occlusion is ischemia affecting the entirety or part of the retina. This is usually due to arterial emboli, but may be due to temporal arteritis.

PRESENTATION is usually abrupt onset of monocular visual loss affecting the entirety (central retinal artery) or part (branch retinal artery) of the visual field. There are typically no other neurologic deficits.

If the occlusion is associated with temporal arteritis, additional findings can be headache with temporal predominance, jaw claudication, and temporal artery tenderness.

DIAGNOSIS is suspected with monocular visual loss with an afferent pupil defect. Branch occlusions may not produce an afferent pupil. Retinal exam shows arterial ischemia. Studies include:

- Imaging of the carotid distribution with CTA or MRA is recommended. carotid duplex sonography (CDS) can be done but, because of the limited field of view, is not the preferred study.
- Lab should include ESR in addition to routine labs for stroke/TIA, and clinical symptoms and findings of temporal arteritis should be looked for.

MANAGEMENT in the absence of temporal arteritis includes secondary stroke prevention; antithrombotic agents plus statins is appropriate if not contraindicated. Interventional radiology approaches to restoration of flow are sometimes considered, but this is not routine practice.

CENTRAL OR BRANCH RETINAL VEIN OCCLUSION

Central or branch retinal vein occlusion is due to thrombotic occlusion. Etiology is usually related to risk factors for thrombotic disease such as hypertension, diabetes, or hypercoagulable state.

PRESENTATION is most commonly acute or subacute (up to days) onset of monocular visual loss. Branch occlusions often produce visual field defects that are in a quadrant. Fundus shows hemorrhages and venous engorgement of a distribution appropriate to the vessel affected. The affected eye is typically painful and red. Pupil response may be normal or reduced if visual loss is severe. Corneal edema may obscure visualization of the fundus.

DIAGNOSIS is considered with acute to subacute monocular visual loss associated with pain and redness. Fundi with hemorrhages help make the diagnosis.

- *Lab*: In addition to routine labs to look for diabetes and other risk factors, ESR, serum protein electrophoresis, and other studies for coagulopathy may be performed, especially in younger patients.
- *Imaging*: Fluorescein angiography can show ischemia. Optical coherence tomography (OCT) can detect macular edema in the presence of hemorrhages that would otherwise obscure fluorescein angiography.
- *Consultation* with ophthalmology is recommended urgently for diagnosis and consideration of treatment options.

MANAGEMENT options are limited. No specific treatment has become standard other than best management of risk factors. Treatments that might be considered include systemic or intravitreal corticosteroids, intravitreal triamcinolone, and intravitreal ranibizumab (neutralizing antibody to vascular endothelial growth factor [VEGF]). Laser photocoagulation is performed for selected patients. Ophthalmology should be consulted urgently for patients with this suspected diagnosis.[1]

32 Neuro-Otology

Karl E. Misulis, MD, PhD and
E. Lee Murray, MD

CHAPTER CONTENTS

- Overview
- Vestibulopathies
  - Benign Paroxysmal Positional Vertigo
  - Vestibular Neuropathy
  - Labyrinthitis
  - Ménière Disease
- Tinnitus
- Acoustic Neuroma

OVERVIEW

Hospital neurology consultation in the field of neuro-otology is usually for the following scenarios:

- Vertigo
- Hearing loss
- Tinnitus

Most central causes of these symptoms are usually associated with other clinical findings that eclipse these complaints. The role of the neurologist is to ensure that neurologic causes are considered and to promote appropriate ENT evaluation and treatment as needed.

VESTIBULOPATHIES

Vestibulopathies are common, with the *idiopathic* variety being the most common diagnosis. Here we consider primary vestibulopathies; also considered in the differential diagnosis are central causes. In general, central causes are less likely to produce sustained nystagmus and are more likely to have associated nonvestibular symptoms. Diagnoses to be considered may be multiple sclerosis, stroke, brainstem tumor, and infections affecting the brainstem. Vestibulopathies include:

- *Benign paroxysmal positional vertigo*
  - Episodes of vertigo and nystagmus with change in head position or specific head position, especially turning or bending over

- o Diagnosed by clinical exam with maneuvers discussed below
- o Imaging often not needed especially with classic presentation and examination
- o Treated by repositioning maneuvers, as discussed below. Medical treatment may include antihistamines, benzodiazepines, and/or antiemetics.
- **Post-traumatic vertigo**
  - o While most causes of vestibulopathy are idiopathic, head trauma can cause vestibular symptoms by injury directly to the labyrinth or CN 8. Hearing loss is common.
- **Ménière disease**
  - o Episodes of vertigo with tinnitus and ultimately hearing loss
  - o Diagnosis is by clinical exam. MRI may be necessary to evaluate for acoustic nerve lesion but often is not needed with classic presentation.
  - o Treatment of acute attacks is with antihistamines, benzodiazepines, and/or antiemetics. Prevention of attacks with diuretics and diet is often prescribed but limited in established efficacy
- **Otosclerosis**
  - o Progressive hearing loss often with vertigo that may be positional. Distinguished from many other causes by the conductive nature of the hearing loss.
  - o Diagnosis is clinical with the conductive loss. Differentiation from Ménière disease is most important.
  - o Treatment is often with surgery.

Regardless of cause, some of the most effective agents for vertigo include antihistamines, anticholinergics, benzodiazepines, and antiemetics. Some representative individual agents include:

- *Antihistamine*: Meclizine.
- *Anticholinergic*: Scopolamine
- *Benzodiazepine*: Diazepam
- *Antiemetic*: Promethazine

Benign Paroxysmal Positional Vertigo

Benign paroxysmal positional vertigo (BPPV) is the most common cause of vertigo but is an uncommon cause of hospital admission; but because this can occur in patients with vascular risk factors, admission sometimes occurs for rapid evaluation and treatment. Patients often reports gait difficulty so posterior circulation stroke is often considered in the differential diagnosis.[1]

PRESENTATION is with abrupt onset of vertigo with change in head position. Symptoms are often noted on waking, especially with sitting up or turning over in bed. Symptoms often abate within 30 secs or less, and symptoms are minimal if the head is still.

DIAGNOSIS is suspected with positional vertigo in the absence of other neurologic symptoms. Differential diagnosis includes stroke, demyelinating disease, and intoxication. Dix-Hallpike maneuvers are diagnostic for many patients. If there is still any doubt or if the maneuvers are inconclusive, then magnetic resonance imaging (MRI) of the brain is appropriate to look for infarction or other structural or inflammatory lesion. MR angiography (MRA) or computed tomography angiography (CTA) may not be needed if no vascular changes are seen on the MRI, but small posterior circulation infarctions may be missed on MRI.

MANAGEMENT usually includes vestibular rehab and medications for vertigo such as meclizine and benzodiazepines, which are often of only modest effectiveness. The Epley canalith repositioning procedure is curative for many patients,[2] but symptoms may recur.

Vestibular Neuropathy

Vestibular neuropathy is a dysfunction of the vestibular system giving symptoms related to incongruent signals from the vestibular apparatuses. The cause is idiopathic in most patients, but some etiologies that have been implicated include HSV-1[3] and trauma. This category might have been labeled *vestibular neuronitis*, but since there is not documentation of an inflammatory component for most patients, the present term is preferred.

PRESENTATION is typically with vertigo that is often severe, lasting for hours or days. Symptoms increase with head movement but are always present during the episode and do not have the degree of exacerbation with movement that would be expected with BPPV. Nausea and vomiting are common. Exam shows nystagmus with the fast phase away from the affected side, although the nystagmus may only be visible with provocation. Gait is often impaired but appendicular coordination is normal.

DIAGNOSIS is suggested by vertigo with more of a steady symptomatology than BPPV. Gait ataxia and nystagmus are supportive. The Hallpike maneuver is especially helpful for patients who do not have characteristic nystagmus on examination.

Specific negatives should include:

- Hearing loss (consider Ménière disease)
- Appendicular or truncal ataxia (consider stroke or demyelinating disease)
- Headache (consider migraine)
- Fever (consider labyrinthitis)

In the absence of signs of other diagnoses, imaging is usually not needed, but if stroke is considered, then MRI brain with MRA or CTA is warranted.

MANAGEMENT begins with reassurance. Hospitalization is usually not needed unless the patient is nonambulatory or in such distress that home management is unrealistic, or for further diagnostic study.

Medical treatment is often needed. No one medication stands out as superior, but among the most commonly considered meds are antihistamines, antiemetics, and benzodiazepines as in the previous section. Corticosteroids, especially prednisone, are also used.

Follow-up as outpatient is especially recommended since symptoms persist for some patients and there also should be surveillance for other diagnoses.

Labyrinthitis

Labyrinthitis is inflammation of the inner ear. The cause is usually bacterial or viral with uncommon cases presumptively autoimmune. Among the viral causes are influenza, HSV-1, VZV, adenovirus but many others. Bacterial etiologies can include *Streptococcus pneumoniae* and other *Streptococci, Staphylococcus, E. coli, Haemophilus influenzae,* and others. Bacterial labyrinthitis can be associated with meningitis.

PRESENTATION is most commonly with vertigo, which can be worse with change in head position. Hearing loss and tinnitus can develop. Patients often have a pressure sensation in the affected ear region. Nausea and vomiting may accompany the vertigo.

- *Viral labyrinthitis* produces usually a very acute onset of vertigo with nausea and vomiting. Symptoms may last days to weeks with gradual resolution.
- *Bacterial labyrinthitis* produces similar vestibular symptoms but is associated with fever and local pain.

DIAGNOSIS is suspected with acute onset of vertigo especially with pain and/or hearing loss. Viral etiology is presumed unless fever or significant pain develops that suggests a bacterial etiology.

- Imaging is often necessary to evaluate for structural pathology. MRI is the study of choice; inflammation may be seen on contrasted scan.
- Labs including CBC and inflammatory markers can be considered if bacterial cause is suspected.
- CSF analysis should be obtained if meningitis is suspected on the basis of fever or other associated neurologic issues, including confusion or neck pain.

Differential diagnosis includes especially vestibular neuropathy, but this is not associated with hearing loss. Ménière disease is considered. Anterior inferior cerebellar artery (AICA) infarction can produce similar symptoms, including hearing loss.[4]

MANAGEMENT depends on whether the etiology is viral or bacterial.

- *Viral labyrinthitis* treatment is supportive, including fluids plus medications for symptomatic improvement, particularly antiemetics and benzodiazepines, and corticosteroids. Antivirals have not been proved to show benefit.[5]
- *Bacterial labyrinthitis* is treated with antibiotics in addition to symptomatic management. Selection of antibiotic depends on the presumed organism and on whether there is meningeal involvement.

Consultation with ENT is appropriate especially for uncertain diagnosis, for refractory cases, or if bacterial infection is suspected.

Ménière Disease

Ménière disease is *idiopathic endolymphatic hydrops* (i.e., increased fluid pressure), a disorder of the endolymph in the labyrinth. Rarely, the increased endolymphatic pressure is due to an identified cause, such as autoimmune or trauma.

PRESENTATION is typically episodes of vertigo, nausea, and vomiting usually associated with tinnitus. There is often a pressure sensation in the ear on the affected side. Symptoms spontaneously remit and then may recur weeks to months later. Hearing loss is often evident and persists between attacks. Exam during an attack usually shows persistent nystagmus.

DIAGNOSIS is suspected with episodes of vertigo, nausea, vomiting, tinnitus, often with acute deterioration in hearing that is preceded by aural fullness. Recurrent attacks reinforce the clinical diagnosis.

- *Imaging*: Patients with a classic presentation and a history of similar events usually do not need imaging, but with a first attack or atypical or incomplete features then MRI brain with additional attention to the inner ear should be considered. CT is performed for patients who cannot have MRI.
- *Audiometry*: Assessment of hearing can be helpful for initial diagnosis but is not necessary acutely. However, follow-up testing is important and can guide treatment decisions.
- *Electronystagmography*: ENG can be helpful but is not necessary and usually not available in a hospital setting.
- *Electrocochleography*: ECOG can aid with assessment of inner ear pressure, but usually is not done in hospitalized patients.
- *ENT consultation* should be requested if this diagnosis is suspected.

MANAGEMENT is initially symptomatic and while most patients can be treated as outpatients, some patients have to be admitted for symptom control and possibly additional study if the diagnosis is uncertain. Medical treatment is generally as follows:

- Symptomatic treatment is often offered, including antiemetics, antihistamines, and/or benzodiazepines.
- Corticosteroids are often used urgently, usually parentally to start, followed by an oral taper.
- Diuretics are often used but benefit is not proved.[6]

Evaluation and follow-up with ENT is recommended.

TINNITUS

Tinnitus is a symptom of several disorders including acoustic neuroma, Ménière disease, age-related hearing loss (presbyacusis), and noise-related hearing loss. Tinnitus is divided into two subgroups: *subjective* and *objective*. Hospital neurology consultation for tinnitus in the absence of other neurologic deficits is not expected.

- *Subjective* is where the examiner cannot hear the sound even with a stethoscope and is by far the most common. Primary neural or cochlear pathology is most likely.
- *Objective* is where the examiner can hear the sound. This is usually due to a vascular flow sound and not primarily originating in neural structures.

PRESENTATION is usually a continuous though variable sound in one or both ears, which can be of various frequencies and have a buzzing, hissing, or ringing character.

DIAGNOSIS usually begins with audiometry, which can document and classify hearing loss. If symptoms are unilateral or if the onset and severity of the symptoms does not suggest a benign cause, then imaging with MRI of the brain with particular attention to the cerebellopontine angle (CPA) is appropriate.

MANAGEMENT is usually supportive with reassurance if there is no reason to suspect serious pathology. Correcting the hearing loss may improve the subjective tinnitus. Medications have an uneven response rate. Among those that have been used are tricyclic antidepressants (TCAs) and benzodiazepines. Transcranial magnetic stimulation has also been tried with some limited success.[7] Sound generators for masking are helpful for some patients who are disturbed by tinnitus.

ACOUSTIC NEUROMA

Acoustic neuroma, also known as *vestibular schwannoma*, is a tumor of CN 8 involving either the cochlear or vestibular portion of the nerve. This is the most common tumor in the CPA. Neurofibromatosis type 2 (NF2) is responsible for some unilateral and most bilateral acoustic neuromas.

PRESENTATION is usually with hearing loss as the most common symptom, present in almost all patients (84%[8]). Tinnitus (40%) and imbalance (51%) are common symptoms. Symptoms are unilateral in most patients but can be bilateral, most notably with NF2. NF1 patients may show acoustic neuroma but bilateral involvement is not expected. Other symptoms included vertigo, gait ataxia, facial pain, headache, and a pressure sensation in the ear. Isolated tinnitus without a perceived hearing loss is an uncommon but possible presentation. Facial weakness is less common.

DIAGNOSIS is suspected with progressive unilateral hearing loss and/or tinnitus. Bilateral symptoms should trigger an examination for other features of NF. Diagnostic studies usually include imaging.

- MRI brain with contrast with attention to the CPA is most sensitive for revealing acoustic neuromas.
- CT brain with contrast with attention to the CPA can show most larger acoustic neuromas but may miss small lesions.
- Brainstem auditory evoked potential can show delay or absence of early waves and delay in wave V absence if severe.
- Audiometry often shows high-frequency hearing loss.

MANAGEMENT can include observation, microsurgical treatment, or stereotactic radiotherapy.

- Observation is appropriate for some patients, especially with advanced age, elevated surgical risk, small tumors, and especially with incidental discovery. Also, if the affected ear is the only hearing ear then observation should be considered.
- Surgery by open microsurgical approach is commonly used.
- Stereotactic radiotherapy is an alternative to surgery, but may predispose to tumor regrowth. Generally, this is used for patients with increased surgical risk who need more than observation.

33 Cranial Nerve Disorders

Karl E. Misulis, MD, PhD and
E. Lee Murray, MD

CHAPTER CONTENTS

- Overview
- Bell Palsy and Ramsay-Hunt Syndrome
- Diabetic Ophthalmoplegia
- Abducens Nerve Palsy
- Horner Syndrome
- Herpes Zoster Ophthalmicus
- Glossopharyngeal Neuralgia
- Multiple Cranial Nerve Palsies

OVERVIEW

The most common primary cranial nerve deficits to come to the attention of the hospital neurologist are listed below. Not discussed here are other medical disorders which produce cranial nerve deficits as part of their clinical presentation including vascular disease (Chapter 16), demyelinating disease (Chapter 22), infectious diseases (Chapter 17) and tumors (Chapter 25). The disorders with primary cranial nerve manifestations include:

- Bell palsy
- Ramsay-Hunt syndrome
- Hemifacial spasm (Chapter 23)
- Herpes zoster ophthalmicus
- Vestibulopathies (Chapter 32)
- Trigeminal neuralgia (Chapter 20)
- Glossopharyngeal neuralgia
- Multiple cranial nerve palsies

Some of these are discussed in the chapters indicated. The remainder are discussed in this chapter.

BELL PALSY AND RAMSAY-HUNT SYNDROME

Bell palsy is the most common cause of unilateral facial weakness. The most common causes are herpes simplex virus (HSV) and varicella zoster virus (VZV); less likely are autoimmune and other infections. *Ramsay-Hunt syndrome* is peripheral facial palsy with *herpes zoster oticus*.

PRESENTATION is with subacute onset of unilateral facial palsy, typically involving upper and lower face (peripheral palsy), although early in the course or with milder symptoms the upper face involvement may be difficult to determine and the lesion might be thought to be central. Pain in or around the ipsilateral ear may be present before, contemporaneous with, or after the onset of the weakness. Bilateral involvement is uncommon and when present suggests diagnoses other than idiopathic facial palsy.

DIAGNOSIS is considered in all patients with unilateral facial weakness. Classic clinical features can make the diagnosis with sufficient accuracy to avoid extensive evaluation. With atypical presentation or other associated symptoms, additional study may be needed. The main differential diagnoses are stroke and demyelinating disease, although diabetes, cerebellopontine angle (CPA) tumor, Lyme disease, and infectious or neoplastic meningitis are considered. Magnetic resonance imaging (MRI) of the brain with special attention to the facial nerve can show inflammatory change but is of most value in ruling out other lesion such as tumor, stroke, or demyelinating plaque.

MANAGEMENT includes protection of the eye from exposure if eye closure and blinking are incomplete. Corticosteroids and antiviral agents are considered.[1]

- *Corticosteroids* can hasten recovery and reduce residual damage. These are usually used unless contraindicated by comorbid condition (e.g., uncontrolled diabetes).
- *Antivirals* have been used but their benefit is unproved. They may be considered especially for patients with severe deficit.

DIABETIC OPHTHALMOPLEGIA

Diabetic ophthalmoplegia is a common cause for hospital neurology consultation because of concerns over stroke syndrome or aneurysm. Etiology is likely ischemia affecting the central portion of the nerve, sparing the peripheral fibers innervating the pupil.

PRESENTATION is most commonly with pupil-sparing CN 3 palsy producing diplopia but without anisocoria unless there is another reason for that. Ptosis can occur. Pain can occur in a peri-orbital distribution. CN 6 or 4 palsies can occur but with lower incidence.

DIAGNOSIS is suspected in a diabetic with pupil-sparing CN 3 palsy. However, imaging with MRI and MR angiography (MRA) is almost always needed to look for aneurysm, cavernous sinus lesion, or other lesion. Brainstem ischemia or demyelination would be unlikely to produce an isolated cranial nerve palsy.

MANAGEMENT is supportive. The key is to rule out more concerning lesions. Most patients improve.

ABDUCENS NERVE PALSY

Abducens palsy in adults is usually due to ischemic neuropathy. Typical vascular risk factors predispose to this.

PRESENTATION is with horizontal diplopia, worse with lateral gaze to the affected side. With complete lesions, the eye does not abduct beyond the midline. If the abducens palsy is vascular, no other deficit is expected. If the lesion is in the cavernous sinus, CSF, or elsewhere in the brain, then additional deficits would be expected.

DIAGNOSIS is suspected by horizontal diplopia in the absence of other findings.

- MRI of the brain is appropriate to look for vascular disease, structural abnormality, or demyelinating disease.
- MRA or computed tomography angiography (CTA) can be performed to look for aneurysm.
- CSF is obtained if no other cause identified and microvascular etiology is not suspected (e.g., young patient, no risk factors).
- Lab may include myasthenia panel, but monocular abduction deficit in with myasthenia gravis (MG) would be uncommon in the absence of other ocular motor deficits. Labs to be considered may include studies for diabetes, syphilis, or vasculitis.

MANAGEMENT is usually supportive; most cases improve spontaneously within weeks to months.

- Patching of the eyes alternately is needed by some patients to allow for functional vision.
- Ocular prisms are used mainly for patients who have not recovered well after several months of follow-up.
- If symptoms of giant cell arteritis are seen with abducens palsy, then corticosteroids are started urgently while the evaluation is completed.

HORNER SYNDROME

Horner syndrome is dysfunction of sympathetic innervation to the eye. Anisocoria is an occasional trigger for neurologic consultation in the hospital. There are multiple potential central and peripheral causes. A few of the causes include:

- Central
  - Brainstem ischemia
  - Multiple sclerosis
  - Transverse myelitis
  - Syrinx
- Peripheral
  - Carotid artery damage (e.g., trauma, surgery, occlusion)
  - Tumor anywhere in the pathway

PRESENTATION is with ptosis and miosis on the affected side, often with anhydrosis. Other associated findings can be clues to localization and diagnosis (e.g., other cranial nerve deficits or ataxia with a brainstem lesion, or limb weakness and corticospinal tract signs with myelopathy).

DIAGNOSIS is clinical. Further study is guided by localization: is this cerebral, spinal, or peripheral? If there is no known inciting factor such as neck trauma, then vascular imaging for carotid lesion should be considered.

MANAGEMENT depends on etiology. For most patients, the task for the hospital neurologist is making the etiologic diagnosis.

HERPES ZOSTER OPHTHALMICUS

Herpes zoster ophthalmicus is reactivation of VZV with involvement of the upper division of the trigeminal nerve (V1 of CN 5). This is most commonly seen in older patients and in those with immune deficiency such as lymphoma.

PRESENTATION usually begins with dysesthesias on the forehead. This is followed by a vesicular rash in a V1 distribution. Periorbital edema with an inflammatory appearance may develop, including corneal edema. Late features may be corneal scarring, retinitis, episcleritis, and ultimately postherpetic neuralgia.

DIAGNOSIS is suspected by the clinical presentation of the prodromal sensory symptoms followed by the rash. This usually makes the diagnosis. Additional studies are usually not needed unless there are atypical features.

MANAGEMENT includes antiviral agents—usually acyclovir, famciclovir, or valacyclovir. Topical corticosteroids are used for uveitis or keratitis. Oral corticosteroids are often used but of unproved benefit.

GLOSSOPHARYNGEAL NEURALGIA

Glossopharyngeal neuralgia is neuropathic pain affecting CN 9. It is usually idiopathic but occasionally due to local tumor. Some patients have symptoms due to cardiodepressant effects in a portion of the vagus.

PRESENTATION is with brief episodes of severe pain in the throat. The pain is activity-dependent, often triggered by chewing, talking, or yawning. The cardiodepressant effects can produce bradycardia and syncope.

DIAGNOSIS is made by clinical presentation. However, because of the possibility of a structural abnormality, imaging if often necessary with MRI or CT studying the throat and lower cranial nerves.

MANAGEMENT of the pain begins with medical therapy but may require surgery.

- Medical management is with anticonvulsants (especially oxcarbazepine, carbamazepine, and gabapentin) or baclofen, sometimes in combination.
- Surgery may be needed and includes decompression of the glossopharyngeal nerve or section of the glossopharyngeal nerve and upper aspect of the vagus nerve.

MULTIPLE CRANIAL NERVE PALSIES

A wide variety of disorders can be associated with clinical presentation of multiple cranial nerve palsies:

- *Herpes zoster*: CN 5 or CN 7 can both be affected. Also possible is CN 8, 9, or 10. Associated with ear pain and then peripheral facial palsy.
- *Sarcoidosis*: Multiple cranial nerve palsies are possible with aseptic meningitis with lymphocytic predominance.
- *Wegener granulomatosis*: Multiple cranial nerve palsies; can develop mononeuritis multiplex and/or polyneuropathy.
- *Intracranial aneurysm*: Unruptured aneurysm can produce multiple cranial nerve palsies by compression of adjacent cranial nerves. Ruptured aneurysm, with subarachnoid hemorrhage can produce more distant cranial nerve palsies.

- *Neoplastic meningitis*: Confusion is the most common symptom but also can produce multiple cranial neuropathies and radiculopathies.
- *Lyme disease*: Suggested by bilateral facial palsies. Can also develop disparate multiple cranial neuropathies. Meningitis may present with multiple cranial nerve palsies and polyradiculopathies.
- *CPA tumors*: Involvement and/or compression can affect CN 8, CB 5, CN 7 especially. With brainstem compression, lower cranial nerves can be affected.
- *Neurofibromas*: NF2 is especially likely to not only have bilateral acoustic neuromas but also to have involvement of other cranial nerves from local compression.
- *Nasopharyngeal carcinoma*: Cranial nerve palsies can develop, with CN 5 being most commonly affected, CN 6 next most common; it can also affect CN 3 and CN 4 in the cavernous sinus. Can also affect other cranial nerves by extension and invasion into the skull base.
- *Chiari malformation*: Hydrocephalus is the most common serious neurologic consequence. Lower cranial nerve palsies can develop.
- *Chronic meningitis*: Multiple cranial nerve palsies can develop, but presentations differ depending on etiology. Hearing loss, facial weakness, and ocular motor deficits are most common at presentation.
- *Cavernous sinus thrombosis*: Involves CN 3 most commonly, but CN 6 and/or CN 4 also may be affected. Headache is the most common and earliest symptom.
- *Tolosa-Hunt syndrome*: CN 5 (especially V1), CN 3, CN 6 are most commonly affected.
- *Stroke*: Multiple stroke syndromes produce cranial nerve palsies, but these are combined with signs of other neurologic dysfunction (e.g., cerebellar or corticospinal).

34 Autonomic Disorders

Karl E. Misulis, MD, PhD and
E. Lee Murray, MD

CHAPTER CONTENTS

- Overview
- Idiopathic Orthostatic Hypotension
- Diabetic Autonomic Insufficiency
- Multiple System Atrophy
- Paraneoplastic Autonomic Neuropathy
- Hereditary Sensory and Autonomic Neuropathy

OVERVIEW

Autonomic difficulty is usually a component of a systemic disease with other neurologic manifestations. A commonality is orthostatic hypotension for most of these. Once the diagnosis of autonomic insufficiency has been made, the differential diagnosis includes the following:

- *Idiopathic orthostatic hypotension*: Pure autonomic failure without other deficits
- *Diabetic autonomic insufficiency*: Most common autonomic disorder. Autonomic neuropathy is typically a component of a multimodal neuropathy.
- *Multiple system atrophy*: Autonomic failure associated with other neurologic deficits including extrapyramidal, corticospinal, or cerebellar dysfunction
- *Paraneoplastic autonomic neuropathy*: Autonomic neuropathy before or after diagnosis of cancer. Often with other neurologic deficits from peripheral neuropathy, cognitive change, seizures, or Lambert-Eaton myasthenic syndrome.
- *Hereditary autonomic neuropathy*: Family of disorders of which autonomic involvement is a component. Type 3 is familial dysautonomia.

IDIOPATHIC ORTHOSTATIC HYPOTENSION

Idiopathic orthostatic hypotension (IOH) is prominent orthostasis with no other associated neurologic or medical disease.

PRESENTATION is with presyncopal sensation on standing. There may also be noticeable anhydrosis. Erectile dysfunction can occur also. The orthostasis can be disabling.

DIAGNOSIS is suspected with a history and exam compatible with orthostasis. Electromyogram (EMG) is done if the autonomic difficulty is believed to be a component of a peripheral neuropathy. Labs for other causes may include Hgb A1C (diabetes), paraneoplastic antibodies, VGCC antibodies (LEMS), and porphyrins if these disorders are suspected.

MANAGEMENT includes use of agents to reduce the orthostasis, including especially midodrine and fludrocortisone. Fluid and salt management is important also. Cessation of drugs that can contribute to autonomic insufficiency is recommended.

DIABETIC AUTONOMIC INSUFFICIENCY

Diabetic autonomic neuropathy can have a wide range of effects; these can include:

- *Orthostatic hypotension*: Hypotension on standing
- *Cardiovascular autonomic dysfunction*: Tachycardia, predisposition to myocardial ischemia
- *Peripheral autonomic dysfunction*: Defect in sweating, edema
- *Gastrointestinal autonomic dysfunction*: Defect in gastric emptying and GI motility

PRESENTATION is usually with a combination of these elements. With improved control of diabetes, the severity of diabetic autonomic neuropathy is lessened. Diabetic autonomic neuropathy is typically combined with sensory neuropathic findings of distal pain and sensory loss.

DIAGNOSIS is clinical. Autonomic testing can document the autonomic disorder. EMG can evaluate the neuropathy. Skin biopsy can be done, but this is seldom needed.

MANAGEMENT includes treatments for orthostatic hypotension as with IOH. Optimal management of diabetes improves the outcome of the autonomic neuropathy.

MULTIPLE SYSTEM ATROPHY

Multiple system atrophy (MSA) is a family of disorders with combinations of autonomic dysfunction plus extrapyramidal, pyramidal, and cerebellar deficits. There are two general categories: MSA-P and MSA-C indicating whether the patient has predominant Parkinsonism or Cerebellar ataxia. These were discussed in detail in Chapter 23.

PARANEOPLASTIC AUTONOMIC NEUROPATHY

Paraneoplastic autonomic neuropathy is seen in patients with a variety of cancers, but the predominate associations are with small-cell lung, breast, and ovarian cancers.

PRESENTATION is with orthostatic hypotension that can be very severe, other autonomic dysfunctions including GI motility, dry mouth, dry eyes, and impaired sweating. Nonautonomic manifestations can be predominant sensory neuropathy with neuropathic pain and sensory loss, and cerebral findings of confusion, personality change, seizures, or ataxia. Lambert-Eaton myasthenic syndrome (LEMS) is a component of this with autonomic and neuromuscular manifestations (see Chapter 25).

DIAGNOSIS is suspected with orthostatic hypotension and a known or suspected cancer. Antineuronal antibodies can be assayed. CSF often shows a mononuclear pleocytosis and increased protein. Survey for malignancy is performed.

MANAGEMENT is generally supportive. Treatment of orthostatic hypotension is as described for IOH. If a malignancy is diagnosed, aggressive treatment might help the paraneoplastic syndrome. If the patient is found to have LEMS, immunosuppressants can be helpful. When a patient is believed to have an occult malignancy, the decision on treatment in the absence of a definite diagnosis is complex, and oncology consultation is recommended.

HEREDITARY SENSORY AND AUTONOMIC NEUROPATHY

Hereditary sensory and autonomic neuropathies (HSAN) is a family of disorders of multiple types. Type 3 is familial dysautonomia, or Riley-Day syndrome.

- Type 1: Hereditary sensory and autonomic neuropathy
- Type 2: Congenital sensory neuropathy
- Type 3: Familial dysautonomia
- Type 4: Congenital insensitivity to pain with anhydrosis
- Type 5: Congenital insensitivity to pain with partial anhydrosis

Type 1 Hereditary sensory and autonomic neuropathy is an autosomal dominant condition in which sensory neuropathic symptoms predominate; autonomic manifestations are not prominent.

Type 3 Familial dysautonomia is an autosomal recessive condition that produces sensory as well as autonomic deficits. Patients may have some insensitivity to pain. Autonomic deficits start in childhood and can include orthostatic hypotension, GI motility issues, labile blood pressure, keratoconjunctivitis sicca, and defective thermoregulation. Nonautonomic deficits may include impaired cognitive development and ataxia.

DIAGNOSIS of familial dysautonomia is suspected in young patients with orthostatic hypotension and other signs of autonomic insufficiency. Exam shows no fungiform papillae on the tongue. Sensory nerve involvement produces reduced tendon reflexes. Paucity of tearing is supportive. Genetic testing can be done, including prenatal testing.

MANAGEMENT is supportive. There are no specific treatments. Premature death is common, with a prominent cause being aspiration pneumonia.

35 Traumatic Brain Injury

Karl E. Misulis, MD, PhD and
E. Lee Murray, MD

CHAPTER CONTENTS

- Overview
- Concussion
- Contusion
- Intracerebral Hemorrhage
  - Intraparenchymal Hemorrhage
  - Subdural Hematoma
  - Epidural Hematoma
  - Subarachnoid Hemorrhage
- Diffuse Axonal Injury
- Seizure After Head Injury
- Repetitive Head Injuries
- Post-Concussive Syndrome
- Return-to-Play Criteria

OVERVIEW

Hospital neurologists play a varied role in evaluation and management of patients with traumatic brain injury (TBI). Facilities with well-developed trauma programs or good neurosurgical coverage often involve neurology only at times of specific need, such as seizures or secondary infarction. Here, we discuss some of the conditions that neurologists may be asked to address.

The terms *concussion* and *contusion* have become matters of some debate, but since they are useful in practice and still in widespread use, they will be used here.

CONCUSSION

Concussion is identified as head injury with transient loss of consciousness followed by confusion. This is the most common diagnosis for patients with head injury reaching medical attention. This is classified as mild TBI (MTBI).

PRESENTATION to the ED is usually after the phase of initial recovery. Patients usually have headache, dizziness, and mild confusion. Exam immediately after the injury, during a phase of unconsciousness, shows no focal signs and good brainstem reflexes. Prolonged unconsciousness or focal signs suggests that the injury is beyond concussion.

Diagnosis is clinical. Computed tomography (CT) of the brain is usually done but may be able to be avoided if the patient is beyond childhood, not elderly, had rapid return of function, is neurologically normal, and is on no anticoagulants. CT should not show findings of acute intracranial injury.

Management is conservative. Symptoms improve over hours. Hospital admission is often not needed. Post-concussive syndrome may follow (discussed later). However, observation and return-to-ED instructions should be given since approximately 1% of patients with MTBI ultimately need neurosurgery.[1]

CONTUSION

Contusion is often categorized with *intracerebral hemorrhage,* but in this context refers to injury to the brain more severe than that of concussion, with microhemorrhages and development of edema.

Presentation is with headache, confusion, and dizziness, as with concussion, but additionally there may be prolonged unconsciousness, seizures, and focal neurologic signs. Extensive contusions with edema can cause critical increase in intracranial pressure (ICP).

Diagnosis is clinical and supported by brain imaging. There is a continuum between contusion with petechial hemorrhage and large intraparenchymal hemorrhage, discussed later.

Management depends on the size and extent of the injuries. Edema with increased ICP is managed with osmotherapy and sedation. Surgical decompression is tried for critical increase in ICP refractory to medical measures. Hypothermia has not been proved to improve outcome for most patients. Seizure treatment is discussed below.

INTRACEREBRAL HEMORRHAGE

Intracerebral hemorrhage (ICH) is indicative of more severe TBI. ICH is more likely in the elderly and in patients on anticoagulants and other antithrombotics. Location of the bleeding can be subarachnoid, subdural, epidural, or intraparenchymal. ICH is discussed also in Chapter 16. Neurosurgery should be consulted for these disorders.

Intraparenchymal Hemorrhage

Intraparenchymal hemorrhage may have direct effects on neuronal function but also increase ICP and produce global symptoms.

Presentation is with persistent cognitive change and headache after an injury. Consciousness may not have been restored. Seizures and focal signs may be seen.

Diagnosis is suspected by prolonged unconsciousness, focal signs, or seizures after a severe head injury, or after a milder head injury in a patient with coagulopathy. CT brain shows the hemorrhage. Magnetic resonance imaging (MRI) may also show the blood.

Management is supportive with ICU observation. Coagulation studies are checked and corrected if abnormal. Increased ICP is generally treated as discussed in Chapter 13. Corticosteroids are of no benefit. Seizures are treated as discussed later.

Surgery for intraparenchymal hemorrhage does not generally have a good outcome, but some patients may benefit from craniectomy or drainage.

Subdural Hematoma

Subdural hematoma (SDH) is blood accumulated between the inner layer of the dura and the arachnoid membrane. In general, SDH is indicative of a severe head injury, but it can develop with more mild head injuries, especially if the patient is on anticoagulants or other antithrombotics or is elderly. In these latter cases, the onset may be more insidious.

PRESENTATION can span a spectrum. Some presentations can be:

- Coma since the injury
- Initial improvement then deterioration
- Gradual development of deficits (confusion, focal signs) over days or weeks
- Seizures

Gradual development after the injury is particularly common in the elderly and with anticoagulation. The trauma may have seemed trivial and may have been forgotten.

DIAGNOSIS is suspected when, after injury, a patient has cognitive change or focal symptoms or signs. CT brain shows the SDH in most cases. If the SDH is very thin, it may be missed on CT but then be detected on MRI. Restudy is warranted if there is deterioration in function. If the SDH is easily visualized on CT, then MRI is usually not needed unless the patient has focal signs that might suggest secondary infarction (e.g., from dissection). Sometimes, acute on chronic SDH is identified.

MANAGEMENT of small SDH can be conservative, with follow-up to ensure that more blood or fluid does not accumulate. If there is progressive accumulation, surgical drainage is often needed. Seizures are treated as discussed later. Patients and families should be advised that surgical removal of the SDH does not reverse the traumatic brain damage.

Epidural Hematoma

Epidural hematoma is accumulation of blood above the dura. Although this is less common than SDH, it often has a more rapid development and progress, so rapid evaluation and management is essential.

PRESENTATION is usually with significant cognitive impairment from confusion to coma. Headache is expected if the patient is awake. Classic teaching speaks of a lucid interval between the injury and later deterioration, but this occurs in a minority of patients. Focal signs are common, which may be evident whether arousable or comatose.

DIAGNOSIS is suspected when a patient presents with marked encephalopathy after head injury. CT brain is performed emergently. Coags are checked for coagulopathy.

MANAGEMENT is usually surgical. There are occasional patients with small epidural hematomas who can be managed conservatively, but Neurosurgery guides management.

Subarachnoid Hemorrhage

Traumatic subarachnoid hemorrhage (SAH) can develop from significant head injury and can be in a spectrum from a small amount of blood without evident direct clinical consequences to marked hemorrhage. While aneurysmal SAH is discussed in Chapter 16, traumatic SAH is much more common.

PRESENTATION can be subtle to devastating. Headache is the most common symptom. Confusion, focal deficits, or seizures can develop. Symptoms can be directly caused by the subarachnoid blood, or due to secondary effects of hydrocephalus, vasospasm, or even pituitary dysfunction.

DIAGNOSIS and *MANAGEMENT* are similar to that described in Chapter 16 for aneurysmal SAH. The incidence of vasospasm is less with traumatic hemorrhage.

DIFFUSE AXONAL INJURY

Diffuse axonal injury (DAI) usually develops from rapid acceleration and/or deceleration injuries. Classic presentation is shaken baby syndrome, but it develops in adults from a variety of injuries. The most common is motor vehicle accident.

PRESENTATION is usually encephalopathy and is suspected when unconsciousness persists for hours. Subsequently, complications from cerebral edema develop. DAI can ultimately result in coma or persistent vegetative state.

DIAGNOSIS is suspected when a patient with head injury has prolonged unconsciousness in the absence of significant abnormality on CT brain. Early changes are often invisible on CT. Subsequently, cerebral edema and perhaps microhemorrhages can be seen on CT. MRI brain can show changes early, with multifocal regions of increased T2 signal. Gradient echo can show microhemorrhages.

MANAGEMENT of DAI consists of support and treatment of cerebral edema. Osmotic agents and hyperventilation are considered for control of edema. Corticosteroids are not used.[2] Hypothermia has been tried but benefit is unproved.

SEIZURES AFTER HEAD INJURY

Seizures are more common with increasing severity of head injury and especially when there are structural abnormalities of the brain: hemorrhage, contusion, edema.

PRESENTATION can be seizures that are focal, generalized, or mixed. Focal seizures with secondary generalization can occur. Seizures are classified as *early* (within 1 week) or *late* (beyond 1 week).

DIAGNOSIS is evident with clinical seizure activity. If seizures occur in a patient who did not have them earlier in the hospital course, reimaging is recommended to look for expanding bleeding or edema. Electroencephalogram (EEG) is performed to look for nonconvulsive seizures, especially if mental status is significantly depressed.

MANAGEMENT with post-traumatic seizures is classically with phenytoin, although carbamazepine and levetiracetam have been used.[3] Treatment reduces the chance of recurrent early seizures but does not appear to reduce the rate of late seizures or *post-traumatic epilepsy* (PTE). Routine seizure management should include advising the patient and family of seizure precautions including self-care and driving restrictions appropriate to the regional laws, regulations, and best practices.

REPETITIVE HEAD INJURIES

Repetitive head injuries are implicated in a variety of chronic neurologic problems. Repeated concussions predispose to dementia and *chronic traumatic encephalopathy* (CTE). CTE is a cognitive difficulty after repeated head injury that can look similar clinically and even pathologically to Alzheimer's disease.

PRESENTATION is with deficits in memory, orientation, attention, and concentration. A history of head injuries is often elicited. Although most people can produce a history of at least one head injury, patients with CTE have usually had multiple concussions.

DIAGNOSIS is suspected with apparent dementia and a history of concussions. Brain imaging with MRI or CT is performed that may not show signs of previous injury. Labs for other reversible causes are warranted.

MANAGEMENT is supportive. There is a small amount of evidence supporting the benefits of rivastigmine.

POST-CONCUSSIVE SYNDROME

Post-concussive syndrome (PCS) occasionally but not invariably follows nontrivial head injuries.

PRESENTATION is typically with core symptoms of headache, dizziness, and cognitive disturbance. Other symptoms that may develop include fatigue, irritability, sleep difficulty, and photophobia.

DIAGNOSIS is suspected when patients are still symptomatic a week or more after injury. The duration of symptoms to qualify for the diagnosis has not been established by consensus. CT or MRI brain is performed if there has not been imaging already or if there was worsening symptoms after initial presentation.

MANAGEMENT is supportive. No specific treatments are helpful. Patients should avoid activities that can result in another head injury, but activity should be maintained, achieving as normal a lifestyle as possible. Education and reassurance are essential. Part of this should be an explanation that normal imaging does not mean they were not injured.

RETURN-TO-PLAY CRITERIA

Athletes who have had a concussion should be removed from the game and not be returned until they have been evaluated by a medical provider well-trained in the evaluation and management of head injuries. Recent revisions in guidelines for management have been published.[4] Quantitative scores to guide management are no longer given; treatment and management must be individualized. Free access to the guidelines is available through PMC and should be in the library of all physicians caring for concussions.

In general, patients with concussion should not be returned to full activity until they have complete recovery from their injury. Patients with one concussion are more likely to have another.

36 Sleep Disorders

Karl E. Misulis, MD, PhD and
E. Lee Murray, MD

CHAPTER CONTENTS

- Overview
- Obstructive Sleep Apnea
- Narcolepsy
- Periodic Limb Movement Disorder
- Insomnia and Sleep Deprivation

OVERVIEW

Sleep disorders are rarely a reason for hospital admission, but they may become an issue during hospitalization for other reasons. Also, many hospitals routinely screen patients for risk of sleep apnea, especially if anesthesia is contemplated. These disorders are detailed below but are briefly described as follows:

- *Obstructive sleep apnea (OSA)*: Episodes of apnea while sleeping resulting in frequent arousals. Predisposes to respiratory difficulty in the hospital and after discharge.
- *Narcolepsy*: Excessive daytime sleepiness typically with episodes of weakness or paralysis (cataplexy) which can be mistaken for seizure or stroke.
- *Periodic limb movement disorder*: Repetitive movements during sleep which cause arousals. Can be mistaken for seizure or myoclonus.
- *Insomnia and Sleep Deprivation*: Almost universal among hospital patients, predisposes to confusion and possibly hospital psychosis.

OBSTRUCTIVE SLEEP APNEA

Obstructive sleep apnea (OSA) is a common and often undiagnosed disorder. It is most common in middle age, in males, and in patients with elevated BMI. OSA increases the risk of respiratory compromise with sedation and anesthesia.

PRESENTATION is with episodes of apnea while sleeping. Patients often have prominent snoring, frequent arousals during sleep, and excessive daytime sleepiness (EDS). OSA can exacerbate headaches, hypertension, and promote cognitive difficulty.

DIAGNOSIS is considered when a patient has a history of snoring, has elevated BMI, and, in the hospital setting, is being evaluated for a condition with OSA implications such as preoperative evaluation or hypertension. Polysomnography (PSG) is indicated but is seldom performed on acute hospitalization.

Screening for OSA in the hospital setting is usually by a simple evaluation described by the acronym STOP-BANG. If more than two questions in either group are positive, then the risk is substantially increased. If more than two questions are positive in both groups, then the risk of mild sleep apnea is at least 90% and moderate or worse is at least 80%.

- *STOP*
  - ○ Snoring
  - ○ Tired
  - ○ Observed to stop breathing
  - ○ High Blood Pressure
- *BANG*
  - ○ BMI >35
  - ○ Age >50 years
  - ○ Neck circumference >17 inches
  - ○ Gender = male

MANAGEMENT of OSA consists of continuous positive airway pressure (CPAP) for most patients. Weight loss can lower the necessity for CPAP, but the success at persistent weight loss is less than desired. If OSA is suspected on the basis of inhouse consultation, sleep lab referral is strongly recommended.

NARCOLEPSY

Narcolepsy is occasionally diagnosed in the acute hospital setting, usually presenting to the ED with sleep attacks or cataplexy, although they are usually not recognized as such by observers.

PRESENTATION in the hospital setting is usually with observed episodes of sleep attack, or cataplexy—sudden loss of muscle tone. Patients may be thought to have had syncope, seizure, or transient ischemic attack, but there is no focal deficit, no loss of consciousness with cataplexy, and, upon further questioning, associated symptoms are usually noted including excessive daytime sleepiness, sleep paralysis, and hypnagogic hallucinations—sensory experiences during the transition from wake to sleep. In the outpatient arena, excessive daytime sleepiness is often the principal complaint.

DIAGNOSIS is suspected when a patient evaluated for "spell" is felt to have sleep attack or cataplexy. Clinical diagnosis is quite accurate when the other associated features are present. Sleep studies including PSG and MSLT are performed for diagnosis, but can seldom be performed during an acute hospitalization. Once the diagnosis is suspected to the exclusion of life-threatening conditions, prompt referral to a sleep specialist for diagnosis and treatment is recommended.

MANAGEMENT is usually referred to a sleep specialist and includes stimulants such as methylphenidate, modafinil, and use of sodium oxybate for the cataplexy.

PERIODIC LIMB MOVEMENT DISORDER

Periodic limb movement disorder (PLMD) is repetitive movements during sleep that can cause arousals and interfere with sleep. PLMD is related to restless leg syndrome (RLS), and is seldom a reason for hospital consultation.

PRESENTATION in the hospital setting is usually with jerking of the legs, which can be interpreted by family as possible seizure.

DIAGNOSIS is confirmed by PSG, although this is usually not available during acute hospitalization.

MANAGEMENT is usually with dopaminergic agents, especially ropinirole, pramipexole, or levodopa preparations.

INSOMNIA AND SLEEP DEPRIVATION

Insomnia seldom triggers inpatient neurology consultation, but the effects of sleep deprivation often do. Insomnia and sleep deprivation in the hospital setting predisposes to delirium, and sometimes hospital psychosis. Reasons for insomnia in the hospital setting can include:

- *Environmental insomnia*: Sleep is disturbed by frequent awakenings from monitors, medical treatments, and evaluations. Change in sleep venue also worsens the quality of sleep.
- *Stress insomnia*: Stresses of many types can cause or exacerbate insomnia; in this context, the stress of hospitalization and concern over the medical condition.
- *Medical condition*: Innumerable medical conditions are associated with insomnia or sleep fragmentation. Medications also can exacerbate this, not only stimulants but also, from a neurologic perspective, anticonvulsants and sedatives.

MANAGEMENT of insomnia in a hospital setting is difficult. The situation is dynamic and temporary. Elements that can be helpful include:

- *Sedative-hypnotics* should be avoided if possible. Chronic therapy can exacerbate insomnia, and patients often have cognitive changes and a predisposition to falls exacerbated by sedatives.
- *Sleep hygiene* should be the first choice for most hospitalized patients. Among these recommendations are:
  - Turn off the lights and TV at sleep-time.
  - Keep patient awake during the day. If possible, the patient should spend time sitting or walking during the day.
  - Minimize night-time awakening for vital signs, phlebotomy, and medication administration.

37 Developmental and Genetic Disorders

Karl E. Misulis, MD, PhD and
E. Lee Murray, MD

CHAPTER CONTENTS

- Developmental Disorders
  - Chiari Malformation
  - Syringomyelia and Syringobulbia
  - Disorders of Neuronal Migration
- Genetic Disorders
  - Hereditary Neuropathies
  - Hereditary Neuropathy with Pressure Palsy
  - Neurofibromatosis
  - Hereditary Spastic Paraparesis
  - Down Syndrome

DEVELOPMENTAL DISORDERS

There are innumerable developmental disorders; this chapter does not address disorders that primarily affect children, because of the adult focus of this book. Instead, we focus here on developmental or genetic disorders that are likely to come to the attention of the hospital neurologist.

Chiari Malformations

Chiari malformations are a family of disorders affecting the brainstem, upper cervical spinal cord, and craniocervical junction. In hospital practice, only Chiari type 1 is commonly encountered; the other types are rarer and/or usually diagnosed in childhood. The types are:

- *Chiari-1*: Cerebellar tonsils extending below the foramen magnum
- *Chiari-2*: Cerebellar tonsils and vermis extending below the foramen magnum, with myelomeningocele
- *Chiari-3*: Cerebellum and brainstem protrude through the foramen magnum, as can the 4th ventricle; may be associated with occipital encephalocele
- *Chiari-4*: Cerebellar hypoplasia, without displacement of the tonsils

PRESENTATION of Chiari-1 is varied. This is often a diagnosis made after magnetic resonance imaging (MRI) is performed for symptoms unrelated to the finding. Chiari has been theorized to be implicated in a variety of disorders for which it has no consistent responsibility, such as fibromyalgia and chronic fatigue syndrome. When Chiari-1 has neurologic symptoms, presentation is usually with headache, which is often worse with movement of the head and neck, cough, or Valsalva maneuver. Neurologic deficits may include cerebellar ataxia, myelopathy, nystagmus, dysarthria, or dysphagia.

DIAGNOSIS is considered when a relatively young patient, usually young adult, has cerebellar and/or corticospinal findings, especially when there are other bulbar deficits. MRI brain shows the anatomical change, with the degree of cerebellar displacement and craniocervical compression appropriate to the symptoms. Mild Chiari-1 unrelated to the presentation is common, and other causes of the symptoms need to be considered. If Chiari is diagnosed, MRI of the spine should be considered to look for syringomyelia.

MANAGEMENT depends on the severity. If symptoms are minimal, only symptomatic treatment is needed. Neurologic deficits should prompt consideration of neurosurgical consultation. Suboccipital decompression can be performed, but more extensive surgery is sometimes needed.

The role of the neurologist is usually to determine whether a newly diagnosed Chiari seen on MRI explains the symptoms and needs further evaluation or treatment. Often, the finding is incidental, and the search for a cause of the neurologic complaints should continue.

Syringomyelia and Syringobulbia

Syringomyelia is a fluid-filled cavity within the spinal cord, and syringobulbia is a similar cavity in the brainstem. Many of these are associated with Chiari malformations or other developmental abnormalities.

PRESENTATION depends on the anatomy:

- Syringomyelia can produce a central cord syndrome with segmental motor deficit at the levels of the lesion. and often relative preservation of descending corticospinal tracts. There may be dissociated sensory loss with deficits in pain and temperature with relative preservation of vibration and proprioception.
- Syringobulbia produces lower brainstem deficits including nystagmus, vertigo, facial sensory loss, and/or motor deficit affecting the tongue, palate, and vocal cord. Corticospinal tracts may be affected by medullary compression.

DIAGNOSIS is considered when a patient presents with multiple neurologic deficits referable to the brainstem, cerebellum, and cervical spine. MRI of the brain and cervical spine shows the abnormal anatomy.

MANAGEMENT of significant compression is usually surgical. Although this can relieve further damage due to anatomic compression, this does not reverse much of the neurological deficit.

The role of the hospital neurologist is usually to identify the cause of complex deficits and determine whether the findings on the imaging explain the clinical findings.

Disorders of Neuronal Migration

Disorders of neuronal migration are a heterogeneous group of conditions that are usually identified in childhood, so the hospital neurologist is aware of them at the time of consultation. We are asked to address neurologic complications. Occasionally, patients reach adult life without the diagnosis. The spectrum of disorders is huge and includes schizencephaly, porencephaly, lissencephaly, agyria, macrogyria, polymicrogyria, pachygyria, microgyria, micropolygyria, neuronal heterotopias, agenesis of the corpus callosum, and agenesis of the cranial nerves.[1]

PRESENTATION to the hospital neurologist is usually with seizures. Otherwise, static deficits can include developmental delay, motor deficit, cognitive deficit, and associated microcephaly. Adults with seizures are occasionally identified as having heterotopias, which can cause a spectrum of seizures including those with focal-onset of various types.[2]

MANAGEMENT of seizures is with typical antiepileptic drugs (AEDs). However, adults with medically refractory epilepsy with identified heterotopia of an appropriate location may be amenable to surgery. Seizure management is discussed in detail in Chapter 19.

GENETIC DISORDERS

Most hereditary disorders seldom result in hospital neurology consultations because of the lack of acuity. In the present climate of efficient medical care, neurologic consultation should address those acute condition(s) that contribute to and complicate the reasons for admission and ongoing hospital care.

Huntington disease (HD) is discussed in Chapter 23.

Hereditary Neuropathies

There are a host of hereditary neuropathies that seldom significantly impact hospitalization. Occasionally, patients may develop mononeuropathy due to compression during hospitalization.

Hereditary Neuropathy with Pressure Palsy

Patients with this condition have a clinically and electrophysiologically mild sensorimotor neuropathy, but the main issue for hospital neurology consultation is an acute pressure neuropathy.

PRESENTATION is with mononeuropathy affecting a susceptible nerve, such as peroneal, ulnar, median, and radial. With persistent arm or leg positioning, plexus involvement can occur. The reason for consultation is usually limb weakness. Examination localizes the lesion.

DIAGNOSIS is suspected when a patient has a mononeuropathy and has a history of similar transient pressure palsies. Electromyogram (EMG) usually does not need to be done acutely, but often shows a mild demyelinating sensorimotor polyneuropathy with focal slowing affecting even asymptomatic areas.

MANAGEMENT is supportive, including counseling on positioning and shifting position to avoid sustained compression. Counseling on the condition should emphasize the relatively benign course for most patients and the inheritance being autosomal dominant with variable penetrance.

Neurofibromatosis

Neurofibromatosis (NF) is usually diagnosed before hospitalization; hospital neurologists are usually asked to address neurologic complications. These are usually seizures or tumors such as acoustic neuromas, meningioma, gliomas that can involve the optic nerve, and spinal cord tumors. NF is autosomal dominant but with spontaneous mutations.

- *NF Type 1* (NF1) is the most common form and presents to the neurologist usually with symptoms related to CNS tumors—seizures, focal deficits, or visual loss. Non-neurologic manifestations are café-au-lait spots, axillary freckles, cutaneous neurofibromas, and Lisch nodules. Most patients have a family history of NF or at least similar cutaneous manifestations.
- *NF Type 2* (NF2) is less common and presents with neurologic manifestations of acoustic neuromas, meningiomas, gliomas. While NF2 has fewer cutaneous manifestations, it does have more CNS manifestations.

DIAGNOSIS is suspected in a patient with a deficit in hearing or vision or occurrence of seizure who is found to have cutaneous manifestations suggesting NF. MRI reveals the lesions, and special study of the optic and acoustic nerves may be indicated if these structures are clinically affected.

MANAGEMENT of seizures is with typical AEDs as outlined in Chapter 19. Neurofibromas and other tumors may be treated surgically. Decisions are individualized based on size, location, extent of disease, severity and type of deficit, and patient preference.

Hereditary Spastic Paraparesis

Hereditary spastic paraparesis (HSP) is a family of degenerative disorders of variable inheritance—autosomal dominant, recessive, or X-linked.

PRESENTATION is with progressive myelopathy with spasticity. Nonspinal manifestations can be deficits related to cerebral, brainstem, or cerebellar involvement. These can be cognitive dysfunction, visual difficulty, ataxia, and extrapyramidal motor deficits.

DIAGNOSIS is suspected with myelopathy when there is also identified brainstem, cerebral, or cerebellar deficits. Family history supports the diagnosis. MRI is performed to rule out other structural defects but usually shows spinal cord atrophy with no specific cerebral findings. Genetic testing is available to identify the defect in about 40% of patients.

MANAGEMENT is supportive. Spasticity is treated with standard meds (Chapter 41). Expert nursing care for paraplegia is needed, as is physical therapy.

Down Syndrome

Down syndrome presents to the hospital neurologist almost always for complications rather than initial diagnosis. Most patients have trisomy 21; most were diagnosed in infancy.

PRESENTATION to the hospital neurologist is usually with progressive decline in function or with seizure.

- Cognitive decline is manifest as recent deterioration in the setting of life-long cognitive delay. Cognitive function can be markedly decompensated by concurrent illness such as urinary tract infection. In addition, patients can develop a progressive dementia resembling Alzheimer's disease, often presenting around the age of 40.
- Motor decline is common in Down syndrome with increasing age.
- Seizure is not one of the usual cardinal issues with Down syndrome, but the risk is more than doubled. Seizure can be generalized or focal-onset.

DIAGNOSIS of Down syndrome is typically already made.

- Alzheimer's disease diagnosis in patients with Down syndrome rests on brain imaging and psychologic testing.
- Seizure diagnosis in patients with Down syndrome relies on brain imaging to rule out other structural lesions (e.g., stroke, tumor). Electroencephalogram (EEG) looks for interictal or persistent ictal discharge.

MANAGEMENT of Alzheimer's disease in Down syndrome sometimes includes acetylcholinesterase inhibitors (e.g., donepezil, rivastigmine, galantamine)[3] although data proving efficacy are limited. It is appropriate to consider these agents, but there is no proof of benefit of memantine.

MANAGEMENT *of decline in mobility* has no interventions available. *Management of seizure* is Down syndrome is with the typical meds as outlined in Chapter 19.

38 Psychiatric Disorders

Karl E. Misulis, MD, PhD and
E. Lee Murray, MD

CHAPTER CONTENTS

- Overview
- Psychosis
- Hospital Delirium
- Catatonia
- Serotonin Syndrome
- Neuroleptic Malignant Syndrome
- Conversion Disorder

OVERVIEW

Neurology consultation in patients with psychiatric conditions is usually related to ruling out neurologic disease or management of neurologic complications of psychiatric disorders.

PSYCHOSIS

Psychosis presents to the ED with hallucinations and delusions. Etiology can be primarily psychiatric or due to concurrent medical conditions. Some of these are:

- Neurologic disorders
  - Migraine
  - Complex partial seizure
  - Stroke
  - Encephalitis
  - Brain tumor
- Endocrine
  - Thyrotoxicosis
  - Hashimoto encephalopathy
  - Cushing syndrome
  - Hyperparathyroidism with hypercalcemia
- Medication-induced
  - PCP
  - Cocaine
  - Amphetamines
  - Corticosteroids.

Anti-NMDA receptor encephalitis is probably underdiagnosed, which is particularly problematic since it is treatable. Further discussion is found in Chapter 25.

PRESENTATION of psychosis is with hallucinations and/or delusions. Associated symptoms can suggest specific diagnoses. While visual hallucinations are more likely with secondary than primary psychosis, none of the findings is sufficiently specific to make the differentiation on clinical grounds in the absence of prior psychiatric history.

- *Tremor* can suggest thyrotoxicosis, Hashimoto encephalopathy, corticosteroids, Parkinson disease, or cocaine.
- *Seizure* can suggest cocaine, PCP, or encephalitis.

DIAGNOSIS is clinical for psychosis, but determination of secondary psychosis can require imaging with computed tomography (CT) or magnetic resonance imaging (MRI) if structural or inflammatory lesion is suspected. Electroencephalogram (EEG) is performed if seizure develops or if nonconvulsive seizure is considered. CSF analysis may be needed for encephalitis. Paraneoplastic antibodies may be indicated especially if the patient has known cancer. Thyroid studies including those for Hashimoto encephalopathy may be needed. If anti-NMDA-receptor encephalitis is suspected, a search for tumor (e.g., ovarian teratoma) is warranted.

The role of the neurologist is often to look for secondary psychosis. All of the outlined potential evaluation does not need to be done in most cases. However, study is indicated especially if there are cognitive changes or other neurologic deficits other than psychosis.

HOSPITAL DELIRIUM

Delirium is common in the hospital setting, especially among elderly patients and those with dementia. Multiple medications and concurrent medical problems also predispose to hospital delirium. Important causes of note include urinary tract infection (UTI), other infections, metabolic derangements including renal and hepatic insufficiency, withdrawal syndrome, and congestive heart failure (CHF).

PRESENTATION is with difficulty with attention and concentration, confusion, and disorientation. Many have agitation, delusions, or hallucinations. Neurologic findings may include dysarthria and other language difficulty.

DIAGNOSIS is suspected when a hospitalized patient develops agitation or confusion.

- Brain imaging with CT or MRI is performed to look for structural abnormality such as stroke, hemorrhage, subdural hematoma (SDH), or abscess.
- EEG is performed especially if seizure is observed or if there is marked encephalopathy since nonconvulsive seizures can produce altered mental status.
- Lumbar puncture (LP) is performed if there is fever or other signs of infection with new mental status changes.

MANAGEMENT depends on the cause. In the absence of reversible cause, general management of delirium is a combination of behavioral management and meds.

- Treat provoking conditions (e.g., UTI, metabolic disturbance).
- Avoid nonessential meds (e.g., sedative/hypnotics).
- Provide visual cues such as familiar items, pictures.
- Favor good sleep–wake cycles by light–dark cycles, avoid restraints and catheters as much as possible; avoid nonessential stimulation at night.
- If needed, meds can be used; some of the most commonly used include haloperidol or atypical neuroleptics such as risperidone or quetiapine. Benzodiazepines are used if the patient was on similar agents prior to hospitalization.

CATATONIA

Catatonia is occasionally seen by the hospital neurologist. Catatonia can be due to a primary psychiatric disorder or due to medical condition.

PRESENTATION is most commonly with mutism and immobility. There may be rigidity, and this may be associated with waxy flexibility. Other manifestations can be agitation, echolalia (repeating speech), or echopraxia (mimicking movements).

DIAGNOSIS is clinical and suspected when patients present with mutism and rigidity. Additional study is usually necessary.

- *Lab studies* for alternative diagnoses would especially look for elevated WBC, elevated creatine phosphokinase, electrolyte derangement especially hyponatremia, and liver function tests.
- *Brain imaging* with CT or MRI is usually necessary.
- *EEG* is performed if nonconvulsive seizure or encephalitis is considered. EEG background is normal in catatonia of primary psychiatric etiology.
- *CSF* analysis is obtained if encephalitis is considered, especially if febrile, increased WBC, or specific neck rigidity. Brain imaging is performed prior to the LP.

MANAGEMENT of catatonia of primary psychiatric origin should be done with psychiatry consultation. Urgent therapy is typically medical.

- Benzodiazepines are often used especially for patients with rigidity.
- Neuroleptics are often used but because of the risk of neuroleptic malignant syndrome (NMS), newer atypical neuroleptics are used preferentially.
- Anticonvulsants have been used, including carbamazepine.
- Agents that might trigger or exacerbate catatonic activity should be discontinued (e.g., neuroleptics, levetiracetam).

The role of the neurologist is to identify medical conditions that can be associated with the clinical appearance of catatonia, especially NMS, encephalitis, and nonconvulsive seizure.

SEROTONIN SYNDROME

Serotonin syndrome (SS) can develop at therapeutic or toxic doses of selective serotonin reuptake inhibitors (SSRIs). Interaction between drugs can make SS more likely. In addition to SSRIs, other medication classes which can precipitate SS include serotonin norepinephrine reuptake inhibitor (SNRIs), tricyclic antidepressants (TCAs), and monoamine oxidase inhibitors (MAOIs). Less likely are amphetamines, triptans, and some opioids.

PRESENTATION is with any combination of agitation, confusion, ataxia, myoclonus, hyperthermia, diaphoresis, and diarrhea. There are established criteria with combinations of these, but any constellation of like symptoms should prompt query about exposure to any meds that can produce SS. Rhabdomyolysis can develop with resultant renal insufficiency.

DIAGNOSIS is suspected when a patient presents with agitation, confusion, and recent exposure to a possible precipitant med. Brain imaging is performed to rule out structural lesion. LP may be indicated to look for meningitis or encephalitis.

MANAGEMENT begins with discontinuation of precipitant meds even before the diagnosis is certain. If the patient has developed metabolic abnormalities or rhabdomyolysis, these are also addressed as soon as identified. Cyproheptadine is sometimes used for persistent symptoms.

NEUROLEPTIC MALIGNANT SYNDROME

NMS is a reaction to any of multiple meds. This is an idiosyncratic reaction and not a dose-dependent toxicity. Among the meds that can produce NMS are the following classes with representative examples in each class:

- Neuroleptics
  - Typical (e.g., haloperidol, chlorpromazine)
  - Atypical (e.g., risperidone, clozapine, olanzapine)
- Antiemetics (e.g., metoclopramide, promethazine, prochlorperazine)
- Lithium (at high doses)
- Dopaminergic drug discontinuation (e.g., levodopa, dopamine agonists)

PRESENTATION is with confusion progressing to delirium, muscle rigidity, hyperthermia, and autonomic hyperactivity with tachycardia, tachypnea, hypertension, and diaphoresis. Hyperthermia and rigidity are not invariable and, if not present, make the diagnosis difficult.

DIAGNOSIS is suspected with muscle rigidity and fever. More subtle presentations, especially the common occurrence of cognitive changes at onset, may not immediately be considered as possible NMS. Development after neuroleptic administration is key, but in the hospital setting, abrupt discontinuation of dopaminergic meds in a patients with Parkinson disease or other movement disorder has to be considered. Surgery or concurrent illness may preclude PO meds. Brain imaging is essential with cognitive changes. Labs should include renal and liver function tests, coagulation studies, CPK, and urine myoglobin in addition to routine labs. Blood and other cultures are indicated with fever. CSF analysis may be needed to rule out meningitis or encephalitis.

MANAGEMENT begins with discontinuation of the offending med or restarting a dopaminergic agent if withdrawal is the cause. Fever can become critically high, so cooling is performed both by antipyretics and mechanical devices if needed. Dantrolene, bromocriptine, or amantadine are often used, although evidence of effectiveness is limited. Benzodiazepines are often used to control agitation.

CONVERSION DISORDER

Conversion disorder is a common hospital diagnosis. Presentation is usually to the ED with neurologic deficit. Initial evaluation and management has to assume organic pathology. Some patients may unconsciously embellish symptoms of a real neurologic condition, and if we detect inconsistencies suggesting an overlay, we might not offer thrombolytics or other appropriate intervention. Luckily, IV tissue plasminogen activator (tPA) has an extremely low incidence of serious side effects for patients without stroke who otherwise meet inclusion and exclusion criteria, hence most hospital neurologists have given thrombolytics to patients who were later identified as having conversion disorder or migraine.

PRESENTATION to the ED is usually with one of the following:

- *Paralysis*, which may be unilateral or bilateral or a single extremity or face. Often there is a disconnect between movement and tone and often resistance to passive movement. Facial "weakness" is associated with increased tone and tightness of the affected side.
- *Unresponsiveness* that has a few features that appear atypical, including hands folded on the body, forced resistance to eye opening, or resistance to passive movement of the limbs.
- *Clinical seizure activity*, which can look convincing since there is quite a spectrum of genuine seizure semiology.
- *Speech difficulty* with or without inability to understand speech. Total absence of speech is typical, although others include an unusual slurring, stuttering, and a baby-talk type of speech. Long pauses between otherwise articulated words favors functional deficit.
- *Blindness*, which is most often both eyes but can be one eye. Pupil responses are preserved. Patients often decline to move their eyes even though a truly blind person can usually move his or her eyes on command.
- *Confusion*, which often spans hierarchical organization (e.g., the patient may remember nothing including his or her own name, names of relatives, or any historical details). The temporal window of memory loss can be absolute (e.g., no memory from a specified point or might remember all details of a previous marriage but none of the present). Some patients forget all aspects of personal identity and history, a common film script scenario but not suggestive of organic deficit.
- *Movement disorders* can be of a many types, but features that suggest conversion disorder include variation in character, intensity, and direction of the movements; wildly flinging movements; discrepancies in presence at rest or with motion. Note that hemiballismus can appear functional the first time a clinician sees it.
- *Seizures* are discussed in depth in Chapter 19. Psychogenic nonepileptic seizures (PNES) is the present preferred term for *pseudoseizures*. These are difficult to diagnose because of the diverse manifestations of epileptic seizures and the transient and episodic nature of the symptoms.

Clinical signs of conversion disorder include:

- *La belle indifference*: Lack of concern for personal clinical deficit has traditionally been considered evidence of conversion disorder but data show that this is not of clinical value.[1]

- *Hoover sign*: Normal action when lifting one leg is to press the opposite leg into the bed as support. If the patient is not making a genuine effort to lift the leg, there will be no downward pressure of the opposite leg.
- *Forced eye closure*: Patients with functional unresponsiveness often exhibit resistance to eye opening, which is only occasionally seen in patients with organic encephalopathy.
- *Inconsistency between exam and observation*: Often patients have more abilities when not being examined (e.g., inability to move a limb during exam yet does so spontaneously while talking).
- *Clenched fist*: This unusual posture is uncommon and usually nonorganic. If it is true motor overactivity, then it should be released by wrist flexion; the absence of this observed effect argues against organic cause.

DIAGNOSIS depends on identifying the inconsistencies on presentation yet remaining vigilant for signs of organic deficit. Depending on the presentation, imaging with CT or MRI is commonly performed. CT has usually been ordered even prior to neurologic consultation as part of a stroke protocol. The key is to do sufficient study to reasonably rule out organic disease but not so extensive that the behavior is reinforced. We do not want the patient to reach the status of "medical mystery."

Diagnostic criteria established in the Diagnostic and Statistical Manual of Mental Disorders (DSM-5) are summarized here[2]:

- One or more disorders of motor or sensory function
- Findings are not compatible with a neurologic or medical condition.
- Deficits cannot be better explained by another disorder.
- Deficit is of sufficient severity to alter function and/or prompt medical attention.

MANAGEMENT is difficult and complex in a fast-paced hospital setting. We recommend not addressing the suspected diagnosis initially. Allow the required studies to be done. Patients often have to be hospitalized briefly to complete the evaluation. When appropriate, a gentle discussion that their condition might have been triggered by "stress" or "nerves" is often, but not invariably, given audience. Avoid telling the patient or family that there is nothing wrong with them or that it is all "in their head." Being available for discussion and also arranging for post-acute care follow-up very soon is important and should be with a neurologist; psychological or psychiatric referral may be successful only after there has been a good relationship established between the clinician and patient. Try to avoid giving meds for diseases they don't have: stroke, multiple sclerosis, or seizures.

SECTION IV
NEUROLOGY
TOOLKIT

SECTION CONTENTS

39 Toolkit: Assessments
40 Toolkit: Studies
41 Toolkit: Neurologic Management
42 Toolkit: Difficult Encounters

39 Toolkit
Assessments

Karl E. Misulis, MD, PhD and
E. Lee Murray, MD

CHAPTER CONTENTS

- Glasgow Coma Scale
- Stroke Scales
  - NIH Stroke Scale
  - Los Angeles Prehospital Stroke Screen
  - ABCD^2 Score
- Subarachnoid Hemorrhage Scales
  - World Federation of Neurosurgery Grading System
  - Modified Fisher Scale

A variety of assessment tools are used in neurology practice. Some of those that are of particular use to hospital neurologists are discussed. Scales for multiple sclerosis, Parkinson disease, and dementia are not included here because they pertain to the outpatient practice of neurology and are rarely used in the inpatient setting.

GLASGOW COMA SCALE

The Glasgow Coma Scale (GCS) is commonly used in hospital neurology and neurosurgery and is part of core assessment metrics at most institutions. It was initially developed at the University of Glasgow and used predominantly for head injury patients.[1] Since then, it has been used in a variety of neurologic conditions.

Points are assessed in three spheres and the response graded. The score is summed for a total scale score.

Scale ranges from 15 (best, normal) to 3 (worst):

- *Eye opening*
  - Spontaneous: 4 points
  - To verbal command: 3 points
  - To pain: 2 points
  - None: 1 point
- *Best motor response*
  - Obeys verbal command: 6 points
  - Localizes painful stimuli: 5 points

- o Withdrawal from painful stimuli: 4 points
- o Flexion response to painful stimuli: 3 points
- o Extension response to painful stimuli: 2 points
- o None: 1 point
- *Best verbal response*
  - o Oriented conversation: 5 points
  - o Confused conversation: 4 points
  - o Incoherent words: 3 points
  - o Incomprehensible sounds: 2 points
  - o None: 1 point

Brain injury classification depends on the score:

- Severe: GCS ≤8
- Moderate: GCS = 9–12
- Minor: GCS ≥13

Interpretation of the scale is somewhat controversial, but these are generally accepted by most facilities.

STROKE SCALES

National Institutes of Health Stroke Scale (NIHSS) is the most commonly used stroke assessment in hospital neurology. Presently, inclusion and exclusion criteria for use of IV tissue plasminogen activator (tPA) relies on the NIHSS. Likewise, decision-making regarding endovascular therapy also relies in part on the NIHSS.

The *Los Angeles Prehospital Stroke Screen (LAPSS)* is a tool to help identify stroke victims before arrival at the hospital.

The *ABCD score* is used to estimate the risk of stroke following a transient ischemic attack (TIA). The present iteration, the ABCD[2] score, is discussed here.

National Institutes of Health Stroke Scale

The *NIHSS* is routinely used for classifying strokes in the hospital. Performance requires special training.

The scale ranges from 0 (normal) to 42 (most severe stroke). In general, the results of the scoring can be divided into the following bins:

- NIHSS 0: No stroke symptoms
- NIHSS 1–4: Minor stroke
- NIHSS 5–15: Moderate stroke
- NIHSS 16–20: Moderate to severe stroke
- NIHSS 21–42: Severe stroke

The complexity of the exam means that the entirety of the description cannot be presented here. A worksheet with the tasks is available in almost all EDs.

There are a variety of apps available to perform the NIHSS or at least keep track of scoring, and an online calculator is available.[2]

The NIHSS categories include

1: Consciousness
- o 1A: Level of consciousness
- o 1B: Ask month and age
- o 1C: Blink eyes and squeeze hands

2: Horizontal eye movements

3: Visual fields

4: Facial palsy

5: Motor of the arm
- o 5A: Left arm drift
- o 5B: Right arm drift

6: Motor of the leg
- o 6A: Left leg drift
- o 6B: Right leg drift

7: Limb ataxia

8: Sensory

9: Language/Aphasia

10: Dysarthria

11: Extinction and inattention.

A modification of the NIHSS is available to improve interexaminer consistency, but this above is the standard set for most clinical use.

Los Angeles Prehospital Stroke Screen

The LAPSS provides guidance on which patients should be placed on a fast-track to stroke evaluation and treatment before they get to the hospital. The screen is meant to be performed by nonphysicians. Meeting all of the criteria means that the patient should be treated with the presumption of acute stroke.

- Age >45 years
- No prior history of seizure disorder
- New onset of neurologic symptoms within the past 24 hours
- Patient was ambulatory prior to the event.
- Blood glucose is between 60 and 400
- Exam shows obvious asymmetry.
  - o Brief motor exam shows unilateral and not bilateral weakness
  - o Facial droop
  - o Grip asymmetry
  - o Arm weakness

Meeting all the major bullet points meets the LAPSS criteria. Any of the subordinate bullet point conditions found on one side of the body but not the other meets criteria for unilateral deficit.

ABCD² Score

The initial ABCD score was revised with the addition of diabetes-related issues. Therefore, the new scale is ABCD with another D, or ABCD²:

- Age
  - <60 years: 0 point
  - ≥ 60 years: 1 point
- Blood pressure
  - Normal: 0 point
  - ≥ = 140/90: 1 point
- Clinical features
  - No speech disturbance and no unilateral weakness: 0 point
  - Speech disturbance but no unilateral weakness: 1 point
  - Unilateral weakness: 2 points
- Duration
  - <10 min: 0 point
  - 10–59 min: 1 point
  - ≥60 min: 2 points
- Diabetes
  - No diabetes: 0 point
  - Diabetes: 1 point

Interpretation of the risk of stroke depends on the total score:

- Score 1–3 (low): 2-day risk of 1.0%, 7-day risk of 1.2%
- Score 4–5 (moderate): 2-day risk of 4.1%, 7-day risk of 5.9%
- Score 6–7 (high): 2-day risk of 8.1%, 7-day risk of 11.7%

The risk determines the urgency of evaluation: higher risk patients should be evaluated with greater urgency.

SAH SCALES

Scales for subarachnoid hemorrhage (SAH) are clinical and radiographic.

World Federation of Neurosurgeons Grading System for Subarachnoid Hemorrhage

The WFNS Scale is a simple scale used to grade the severity of SAH. It is based on the Glasgow Coma Scale (GCS).

- Grade 1: GCS 15, no motor deficit
- Grade 2: GCS 13–14, no motor deficit
- Grade 3: GCS 13–14, with motor deficit
- Grade 4: GCS 7–12, with or without motor deficit
- Grade 5: GCS 3–6, with or without motor deficit

Prognosis is based on the GCS:

- GCS = 15: Best chance of recovery
- GCS ≥8: Good chance of recovery
- GCS 3–5: Potentially fatal especially if associated with fixed pupils or absent oculo-vestibular responses
- GCS 3: Worse prognosis

Modified Fisher Scale

The Fisher scale is a classification of SAH depending on appearance on brain computed tomography (CT) and the coexistence of intracerebral hemorrhage (ICH) and/or intraventricular hemorrhage (IVH). The present version is the *Modified Fisher Scale*, which classifies SAH and IVH:

- Group 0: No SAH or IVH
- Group 1: Focal or diffuse, thin SAH, no IVH
- Group 2: Focal or diffuse, thin SAH, with IVH
- Group 3: Focal or diffuse, thick SAH, no IVH
- Group 4: Focal or diffuse, thick SAH, with IVH

Definition of thin is less than 1 mm thick, whereas thick SAH is greater than 1 mm. Higher grades have an increased risk of vasospasm.

40 Toolkit
Studies

Karl E. Misulis, MD, PhD and
E. Lee Murray, MD

CHAPTER CONTENTS

- Electroencephalography
  - Indications
  - Clinical Interpretation
- Nerve Conduction Studies and Electromyography
  - Nerve Conduction Studies
  - Electromyography
  - Repetitive Nerve Stimulation
  - Single-Fiber Electromyography
  - Clinical Implications
- Magnetic Resonance Imaging
- Magnetic Resonance Angiography and Venography
- Computed Tomography Angiography and Venography
- Carotid Ultrasonography
- Lumbar Puncture and CSF
- Catheter Angiography
- Echocardiography

ELECTROENCEPHALOGRAPHY

Electroencephalography (EEG) is measurement of electrical activity of the brain, principally the cortex. In most hospital patients, this is performed by scalp recordings but for patients with epilepsy being considered for surgery, intracranial electrodes and special extracranial electrodes (e.g., sphenoidal) are often used.

Indications

Indications for EEG usually include:

- Seizure
- Encephalopathy
- Brain death
- Unexplained focal deficit
- Myoclonus

Some conditions for which EEG is sometimes ordered but *not* usually clinically indicated are:

- Dizziness, vertigo
- Headache
- Most psychiatric disorders, although EEG may be indicated for patients who are felt to have catatonia, psychosis, or other disorder with cognitive implication.

Clinical Interpretation

EEG has been discussed in numerous chapters of this book. Here we present the clinical implications of some important and common EEG findings. A detailed discussion of EEG is found in our recent book, *Atlas of EEG, Seizure Semiology, and Management.*[1]

Normal waking background : Interpretation of a normal waking background is the best laboratory evidence of normal cognitive function. However, normal waking rhythms can be seen in early dementia and very mild encephalopathy. Also, a normal waking EEG does not rule out epilepsy unless the patient had a clinical event during the EEG; in fact, there are some seizure patterns which can have a normal ictal EEG with scalp recordings, but this is rare.

Normal sleeping background : A patient who has a normal sleeping background but no waking state recorded might still have encephalopathy because the background slowing seen with encephalopathy is often not evident during sleep.

Mild generalized slowing in the awake state : This is one of the most commonly encountered findings in hospitalized patients. This can be indicative of mild encephalopathy or dementia but is nonspecific.

Moderate generalized slowing in the awake state : Moderate slowing is usually due to significant encephalopathy; although chronicity cannot be determined, it can be from dementia or encephalopathy and the differential diagnosis can be metabolic, toxic, multifocal infarctions, or almost any cause of encephalopathy.

Triphasic waves : These waves usually appear on a generally slow background. They usually suggest metabolic encephalopathy, usually hepatic or renal failure. However, the finding is not specific, with other causes being hypoxic encephalopathy and some toxic encephalopathies.

Focal slowing : This suggests a focal structural lesion. This association is greater if the appearance is polymorphic—a disorganized appearance to the slow activity. However, absence of focal slowing does not rule out a structural lesion.

Attenuation versus suppression : These terms are sometimes used interchangeably, but they have different appearances and implications. *Attenuation* is a lower amplitude of the recording and is usually due to separation of the cortex from the scalp electrodes (e.g., subdural hematoma). *Suppression* is more severe because it indicates a slowing and disorganization of the activity that is there, clearly indicating damage to the cortex of almost any cause.

Generalized discharge : This suggests seizure activity. If the duration is beyond 1–2 seconds, then a clinical seizure has been observed.

Three-per-second spike-wave : This is typical of absence seizure. Brief discharges can occur without noted clinical symptoms. The background is otherwise normal.

Periodic lateralized epileptiform discharge (PLEDs) : PLEDs are sometimes called *lateralized periodic discharges* (LPDs) and are indicative of significant destructive lesions near the region of the discharge. Classically, temporal destruction of herpes simplex virus (HSV) encephalitis produces PLEDs, but they are not always present so absence does not rule out the diagnosis. Also, the finding is not specific and is often seen with stroke and other destructive processes. Most patients with PLEDs have seizures although the PLEDs may or may not be ictal themselves.

Bilateral periodic lateralized epileptiform discharges (BiPLEDs) : BiPLEDs are the occurrence of PLEDs bilaterally and indicate bilateral destruction. The most common cause is anoxia. This looks different from generalized periodic discharge in that the PLEDs from the two sides are not synchronous.

Generalized periodic discharge : Unfortunately, this is a common pattern seen in hospital neurology. The periodic discharges are synchronous and often anterior in prominence. The most common etiology is anoxia.

Muscle and movement artifact : These artifacts are especially important in that they obscure activity of cerebral origin. In the hospital setting, we often have a patient with clinical seizure activity monitored to document discharge with the clinical events. But if there is marked muscle activity, whether epileptic or nonepileptic (psychogenic), cerebral activity can be obscured, making EEG differentiation sometimes impossible.

No detectable electrocerebral activity : This is a pattern usually seen in patients meeting criteria for brain death. In order for EEG to be used as a confirmatory test, there are stringent criteria governing EEG performance and interpretation in addition to the brain death guidelines discussed in Chapter 15.

NERVE CONDUCTION STUDIES AND ELECTROMYOGRAPHY

Nerve conduction study (NCS) and *electromyography (EMG)* are usually considered as a package that also includes other special studies, but there are different purposes and indications for each. Certain conditions may not be identified on routine NCS and EMG without the special studies, so these need to be requested specifically.

NCS measures the conduction of motor and sensory nerves with the recorded parameters including velocity and amplitude. This assesses the integrity of nerve conduction. Demyelinating lesions cause slowing of conduction. Axonal and neuronal lesions cause reduction in amplitude. These are generalizations because, with demyelination, dispersion of the waveforms causes a somewhat lower amplitude, and with axonal or neuronal damage there can be a mild reduction in velocity.

Clinically, NCS has a specific role in assessing the myelin component primarily. As such, it is indicated for most suspected peripheral neuropathies. In the hospital setting, NCS is used predominantly for patients with progressive weakness where the differential diagnoses are acute inflammatory demyelinating polyneuropathy (AIDP) and critical illness neuromyopathy (CIN). As a component of NCS, F-waves are the only way to evaluate the proximal nerve and are of special importance for assessment of suspected AIDP.

Indications for NCS in the hospital setting include suspected:

- Chronic peripheral neuropathy, especially suspected chronic inflammatory demyelinating polyneuropathy (CIDP)

- Acute and subacute neuropathy, especially suspected AIDP
- CIN
- Mononeuropathy (e.g., median, ulnar, peroneal).
- Myasthenia gravis (MG)
- Lambert-Eaton myasthenic syndrome (LEMS)

Study of suspected MG and LEMS involves repetitive stimulation but with different protocols (described later). If these are suspected, the electromyographer should be informed so that the proper studies are performed.

Electromyography

EMG assesses the electrical activity of skeletal muscle and provides information on the integrity of neural innervation of the muscle and potential defects in the electrical function of the muscle fibers.

Indications for EMG include evaluation of suspected:

- Chronic peripheral neuropathy (e.g., diabetic, CIDP, multifocal motor neuropathy [MMN])
- Chronic mononeuropathy (e.g., median, ulnar)
- Motoneuron degeneration (e.g., amyotrophic lateral sclerosis [ALS])
- Myopathy (e.g., polymyositis, muscular dystrophy)

EMG is usually normal with acute or subacute axonal or neuronal damage because it takes up to 4 weeks for electrical signs of denervation to appear on routine study, especially for distal muscles. However, if there is loss of sufficient neuronal input to reduce muscle activation, a reduction in functioning units will be seen acutely.

Repetitive Nerve Stimulation

Repetitive nerve stimulation (RNS) is used predominantly for the evaluation of suspected neuromuscular transmission disorders, especially MG, LEMS, and botulism.

Symptoms that might suggest that RNS is indicated are:

- Excessive weakness
- Excessive fatigue
- Diplopia and/or ptosis

If a patient has any neuromuscular transmission abnormalities other than for botulism, he or she should be screened for neoplasm. Note that the majority of patients with LEMS do not have malignancy.

Single-Fiber EMG

Single-fiber EMG (SFEMG) is sometimes used for the diagnosis of neuromuscular transmission disorders. A fine electrode is inserted into the muscle, which has the characteristics of being able to record from at least two muscle fibers innervated by the same motoneuron. SFEMG is valuable for neuromuscular junction pathologies; however, its use is limited.

Clinical Implications of Nerve Conduction Studies and Electromyography

Common scenarios of electrodiagnostic abnormalities include:

- *Normal*: Ideal result of an EMG but this does not rule out neuromuscular pathology. Routine NCS can be normal in many disorders including axonal neuropathies or motoneuron diseases when early or mild and in neuromuscular transmission disorders.
- *Demyelinating neuropathy*: Suggests AIDP or CIDP although there are other possibilities.
- *Axonal neuropathy*: Axonal neuropathy is the most common type, and these are usually chronic. However, AIDP does have axonal variants, as discussed in Chapter 31.
- *Lower motoneuron disorder*: Degeneration of the lower motoneurons without other electrodiagnostic findings may suggest a specific lower motoneuron disorder such as progressive muscular atrophy.
- *Chronic sensorimotor neuropathy*: This is the most common finding on EMG in the hospital. Diabetes is the most common etiology, but the differential diagnosis is huge.
- *Conduction block*: This indicates areas of marked reduction in compound motor action potential (CMAP) amplitude. This is most sensitive for acute demyelinating neuropathies (e.g., AIDP).
- *Myopathy*: A wide variety of myopathies can be identified, and there are various types with different implications. Acuity versus chronicity can be determined as well as anatomic distribution. EMG/NCS can help rule out other pathologies, such as neuropathy. EMG is also useful in choosing a suitable site for muscle biopsy.
- *Decremental response to RNS*: This is an abnormal response to repetitive nerve stimulation most commonly seen in patients with MG, but it is not specific for this. Decremental response at low rates of stimulation can also be seen in botulism and LEMS. Decremental response at low frequencies with incremental response at high frequency suggests LEMS or botulism.
- *Incremental response to RNS*: This is an abnormal response to repetitive stimulation typically given at higher frequencies than those used for evaluation of MG. An incremental response is seen in patients with LEMS and botulism.

MAGNETIC RESONANCE IMAGING

Magnetic resonance imaging (MRI) of neural structures is the gold standard for many conditions. A detailed discussion of its uses is beyond the scope of this book; however, there are some general scenarios affecting hospital neurology that deserve special comment.

Intracranial hemorrhage of various types is generally better seen on MRI than on computed tomography (CT) but subarachnoid hemorrhage may be missed on MRI. If intracranial hemorrhage is suspected, urgent CT should usually be done with subsequent MRI as available. Some hemorrhages have underlying ischemia, which is much better visualized on MRI.

Mass lesions are generally better visualized on MRI than CT. Contrast is given if a mass lesion is suspected as long as the patient does not have a contraindication, such as allergy or renal insufficiency. If a contrasted study has to be done with renal failure, CT is preferable to MRI.

Pregnancy has a host of potential neurologic complications. For brain abnormalities, most of us feel that MRI is preferable to CT, especially after the first trimester.

Implanted devices are a contraindication to MRI for most devices. There are some compliant devices, including new versions of MRI-compatible pacemakers and stimulators. Some devices have to be reprogrammed after MRI, so the study should be performed only if this is available and the device is otherwise MRI compliant.

MAGNETIC RESONANCE ANGIOGRAPHY AND VENOGRAPHY

Vascular imaging with MRA and MRV is satisfactory for many patients, although CT angiography and venography (CTA/CTV) generally give better visualization.

- When patients present with acute stroke, we usually perform CTA at the time of the urgent CT brain scan, often with perfusion study. Then we perform MRI brain at a later time.
- If repeated vascular studies need to be done, MRA is preferable.
- If a one-time study is to be done, then CTA is preferable if there is significant reason to believe vascular pathology is present.
- If the patient has a possible but low likelihood for intracranial pathology (e.g., screening for familial predisposition to aneurysm), the MRA has sensitivity that is adequate for most patients.

COMPUTED TOMOGRAPHY ANGIOGRAPHY AND VENOGRAPHY

CTA is used especially in patients with acute ischemic stroke (AIS). This is often done in the ED as part of the emergent intake. A perfusion study (CTP) is performed also to help determine if the patient is a candidate for endovascular therapy. Many stroke centers are moving to direct-to-CT arrival in the ED; if the patient's clinical characteristics are appropriate, CTA and CTP are then considered.

Indications for CTA other than AIS include intracranial hemorrhage, especially to identify aneurysm or vascular malformation. CTA is also done for some tumors before consideration of surgical options. Among patients with stroke, vasculitis might be identified on CTA but is usually better visualized on catheter angiography.

CTV is used for patients with suspected venous thrombosis. CTV may show lesions not seen on MRV.

CAROTID ULTRASONOGRAPHY

Carotid ultrasonography is still performed for select patients but less so than prior to MRA and CTA. Carotid ultrasonography shows the bifurcations fairly well and sometimes can give additional detail regarding carotid bifurcation pathology, but it does not see more proximal and distal vasculature and sees only evidence of flow in the vertebral arteries without anatomic detail.

Scenarios where carotid ultrasonography may be indicated include:

- Patients who should avoid CTA because of renal failure or risk of severe dye reaction and cannot have MRA because of implanted device
- Patients who have difficult visualization of the details at the carotid bifurcation on CTA or MRA
- Patients with possible internal artery occlusion whose studies are not able to rule out small residual flow

Scenarios where carotid ultrasonography is usually not indicated include:

- Syncope
- Acute ischemic stroke where CTA or MRA is of good diagnostic quality
- Intracranial hemorrhage

LUMBAR PUNCTURE AND CEREBROSPINAL FLUID

Lumbar puncture (LP) with CSF sampling is performed routinely in hospital patients, usually for consideration of infectious disease, but the indications are more extensive than this.

LP and CSF sampling is performed usually when at least one of the following conditions is being considered in the differential diagnosis:

- Meningitis
- Encephalitis
- Subarachnoid hemorrhage
- Encephalomyelitis (e.g., ADEM)
- Neoplastic meningitis
- Multiple sclerosis
- Neuromyelitis optica
- Transverse myelitis
- Pseudotumor cerebri syndrome

Normal parameters of LP and CSF can differ between institutions so check local norms. Some general guidelines are:

- Opening pressure = 10–20 cm H_2O
- WBC ≤5 cells/μL
- RBC = 0–5/mm^3 unless pathologic or traumatic

- Glucose >60% of serum glucose
- Protein <45 mg/dL
- Appearance = clear, colorless

Interpretation of some key abnormalities on LP and CSF can be:

- *Appearance*
  - Cloudy: Increased white cells suggestive of meningitis or encephalitis
  - Bloody: Subarachnoid hemorrhage or traumatic tap
- *Opening pressure*
  - Elevated: Multiple causes (e.g., meningitis, pseudotumor cerebri)
  - Low: May be partial obstruction to CSF flow, CSF leak (low pressure).
- *WBC*
  - Increased to less than 100 suggests viral or neoplastic process
  - Increased to more than 100 can be viral or neoplastic, but bacterial meningitis is of concern also
  - Increased to at least 1,000: Seldom viral and rarely neoplastic, suggests a bacterial process
  - Normal: Does not rule out viral or fungal infection or neoplastic meningitis
- *RBC*: Normally there are few, but with a traumatic tap there can be up to thousands. Bloody CSF is less likely to be SAH if there is not xanthochromia on the spun specimen. Mild increase in CSF RBC can be seen in meningitis and encephalitis, especially HSV.
- *Glucose*: Low glucose suggests consumption, and the most likely are bacterial, fungal, and neoplastic processes. Occasionally viral syndromes can produce lowered glucose.
- *Protein*: Elevation to the 100 range can be seen with neuropathies. Modest elevation is common with any destructive or inflammatory process. Elevation in the thousands suggests cord compression or other significant structural lesion.

CSF findings for specific disorders discussed are included in their respective chapters, but for some select common conditions, typical findings are shown in the list. Note that atypical cases exist for almost all conditions, so finding are not absolute.

LP and CSF findings with some important disorders:

- Bacterial meningitis
  - *Appearance*: Cloudy; occasionally clear
  - *Pressure*: Usually elevated, may be normal
  - *Cells*: WBC usually hundreds to thousands; RBCs may be present
  - *Chemistry*: Glucose low, protein high
- Viral meningitis
  - *Appearance*: Clear, colorless
  - *Pressure*: Normal or mildly increased
  - *Cells*: WBC 10–100, occasionally higher; RBC near 0
  - *Chemistry*: Protein usually increased, more than 60; glucose usually normal
- Fungal meningitis
  - *Appearance*: Often clear; can be cloudy
  - *Pressure*: Usually increased

- o *Cells*: WBC 10–500; RBC 0 or low
- o *Chemistry*: Protein increased; glucose often low
- Viral encephalitis
  - o Appearance: Clear
  - o *Pressure*: Usually normal
  - o *Cells*: WBC mildly increased, RBC may be increased, especially with HSV
  - o *Chemistry*: Protein mildly increased; glucose normal
- Subarachnoid hemorrhage
  - o *Appearance*: Bloody or xanthochromic if not acute
  - o *Pressure*: Increased
  - o *Cells*: RBC increased; WBC mildly increased commensurate with RBC (about 1 WBC for every 700–100 RBC depending on peripheral WBC)
  - o *Chemistry*: Protein increased; glucose normal
- AIDP
  - o Appearance: Clear
  - o *Pressure*: Normal or mildly increased
  - o *Cells*: WBC usually normal; RBC normal
  - o *Chemistry*: Protein increased; glucose normal
- Multiple sclerosis
  - o Appearance: Clear
  - o Pressure: Normal
  - o *Cells*: WBC normal or mild increase; RBC normal
  - o *Chemistry*: Protein mildly increased; glucose normal
- Pseudotumor cerebri
  - o Appearance: Clear
  - o *Pressure*: Increased, often markedly
  - o *Cells*: WBC and RBC are normal
  - o *Chemistry*: Glucose and protein are normal
- Neoplastic meningitis
  - o *Appearance*: Clear or possibly cloudy
  - o *Pressure*: Increased usually
  - o *Cells*: WBC increased from mild to marked; RBC usually normal
  - o *Chemistry*: Protein increased; glucose decreased
- NMO
  - o Appearance: Clear
  - o Pressure: Normal
  - o *Cells*: WBC increased in about half of cases; RBC normal
  - o *Chemistry*: Protein increased in the majority but not all; glucose normal

CATHETER ANGIOGRAPHY

Catheter angiography is used most commonly for stroke, but there are other indications. Angiography can be purely diagnostic or as part of endovascular therapy. Scenarios where catheter angiography may be indicated include:

- *Acute ischemic stroke*: Angiography can be a prelude to endovascular therapy. This study should be considered as soon as possible after onset of symptoms.

- *Cerebral aneurysm*: Catheter angiography is an excellent study for suspected cerebral aneurysm either because of proven subarachnoid hemorrhage or incidental finding of aneurysm on MRA or CTA performed for another reason.
- *Vascular malformation*: A host of vascular malformations are evaluated well by catheter angiography including arteriovenous malformation (AVM), dural fistulas.
- *Vasculitis*: Patients with clinical and/or radiological signs of multifocal ischemia are often considered as having possible vasculitis. This can occur in the setting of a known autoimmune disorder or be isolated. Whereas noninvasive vascular imaging can occasionally reveal vasculitis, conventional angiography is superior.

ECHOCARDIOGRAPHY

Echocardiography (echo) as used for hospital neurology consists of trans-thoracic echo (TTE) and trans-esophageal echo (TEE). TTE is performed on most patients with AIS.

Indications to order TTE for AIS include any of the following:

- AIS that might be embolic on the basis of clinical presentation and imaging
- AIS with imaging findings of multiple infarctions in different vascular distributions
- AIS with no signs of responsible etiology on neurovascular imaging of the supplying vessels: carotid or vertebral
- AIS with hemorrhagic transformation, especially without a known neurovascular etiology of embolic source
- Suspicion of right-to-left shunt (e.g., in patient with AIS with known deep venous thrombosis)
- Suspicion of cardiac source (e.g., new murmur, signs of non-neuro emboli, suspicion of septic emboli)
- AIS with cardiac symptoms at the time of onset (e.g., chest pain or palpitations)

TEE is sometimes performed for follow-up of a suspected pathologic finding on TTE. At other times, TEE is performed even if the TTE is negative; in these patients, it typically is appropriate to go right to TEE.

Indications to order TEE for AIS include any of the following:

- Suspicion of cardiac emboli despite a negative TTE
- Suspicion of right-to-left shunt
- Septic emboli suggesting infected cardiac source

TEE is often performed for cryptogenic stroke, but it is not clear that this is always indicated. Recent meta-analysis raised concern over marked differences in the results of TEE in patients with cryptogenic stroke and TIA.[2]

41 Toolkit
Neurologic Management

Karl E. Misulis, MD, PhD and
E. Lee Murray, MD

CHAPTER CONTENTS

- Spasticity
- Increased Intracranial Pressure
  - Sedation
  - Corticosteroids
  - Osmotic Agents
  - Barbiturate Coma
  - Hyperventilation
  - Surgical Therapy
- Immune Therapy
  - Corticosteroids
  - Interferons
  - Intravenous Immunoglobulin
  - Azathioprine
  - Cyclophosphamide
  - Methotrexate
  - Plasma Exchange
  - Rituximab
  - Other Immunosuppressants

SPASTICITY

Spasticity is common with a wide range of neurologic diseases. Management can be difficult and is almost always multimodal, although not all patients need treatment other than maintaining activity. However, management is considered especially when the patient has intractable pain or significant limitation of motion because of the spasticity.

Physical therapy should be considered first-line for almost all patients. The type and extent of therapy depend on the severity of the deficit.

Baclofen is a gamma aminobutyric acid (GABA) agonist commonly used for spasticity. Initial treatment is usually orally, but it is very effective intrathecally, given by continuous pump. Overdose can produce severe encephalopathy. A common starting dose is 5 mg t.i.d.

Benzodiazepines are commonly used, especially diazepam and clonazepam. They often cause sedation; this is most prominent initially and on dose increments.

Dantrolene is an alternative especially to baclofen. Because of the mainly peripheral action, it is less likely to produce cognitive effects at therapeutic doses. Starting dose is usually 25 mg/day.

Tizanidine is a newer agent that may produce less reduction in muscle function than the other agents described. Starting dose is often 2 mg q6-8h prn, max 3 doses/day.

Botulinum toxin injections is used for spasticity and focal spasms. Because of the size of the muscle mass involved, patients with widespread spasticity may not be a candidate for this treatment.

Surgery of various sorts can be done for spasticity. Some of these approaches can include contracture release, osteotomy, and implantation of a pump. Selective dorsal rhizotomy is considered for medically refractory cases.

INCREASED INTRACRANIAL PRESSURE

Intracranial pressure (ICP) can be increased from a wide variety of conditions discussed in this book. Generally, the causes fall into the following categories:

- Mass lesion
- Cerebral edema
- Obstruction of CSF flow
- Obstruction of CSF absorption
- Increased venous pressure

PRESENTATION depends on etiology and acuteness. Common symptoms include headache, nausea, vomiting, visual change including blurring or diplopia, and, ultimately, confusion, lethargy, and pupillary dilation. Diplopia from increased ICP is usually horizontal and due to abducens palsy. Visual change can be blurring to blindness. Papilledema is seen on exam unless the ICP increase is very acute. Additional brainstem findings can be from displacement and compression of neural structures as well as ICP itself.

DIAGNOSIS is discussed in depth throughout this book. Imaging is performed urgently when increased ICP is suspected.

MANAGEMENT is individualized on the basis of cause, acuity, and severity, but some general tools include:[1]

- Corticosteroids
- Osmotic agents
- Barbiturate coma
- Hyperventilation
- Surgical therapy.

Cerebral edema from tumor or infection can be responsive to any of these. Edema from stroke or hypoxia does not respond well to corticosteroids.

Mass lesion without edema, such as large subdural hematoma, responds best to surgical evacuation, and, until this is performed, osmotic agents and hyperventilation can be helpful. Corticosteroids are less likely to be helpful.

Mass lesion with edema, such as from a large tumor with surrounding edema, may respond to corticosteroids, but this is not a replacement for treatment of the mass.

Focal edema from large stroke may have to be treated with craniectomy.

Sedation

Many patients with increased ICP have prominent encephalopathy or are in coma, but others may continue to have motor activity and appear restless.

The most commonly used agents include midazolam and lorazepam. Propofol is also used. Use of these may be limited by hypotension.

Corticosteroids

Corticosteroids are one of the cornerstones of management of increased ICP for many but not all conditions. They are effective for cerebral edema due to infection and tumor, but generally not for edema from stroke, hypoxia, or trauma.

Corticosteroids do not have an immediate effect. In times of critical increase in ICP, mannitol, hyperventilation, and/or surgery should be considered.

Decadron is used often starting at 10 mg IV × 1, followed by 4 mg IV q6h. Higher doses are often used.

Osmotic Agents

Mannitol is the most commonly used agent. This reduces the volume of brain tissue outside the lesioned area. Response occurs within minutes.

A common regimen is a 0.25–1.0 g/kg bolus with the higher dose used when critical ICP needs to be reduced as soon as possible. Maintenance dose is usually 0.25–0.50 g/kg q6h.

Serum osmolarity is measured and maintained typically in the range of 300–320 mOsm. Blood pressure is monitored because of the possibility of hypotension reducing cerebral perfusion pressure. Electrolytes are monitored closely.

When mannitol is no longer needed, it must be tapered to reduce the effects of rebound cerebral edema, since mannitol does open the blood–brain barrier.

Hypertonic saline is sometimes used, but mannitol is the preferred agent for most patients. Hypertonic saline may be preferential especially for patients with hypotension on admission.

Barbiturate Coma

Barbiturates are used less often than the other treatments discussed, but they still may be valuable for select patients. This is usually considered rescue therapy for refractory increased ICP. EEG monitoring is recommended, and the dose is adjusted to burst-suppression.

Hyperventilation

Hyperventilation (HV) reduces cerebral blood volume by vasoconstriction. However, the reduction is temporary. Also, the vasoconstriction may reduce perfusion pressure to areas of the brain. However, HV is still effective for producing an urgent reduction in ICP. HV should be avoided in stroke and head injury if possible.

Surgical Therapy

Ventricular drain is often performed especially when the cause of the increased ICP is at least partly hydrocephalus.

Craniectomy is performed especially when life-threatening cerebral edema needs to be decompressed to maintain perfusion pressure. This is usually unilateral (e.g., over an area of ischemia with edema). Bilateral craniectomy has rarely been performed as an acute life-saving attempt.

IMMUNE THERAPY

Immunosuppression has been discussed in multiple sections of this book. Here, we consider some general principles of immunosuppression. This is a rapidly moving field so current literature should be reviewed. Many uses are not FDA approved.

Neurologic conditions that may require immunosuppression in the hospital setting can include:

- *Myasthenia gravis (MG)*: Especially myasthenic crisis but also for initial presentation
- *Multiple sclerosis (MS)*: Usually as an acute attack in a patient with or without a known diagnosis of MS
- *Acute inflammatory demyelinating polyneuropathy (AIDP)*: With initial presentation
- *Chronic inflammatory demyelinating polyneuropathy (CIDP)*: With initial presentation or more commonly with exacerbation of known disease
- *CNS vasculitis*: Can be an initial diagnosis in a patient with stroke or with an exacerbation in a patient with known CNS vasculitis
- *Temporal arteritis (TA)*: Usually with first diagnosis
- *Optic neuritis (ON)*: For acute visual loss at initial presentation; less likely in a patient with prior demyelination

Neurologic complications of immunosuppression that may trigger neurologic evaluation in the hospital may be:

- Opportunistic infection
- Steroid myopathy
- Cushing syndrome
- Cancer induced by immunosuppressant, with neurologic involvement

Corticosteroids

Corticosteroids reduce the formation of a host of vasoactive substances.

MG is often treated with prednisone. Dose is gradually escalated because of the potential for worsening weakness early in administration. Ultimately, other agents such as azathioprine reduce the need for as much corticosteroids. Corticosteroids principally benefit systemic symptoms and less so ocular manifestations.

MS is often treated with high-dose corticosteroids for acute attacks. A common regimen is 1,000 mg methylprednisolone IV daily for 3–5 days, followed by a brief oral steroid taper. Oral methylprednisolone may be similarly effective for select patients.[2]

CIDP can be treated with corticosteroids, especially prednisone. This is used for chronic therapy rather than pulsed for acute therapy.

AIDP is not treated with corticosteroids. If there is concern that a patient presenting with a demyelinating neuropathy might have AIDP or CIDP, then corticosteroids should likely not be first-line: IV immunoglobulin (IVIg) or plasma exchange (PLEX) should be considered.

Temporal arteritis is treated initially with corticosteroids. A typical regimen starts with 40–60 mg/day prednisone PO. IV solumedrol is sometimes used.

Neuromyelitis optica (NMO) is a demyelinating disease that can be treated with high-dose corticosteroids initially. A common regimen is methylprednisolone as for MS attack.

Acute disseminated encephalomyelitis (ADEM) is an inflammatory disorder that is usually treated with high-dose corticosteroids. A common protocol is 1 g/day methyl-prednisolone IV for 3–5 days followed by an oral taper.

Interferons

Interferons are immune modulators that are used predominantly in neurology for MS. There are a multiplicity of biological actions that can contribute to the immunomodulatory effect.

MS is often treated with interferons as first-line disease-modifying therapy. These are usually not started in the hospital, although arrangements for insurance approval are often begun during the hospitalization.

Intravenous Immunoglobulin

IVIg is used for a host of neurologic diseases, especially for acute worsening of symptoms.

MG is often treated with IVIg for myasthenic crisis or for perioperative treatment.

AIDP can be treated with IVIg and is the first-line selection for many neurologists. Patients with more severe disease are often offered PLEX, although there is no data to indicate that one treatment is superior to the other. Treatment with both does not offer additional advantage.

CIDP can be treated with IVIg as part of initial therapy and for maintenance as pulsed treatment. Transient worsening of weakness can also be treated by IVIg.

MS attacks can be treated with IVIg if the patient cannot take corticosteroids. Supporting data are limited.

Azathioprine

Azathioprine is a purine antagonist antimetabolite used in neurology mainly for MG.

MG is often treated chronically with azathioprine after beginning corticosteroids. Ultimately, as the azathioprine shows sustained benefit, the effective dose of corticosteroids can be reduced.

NMO is often treated with corticosteroids initially, with the simultaneous institution of azathioprine.

Cyclophosphamide

Cyclophosphamide is an alkylating agent that is mainly used for neoplasms but also for select autoimmune diseases.

Primary CNS angiitis is treated with corticosteroids acutely with cyclophosphamide.

Methotrexate

Methotrexate is an antimetabolite that is used for cancers and select autoimmune diseases.

Primary CNS angiitis is usually treated with corticosteroids and cyclophosphamide, but methotrexate is also used.

NMO is sometimes treated by methotrexate, but azathioprine is used more commonly.

Plasma Exchange

PLEX is used for a wide variety of autoimmune diseases, and multiple neurologic conditions respond to plasma exchange:

MG can be treated with plasma exchange especially for myasthenic crisis. PLEX is often used for initial treatment as corticosteroid therapy is begun.

NMO has been treated with PLEX. This is supplemented by meds with a longer immunomodulatory effect such as azathioprine, methotrexate, or rituximab.

AIDP is commonly treated with PLEX. While this might be about equivalent to IVIg in effectiveness, many of us tend to use PLEX for patients more severely and rapidly affected. Combined treatment does not offer additional advantage.

MS can be treated with PLEX especially if symptoms are refractory to or patients cannot take the corticosteroids. Supporting data are limited.

Rituximab

Rituximab is a monoclonal antibody that binds to and destroys B-cells.

MG is not routinely treated with rituximab, but this has been used when patients have failed first- and second-line therapy, especially with anti-MuSK MG.

MS is usually treated with interferons or glatiramer. Rituximab may be effective for some patients and may be considered for patients with refractory disease. This is predominantly for patients with relapsing-remitting disease, although some patients with primary progressive MS may have a reduction in disease activity.

Other Immunosuppressants

There are many other immunosuppressents, and details of these are beyond the scope of this book. Also, this is a constantly changing field. Two agents are of potential importance to hospital neurology practice.

Fingolimod is the first oral med approved for relapsing-remitting MS. A principal risk is cardiac, with bradyarrhythmia and AV block. Because of this risk, the first dose must be administered with cardiac monitoring, potentially involving the hospital neurologist.

Natalizumab is a monoclonal antibody used for MS. This is not a first line treatment; it is usually used for patients with refractory disease. Risk of progressive multifocal leukoencephalopathy (PML) is of concern. When natalizumab is discontinued because of concern for PML, immune reconstitution inflammatory syndrome (IRIS) may develop.

42 Toolkit
Difficult Encounters

Karl E. Misulis, MD, PhD and
E. Lee Murray, MD

CHAPTER CONTENTS

- Brain Death
- Persistent Vegetative State
- End of Life Care
- Lack of Good Working Relationship with Family
- Mistakes

Difficult encounters with patients and patients' family and loved ones are common, but thankfully are usually resolved amicably. Among the most difficult concern the diagnoses of brain death (BD) or persistent vegetative state (PVS). The clinical aspects of BD and PVS are discussed in CHAPTER 15. Here, we discuss interpersonal interactions that may arise in the context of these diagnoses.

Difficult encounters have a variety of origins. Among these are:

- Unfamiliarity with concepts of BD, PVS, and end-of-life care
- Absence of advanced directives
- Conflict within the family about representing patient's wishes
- Guilt on the part of individual(s)
- Concern over quality of care

Unfamiliarity with the concepts can be remedied somewhat by education. When appropriate, a realistic assessment of the patient's status should be presented to the family, and, when appropriate, the relevant concepts of do not resuscitate (DNR) orders, PVS, and BD should be discussed.

Advanced directives are increasingly in use, but many patients still do not have them in place. Most electronic medical record (EMR) systems allow for the easy identification and retrieval of advanced directives; however, families are encouraged to have ready access to the original documents.

Conflict in the family is usually regarding opinions on the aggressiveness of care. Classically, one or more family members express a desire for more aggressive care than the wishes of the rest of the family. One approach we use is to emphasize that the focus is on the wishes of the patient. While there are some data that suggest that proxy decision-makers do not represent the wishes of the patient as well as would be hoped, family should tell us the opinions that they believe the patient would have expressed. Laws in effect at the locale also must be followed because proxy decision-making for patients falls under the legal regulations in effect.

Concern over quality of care can promote more prolonged and more aggressive medical care than might be appropriate. Providers who become aware of quality issues should consider offering a change in provider or facility, depending on the clinical situation.

General principles of communication in this context include:

- *Clinicians on the team must communicate with each other:* Even if they do not all agree on the assessment and prognosis, they need to be aware of each other's opinions and the bases of these. Discussion between the clinicians can often resolve much of the difference. The team should try to come to a general consensus on diagnoses, management, prognosis, and issues to be communicated to the patient and family.
- *Clinicians on the team must communicate with family and patient:* This communication is easiest of there is an open ICU visitation policy so that the clinicians can interact with the family at the bedside. If the patient is able to understand, he or she should be included.
- *Be frank about status and prognosis:* Explanation complexity is tailored to the audience, but generally consensus opinion with only basic supporting clinical information should be presented.
- *Discussions are often easier with small groups at least initially:* Emotionally charged information presented to a large group can provoke a different reaction than the same information presented to a small group.
- *The dataset presented should be limited:* Information overload can result in failure of comprehension and internalization of essential data. This can breed distrust and loss of confidence in the healthcare team.
- *The patient should always be the focus:* We generally recommend that the patient's wishes be followed, if known. In the absence of an advance directive, family should be asked what they believe the patient would want done in the particular clinical situation.

BRAIN DEATH

The BD diagnosis was discussed in depth in Chapter 15. This section discusses some common scenarios. Note that our approaches for consideration are by no means the only methods of dealing with these issues.

Family does not accept the concept of brain death : Brain death is a concept with meaning in both the medical and legal arenas. As providers, we are used to this discussion, but this may be an alien concept to some families. Often, conflict can be resolved by education and a compassionate approach. Most hospitals have consultants who advise on end-of-life care, and these should be used if available. Ethics committees can also be of great assistance.

Family wants to wait for others to come before terminating life supports : We generally are fairly liberal about continuing supports if the family member will arrive within 24 hours or so. Prolonged maintenance on supports is not appropriate for most clinical situations. Gentle explanation that the patient has already died can help with this transition.

Family wants to transfer the patient to another facility : Families may request transfer to another facility because of lack of confidence in the present healthcare or desire for another opinion. Most referral facilities will decline to take in transfer a patient meeting BD criteria. If education does not resolve this issue, we will accommodate the family wishes and ask, but we have never had another hospital accept a patient who is BD. We will offer additional opinions from other providers in our hospitals.

PERSISTENT VEGETATIVE STATE

PVS is often more difficult to deal with than BD since there is some brain activity, and some movements can appear to have a cognitive basis. We explain the physiology of PVS and have a frank but diplomatic discussion about prognosis. Families usually need time to internalize and adjust to the new reality of their loved one's situation. If the family desires or seems to need a second opinion, we offer that.

Disposition of a patient with PVS is usually to a long-term care facility. Families are educated about the roles of acute-care hospitals and the spectrum of long-term care facilities: skilled nursing facilities (SNF), long-term acute care facilities (LTAC), nursing homes, and rehab units. Initially, many families intend on caring for the patient at home, but as they observe the intensity of care required, this often changes.

END-OF-LIFE CARE

End-of-life care includes several facets, some of which include:

- Determination of intensity of ongoing and emergent medical care
- Determination of post-acute care disposition
- Decisions about feeding and hydration

Intensity of care : Discussions usually begin with an explanation of current medical status and prognosis. Then we transition to discussing resuscitation status. There is a spectrum of resuscitation options; those usually used at our large referral hospital are:

- Full resuscitation
- Do not resuscitate (DNR)
- DNR with limited therapy
- Comfort measures only

Then there are various combinations that are occasionally requested by families (including use of antibiotics versus pressors), but generally patients will usually be either full resuscitation or DNR or comfort measures only.

Palliative care and *hospice care* are services that most larger hospitals offer. Palliative care offers symptomatic and comfort care but allows treatment to continue. Hospice is for patients who are terminal and are not continuing to receive disease-modifying therapy.

Donor services are also offered in many larger hospitals. These individuals often are the first to approach families about organ donation, and they do it well. Some physicians feel obligated to discuss these issues themselves, and that is fine, but we recommend using our skilled and experienced colleagues in these arenas.

Most patients at suspected end-of-life are considered for hospice. Prior to that, palliative care is usually offered. Disposition can be to home with home healthcare, an established hospice unit, nursing home, or skilled nursing facility.

Feeding and hydration : These are issues with an emotional charge for many families. Decisions on intravenous and tube feedings for a patient with a terminal disorder necessitates a frank discussion, and our colleagues in palliative care, hospice, and ethics committees can be of benefit. It may be helpful to explain that, in many patients, these treatments do no more than prolong the dying process.

LACK OF GOOD WORKING RELATIONSHIP WITH FAMILY

Lack of a good working relationship may range from disagreements about services to be provided to frank anger. Providers will try to improve the relationship by discussion and education, but often at least some of the family will not accept the providers' opinions and not value the providers' care. The distrust or animosity may not be verbalized, so if the provider detects a trust issue or learns of it from other staff, a change in provider should be requested, whether as attending or consultant.

Methods for establishing credibility with the families should include:

- Clearly and concisely explaining diagnosis(es), condition, management recommendations, and prognosis
- Answering questions and soliciting questions if none is spontaneously forthcoming
- Inviting family to be in the ICU at the time of rounding, if they are not already there

Additional methods for enhancing credibility can be:

- Showing images of scans and electroencephalograms (EEGs) can be very powerful, especially if they are demonstrably abnormal.
- Offer to discuss the situation with the patient's personal physician—this can be of tremendous benefit and can make the newly met specialist part of the family's medical team.

MISTAKES

Medicine is an imperfect science, and, as providers, we are imperfect beings. Mistakes will be made by providers, our associates, ancillary staff, and by the system. While we try to establish mechanisms to minimize mistakes, they are not completely avoidable. Mechanisms to minimize mistakes include:

- *Work within our comfort zone*: Ensure that the conditions being treated are within our expertise and the capabilities of our facility.
- *Control volume*: Mistakes are more likely when we are hurried or fatigued. Except in disaster conditions, we should be able to limit our workload.

- *Control hours*: Long call epochs are disappearing, especially in neurology where the numbers of emergencies has skyrocketed because of the focus on emergent stroke care. Solutions can be recruiting additional permanent or temporary providers, defined shifts, and telemedicine.

When a mistake is identified, severity and impact should be assessed. Discussion with the patient, if possible, and the family should include a truthful discussion of the event, cause, impact, and remedy. Discussion of remedy should first focus on the remedy for this particular patient. In addition, it might be appropriate to include in the discussion what we have learned from this event and how this will change our practice.

When there is a mistake or otherwise a case seems to have potential for litigation, we recommend notification of your hospital's Risk Management department for their review. This accomplishes the following:

- Gather information that can help with defense if a claim is ultimately filed.
- Identify opportunities for improvement that would make similar events less likely.
- Psychologically, for the provider, it is helpful to engage the team that will support our efforts to deliver the best care we can.

References

CHAPTER 1

1. Association of British Neurologists. Neurology Survey. Available at http://www.theabn. org/media/Acute Neurology Survey—FINAL Dec14.pdf.
2. Carter ND, Wade DT. Delayed discharges from Oxford city hospitals: who and why? *Clin Rehabil.* 2002 May;16(3):315–20.

CHAPTER 2

1. Bushnell C, Arnan M, Han S. A new model for secondary prevention of stroke: transition coaching for stroke. *Front Neurol.* 2014 Oct 27;5:219.

CHAPTER 3

1. American Academy of Neurologists. Available at https://www.aan.com/practice/ quality-measures/
2. Shepperd S, Doll H, Angus RM, et al. Admission avoidance hospital at home. *Cochrane Database Syst Rev.* 2008 Oct 8;(4):CD007491.
3. Shepperd S, Doll H, Broad J, Gladman J, Iliffe S, Langhorne P, Richards S, Martin F, Harris R. Early discharge hospital at home. *Cochrane Database Syst Rev.* 2009 Jan 21;(1):CD000356.

CHAPTER 4

1. Misulis KE, Murray EL. (2015). Sensory Abnormalities of the Limbs, Trunk, and Face, from Bradley's Neurology in Clinical Practice. In: Daroff RB, Jankovic J, Maziotta JC, Pomeroy SL (Eds.) Elsevier.
2. Alshekhlee A, Basiri K, Miles JD, Ahmad SA, Katirji B. Chronic inflammatory demyelinating polyneuropathy associated with tumor necrosis factor-alpha antagonists. *Muscle Nerve.* 2010 May;41(5):723–7.

CHAPTER 5

1. Evans RL, Connis RT. Risk screening for adverse outcomes in subacute care. *Psychol Rep.* 1996 Jun;78(3 Pt 1):1043–8.
2. Joray S, Wietlisbach V, Büla CJ. Cognitive impairment in elderly medical inpatients: detection and associated six-month outcomes. *Am J Geriatr Psychiatry.* 2004 Nov–Dec;12(6):639–47.
3. Calvo-Ayala E, Khan B. Delirium management in critically ill patients. *J Symptoms Signs.* 2013;2(1):23–32.
4. Ahmed S, Leurent B, Sampson EL. Risk factors for incident delirium among older people in acute hospital medical units: a systematic review and meta-analysis. *Age Ageing.* 2014 May;43(3):326–33.

5. Zaal IJ, Devlin JW, Peelen LM, Slooter AJ. A systematic review of risk factors for delirium in the ICU. *Crit Care Med.* 2015 Jan;43(1):40–7.

6. Sullivan R, Hodgman MJ, Kao L, Tormoehlen LM. Baclofen overdose mimicking brain death. *Clin Toxicol (Phila).* 2012 Feb;50(2):141–4.

7. Kanjwal K, Kanjwal Y, Karabin B, Grubb BP. Psychogenic syncope? A cautionary note. *Pacing Clin Electrophysiol.* 2009 Jul;32(7):862–5.

8. Meyer MA. Seizure as the presenting sign for massive pulmonary embolism: case report and review of the literature. *Seizure.* 2009 Jan;18(1):76–8.

9. Wang SY, Chen H, Di LG. Caution for acute submassive pulmonary embolism with syncope as initial symptom: a case report. *J Thorac Dis.* 2014 Oct;6(10):E212–6.

10. Miyakoshi N, Hongo M, Kasukawa Y, Shimada Y. Syncope caused by congenital anomaly at the craniovertebral junction: a case report. *J Med Case Rep.* 2014 Oct 8;8:330.

11. Piñol I, Ramirez M, Saló G, Ros AM, Blanch AL. Symptomatic vertebral artery stenosis secondary to cervical spondylolisthesis. *Spine (Phila Pa 1976).* 2013 Nov 1;38(23):E1503–5.

12. Chan-Tack KM. Subclavian steal syndrome: a rare but important cause of syncope. *South Med J.* 2001 Apr;94(4):445–7.

13. Pflaumer A, Davis AM. Guidelines for the diagnosis and management of catecholaminergic polymorphic ventricular tachycardia. *Heart Lung Circ.* 2012 Feb;21(2):96–100.

14. Denis DJ, Shedid D, Shehadeh M, Weil AG, Lanthier S. Cervical spondylosis: a rare and curable cause of vertebrobasilar insufficiency. *Eur Spine J.* 2014 May;23 Suppl 2:206–13.

15. Khadilkar SV, Yadav RS, Jagiasi KA. Are syncopes in sitting and supine positions different? Body positions and syncope: a study of 111 patients. *Neurol India.* 2013 May–Jun;61(3):239–43.

16. Bień B, Wilmańska J, Jańczak W, et al. Syncope and near-syncope as a multifactorial problem in geriatric inpatients: systemic hypotension is an underrated predictor for syncope exclusively. *Adv Med Sci.* 2011;56(2):352–60.

17. Murahara T, Takaya S, Yamaguchi D, et al. Convulsive syncope associated with transient hemodynamic ischemia in the basal ganglia. *Rinsho Shinkeigaku.* 2011 May;51(5):338–44.

18. Kashiwazaki D, Kuroda S, Terasaka S, et al. [Carotid occlusive disease presenting with loss of consciousness]. *No Shinkei Geka.* 2005 Jan;33(1):29–34.

19. Lempert T. Syncope. Phenomenology and differentiation from epileptic seizures. *Nervenarzt.* 1997 Aug;68(8):620–4.

20. Boissonnot L, Herpin D, Neau P, Allal J, Haldenwang P, Gil R. [Brief losses of consciousness of unknown origin. The contribution of echocardiography and of Holter monitoring]. *Ann Cardiol Angeiol (Paris).* 1986 Jul-Sep;35(7):381–5.

21. van der Velde N, Stricker BH, Roelandt JR, Ten Cate FJ, van der Cammen TJ. Can echocardiographic findings predict falls in older persons? *PLoS One.* 2007 Jul 25;2(7):e654.

22. Ergul Y, Tanidir IC, Ozyilmaz I, Akdeniz C, Tuzcu V. Evaluation rhythm problems in unexplained syncope etiology with implantable loop recorder. *Pediatr Int.* 2014 Oct 28:359–366.

23. Edvardsson N, Garutti C, Rieger G, Linker NJ; PICTURE Study Investigators. Unexplained syncope: implications of age and gender on patient characteristics and evaluation, the diagnostic yield of an implantable loop recorder, and the subsequent treatment. *Clin Cardiol.* 2014 Oct;37(10):618–25.

24. Ahmed AS, Foley E, Brannigan AE, Decker PA, Burke PE, Grace PA. Critical appraisal of the application of carotid duplex scanning. *Ir J Med Sci.* 2002 Oct-Dec;171(4):191–2.

25. Sorajja D, Shen WK. Driving guidelines and restrictions in patients with a history of cardiac arrhythmias, syncope, or implantable devices. *Curr Treat Options Cardiovasc Med.* 2010 Oct;12(5):443–56.

CHAPTER 6

1. Lemos J, Eggenberger E. Neuro-ophthalmological emergencies. *Neurohospitalist.* 2015 Oct;5(4):223–33.
2. Bryan BT, Pomeranz HD, Smith KH. Complete binasal hemianopia. *Proc (Bayl Univ Med Cent).* 2014 Oct;27(4):356–8.

CHAPTER 7

1. Toyoda K. Anterior cerebral artery and Heubner's artery territory infarction. *Front Neurol Neurosci.* 2012;30:120–2.

CHAPTER 10

1. Ybarra M, Rosenbaum T. Typical migraine or ophthalmologic emergency? *Am J Emerg Med.* 2012 Jun;30(5):831.e3–5.
2. Gilron I, Baron R, Jensen T. Neuropathic pain: principles of diagnosis and treatment. *Mayo Clin Proc.* 2015 Apr;90(4):532–45.
3. American Pain Society. Available at http://americanpainsociety.org/education/guidelines/overview
4. American Academy of Pain Medicine. Available at http://www.painmed.org/files/use-of-opioids-for-the-treatment-of-chronic-pain.pdf
5. Hung CI, Liu CY, Fu TS. Depression: an important factor associated with disability among patients with chronic low back pain. *Int J Psychiatry Med.* 2015;49(3):187–98.
6. Chapman SL, Wu LT. Associations between cigarette smoking and pain among veterans. *Epidemiol Rev;*2015;37:86–102.
7. Petre B, Torbey S, Griffith JW, et al. Smoking increases risk of pain chronification through shared corticostriatal circuitry. *Hum Brain Mapp.* 2015 Feb;36(2):683–94. PMID: 25307

CHAPTER 11

1. Joseph E. Safdieh. Continuum (Minneap Minn). 2014 Jun;20(3 Neurology of Systemic Disease):511–762.
2. Martin GS. Sepsis, severe sepsis and septic shock: changes in incidence, pathogens and outcomes. *Expert Rev Anti Infect Ther.* 2012 Jun;10(6):701–6.
3. Noy ML, George S. Unusual presentation of a spinal epidural abscess. *BMJ Case Rep.* 2012 Jul 25;2012:pii: bcr0320125956.
4. Fugate JE, Kalimullah EA, Hocker SE, Clark SL, Wijdicks EF, Rabinstein AA. Cefepime neurotoxicity in the intensive care unit: a cause of severe, underappreciated encephalopathy. *Crit Care.* 2013 Nov 7;17(6):R264.
5. Ko K, Sung DH, Kang MJ, et al. Clinical, electrophysiological findings in adult patients with non-traumatic plexopathies. *Ann Rehabil Med.* 2011 Dec;35(6):807–15.
6. Navi BB, Reiner AS, Kamel H, et al. Association between incident cancer and subsequent stroke. *Ann Neurol.* 2015 Feb;77(2):291–300.
7. Kim MH, Hwang MS, Park YK, et al. Paraneoplastic Guillain-Barré syndrome in small cell lung cancer. *Case Rep Oncol.* 2015 Jul 30;8(2):295–300.
8. Antoine JC, Mosnier JF, Absi L, Convers P, Honnorat J, Michel D. Carcinoma associated paraneoplastic peripheral neuropathies in patients with and without anti-onconeural antibodies. *J Neurol Neurosurg Psychiatry.* 1999 Jul;67(1):7–14.

9. Mostoufizadeh S, Souri M, de Sezea J. A case of paraneoplastic demyelinating motor polyneuropathy. *Case Rep Neurol.* 2012 Jan–Apr;4(1):71–76.

10. McKeon A. Paraneoplastic and other autoimmune disorders of the central nervous system. *Neurohospitalist.* 2013 Apr;3(2):53–64.

11. Capek S, Howe BM, Amrami KK, Spinner RJ. Perineural spread of pelvic malignancies to the lumbosacral plexus and beyond: clinical and imaging patterns. *Neurosurg Focus.* 2015 Sep;39(3):E14.

12. Barnholtz-Sloan JS, Sloan AE, Davis FG, Vigneau FD, Lai P, Sawaya RE. Incidence proportions of brain metastases in patients diagnosed (1973 to 2001) in the Metropolitan Detroit Cancer Surveillance System. *JCO* Jul 15, 2004:2865–72.

13. Sawaya R. Considerations in the diagnosis and management of brain metastases. *Oncology (Williston Park),* 2001 Sep;15(9):1144–54, 1157–58.

14. Rohren EM, Provenzale JM, Barboriak DP, Coleman RE. Screening for cerebral metastases with FDG PET in patients undergoing whole-body staging of non-central nervous system malignancy. *Radiology.* 2003 Jan;226(1):181–7.

15. Paholpak P, Sirichativapee W, Wisanuyotin T, Kosuwon W, Jeeravipoolvarn P. Prevalence of known and unknown primary tumor sites in spinal metastasis patients. *Open Orthop J.* 2012;6:440–44.

16. Giglio P, Gilbert MR. Neurologic complications of cancer and its treatment. *Curr Oncol Rep.* 2010 Jan;12(1):50–9.

17. Singh SK, Leeds NE, Ginsberg LE. MR imaging of leptomeningeal metastases: comparison of three sequences. *AJNR Am J Neuroradiol.* 2002 May;23(5):817–21.

18. Fullerton HJ, Stratton K, Mueller S, et al. Recurrent stroke in childhood cancer survivors. *Neurology.* 2015 Sep 22;85(12):1056–64.

19. Wilbers J, Meijer FJ, Kappelle AC, et al. Magnetic resonance imaging of the carotid artery in long-term head and neck cancer survivors treated with radiotherapy. *Acta Oncol.* 2015;54(8):1175–80.

20. Kissela BM, Khoury J, Kleindorfer D, et al. Epidemiology of ischemic stroke in patients with diabetes: the greater Cincinnati/Northern Kentucky Stroke Study. *Diabetes Care.* 2005 Feb;28(2):355–59.

21. Imad H, Johan Z, Eva K. Hypoglycemia and risk of seizures: a retrospective cross-sectional study. *Seizure.* 2015 Feb;25:147–9.

22. Neil WP, Hemmen TM. (2011). Neurologic manifestations of hypoglycemia, diabetes. In: Rigobelo E, ed., *Diabetes: Damages and Treatments.* InTech. Available at: http://www.intechopen.com/books/diabetes-damages-and-treatments/neurologic-manifestations-of- hypoglycemia

23. Jones R, Redler K, Witherick J, Fuller G, Mahajan T, Wakerley BR Posterior reversible encephalopathy syndrome complicating diabetic ketoacidosis: an important treatable complication. *Pediatr Diabetes.* 2016 Jan 14.

24. Cohen MB, Mather PJ. A review of the association between congestive heart failure and cognitive impairment. *Am J Geriatr Cardiol.* 2007 May–Jun;16(3):171–4.

25. Cannon JA, McMurray JJ, Quinn TJ. "Hearts and minds": association, causation and implication of cognitive impairment in heart failure. *Alzheimers Res Ther.* 2015 Feb 27;7(1):22.

26. Witt BJ, Ballman KV, Brown RD Jr, Meverden RA, Jacobsen SJ, Roger VL. The incidence of stroke after myocardial infarction: a meta-analysis. *Am J Med.* 2006 Apr;119(4):354.e1–9.

27. Bamalwa M, Mahmood SN, Praharaj SK. Delirium in cardiac ICU patients. *Ann Clin Psychiatry.* 2016 Feb;28(1):51–5.

28. Kocabay G, Karabay CY, Kalayci A, et al. Contrast-induced neurotoxicity after coronary angiography. *Herz*. 2014 Jun;39(4):522-7.

29. Lu R, Kiernan MC, Murray A, Rosner MH, Ronco C. Kidney-brain crosstalk in the acute and chronic setting. *Nat Rev Nephrol*. 2015 Dec;11(12):707-19.

30. Patel N, Dalal P, Panesar M. Dialysis disequilibrium syndrome: a narrative review. *Semin Dial*. 2008 Sep-Oct;21(5):493-8.

31. Sureka B, Bansal K, Patidar Y, Rajesh S, Mukund A, Arora A. Neurologic manifestations of chronic liver disease and liver cirrhosis. *Curr Probl Diagn Radiol*. 2015 Sep-Oct;44(5):449-61.

32. Goldstein JM. Neurologic complications of rheumatic disease. *Continuum (Minneap Minn)*. 2014 Jun;20(3 Neurology of Systemic Disease):657-9.

33. Zha AM, Di Napoli M, Behrouz R. Prevention of stroke in rheumatoid arthritis. *Curr Neurol Neurosci Rep*. 2015 Dec;15(12):77.

34. Jeong HN, Suh BC, Kim YB, Chung PW, Moon HS, Yoon WT. Posterior reversible encephalopathy syndrome as an initial neurological manifestation of primary Sjögren's syndrome. *Clin Auton Res*. 2015 Aug;25(4):259-62.

35. Colaci M, Cassone G, Manfredi A, Sebastiani M, Giuggioli D, Ferri C. Neurologic complications associated with Sjögren's disease: case reports and modern pathogenic dilemma. *Case Rep Neurol Med*. 2014;2014:590292.

36. Ladwa R, Peters G, Bigby K, Chern B. Posterior reversible encephalopathy syndrome in early-stage breast cancer. *Breast J*. 2015 Nov;21(6):674-77.

37. Granata G, Greco A, Iannella G, et al. Posterior reversible encephalopathy syndrome--Insight into pathogenesis, clinical variants and treatment approaches. *Autoimmun Rev*. 2015 Sep;14(9):830-6.

CHAPTER 12

1. Boardman ND 3rd, Cofield RH. Neurologic complications of shoulder surgery. *Clin Orthop Relat Res*. 1999 Nov;(368):44-53.

2. Cornwall R, Radomisli TE. Nerve injury in traumatic dislocation of the hip. *Clin Orthop Relat Res*. 2000 Aug;(377):84-91.

3. Thompson K, Pohlmann-Eden B, Campbell LA, Abel H. Pharmacological treatments for preventing epilepsy following traumatic head injury. *Cochrane Database Syst Rev*. 2015 Aug 10;8:CD009900.

4. Biller J, Ferro JM. Neurologic aspects of systemic disease. In: Part III *Handbook of Clinical Neurology* (Part III, Vol. 121). City: Elsevier, 2014: 2-1828.

5. Mour G, Wu C. Neurologic complications after kidney transplantation. *Semin Nephrol*. 2015 Jul;35(4):323-34.

6. White H. Neurologic manifestations of acute and chronic liver disease. *Continuum (Minneap Minn)*. 2014 Jun;20(3 Neurology of Systemic Disease):670-80.

CHAPTER 13

1. Koton S, Eizenberg Y, Tanne D, Grossman E. Trends in admission blood pressure and stroke outcome in patients with acute stroke and transient ischemic attack in a National Acute Stroke registry. *J Hypertens*. 2016 Feb;34(2):316-22.

2. Jauch EC, Saver JL, Adams HP Jr, et al.; American Heart Association Stroke Council; Council on Cardiovascular Nursing; Council on Peripheral Vascular Disease; Council on Clinical Cardiology. Guidelines for the early management of patients with acute ischemic stroke: a guideline for healthcare professionals from the American Heart Association/American Stroke Association. *Stroke*. 2013 Mar;44(3):870-947.

3. Activase. Available at: https://www.activase.com/iscstroke/patient-selection-for-activase/contraindications

4. James PA, Oparil S, Carter BL, et al. 2014 evidence-based guideline for the management of high blood pressure in adults: report from the panel members appointed to the Eighth Joint National Committee (JNC 8). *JAMA*. 2014 Feb 5;311(5):507–20.

5. Godoy DA, Piñero GR, Koller P, Masotti L, Di Napoli M. Steps to consider in the approach and management of critically ill patient with spontaneous intracerebral hemorrhage. *World J Crit Care Med*. 2015 Aug 4;4(3):213–29.

6. Lamy C, Oppenheim C, Mas JL Posterior reversible encephalopathy syndrome. *Handb Clin Neurol*. 2014;121:1687–701.

7. Diaz A, Deliz B, Benbadis SR. The use of newer antiepileptic drugs in patients with renal failure. *Expert Rev Neurother*. 2012 Jan;12(1):99–105. PMID: 22149658

8. Lacerda G, Krummel T, Sabourdy C, Ryvlin P, Hirsch E. Optimizing therapy of seizures in patients with renal or hepatic dysfunction. *Neurology*. 2006 Dec 26;67(12 Suppl 4):S28–33.

9. Zepeda-Orozco D, Quigley R. Dialysis disequilibrium syndrome. *Pediatr Nephrol*. 2012 Dec;27(12):2205–11.

10. Hirsch KG, Spock T, Koenig MA, Geocadin RG. Treatment of elevated intracranial pressure with hyperosmolar therapy in patients with renal failure. *Neurocrit Care*. 2012 Dec;17(3):388–94.

11. Soomro A, Al Bahri R, Alhassan N, Hejaili FF, Al Sayyari AA. Posterior reversible encephalopathy syndrome with tactile hallucinations secondary to dialysis disequilibrium syndrome. *Saudi J Kidney Dis Transpl*. 2014 May;25(3):625–9.

12. Aydin OF, Uner C, Senbil N, Bek K, Erdoğan O, Gürer YK. Central pontine and extrapontine myelinolysis owing to disequilibrium syndrome. *J Child Neurol*. 2003 Apr;18(4):292–6.

13. Herrington W, Haynes R, Staplin N, Emberson J, Baigent C, Landray M. Evidence for the prevention and treatment of stroke in dialysis patients. *Semin Dial*. 2015 Jan–Feb;28(1):35–47. PMID: 25040468

14. Saeed F, Adil MM, Piracha BH, Qureshi AI. Outcomes of endovascular versus intravenous thrombolytic treatment for acute ischemic stroke in dialysis patients. *Int J Artif Organs*. 2014 Oct;37(10):727–33. PMID: 25262635

15. Lam S, Gomolin IH. Cefepime neurotoxicity: case report, pharmacokinetic considerations, and literature review. *Pharmacotherapy*. 2006 Aug;26(8):1169–74.

16. Thabet F, Al Maghrabi M, Al Barraq A, Tabarki B. Cefepime-induced nonconvulsive status epilepticus: case report and review. *Neurocrit Care*. 2009;10(3):347–51.

17. Blei AT, Córdoba J. Practice parameters committee of the American College of Gastroenterology. Hepatic Encephalopathy. *Am J Gastroenterol*. 2001 Jul;96(7):1968–76.

18. Corrêa Borges de Lacerda, G. Treating seizures in renal and hepatic failure. *J Epilepsy Clin Neurophysiol*. 2008;14(Suppl 2):46–50.

19. Jones R, Redler K, Witherick J, Fuller G, Mahajan T, Wakerley BR. Posterior reversible encephalopathy syndrome complicating diabetic ketoacidosis: an important treatable complication. *Pediatr Diabetes*. 2016 Jan 14;.

20. Jovanovic A, Stolic RV, Rasic DV, Markovic-Jovanovic SR, Peric VM. Stroke and diabetic ketoacidosis—some diagnostic and therapeutic considerations. *Vasc Health Risk Manag*. 2014;10:201–4.

21. Goldstein JM. Neurologic complications of rheumatic disease. *Continuum (Minneap Minn)*. 2014 Jun;20(3 Neurology of Systemic Disease):657–69.

22. Kasama T, Maeoka A, Oguro N. Clinical features of neuropsychiatric syndromes in systemic lupus erythematosus and other connective tissue diseases. *Clin Med Insights Arthritis Musculoskelet Disord*. 2016 Jan 18;9:1–8.

23. Sternlicht H, Glezerman IG. Hypercalcemia of malignancy and new treatment options. *Ther Clin Risk Manag.* 2015 Dec 4;11:1779–88.

CHAPTER 14

1. Lascarrou JB, Meziani F, Le Gouge A, et al.; Clinical Research in Intensive Care and Sepsis (CRICS) Group and HYPERION Study Group. Therapeutic hypothermia after nonshockable cardiac arrest: the HYPERION multicenter, randomized, controlled, assessor-blinded, superiority trial. *Scand J Trauma Resusc Emerg Med.* 2015 Mar 7;23:26.
2. Hessel EA 2nd. Therapeutic hypothermia after in-hospital cardiac arrest: a critique. *J Cardiothorac Vasc Anesth.* 2014 Jun;28(3):789–99.
3. Wijdicks EF, Hijdra A, Young GB, Bassetti CL, Wiebe S. Quality standards subcommittee of the American Academy of Neurology. Practice parameter: prediction of outcome in comatose survivors after cardiopulmonary resuscitation (an evidence-based review): report of the Quality Standards Subcommittee of the American Academy of Neurology. *Neurology.* 2006 Jul 25;67(2):203–10.

CHAPTER 15

1. Guidelines for the determination of death. Report of the medical consultants on the diagnosis of death to the President's Commission for the Study of Ethical Problems in Medicine and Biomedical and Behavioral Research. *JAMA.* 1981 Nov 13;246(19):2184–6.
2. Practice parameters for determining brain death in adults (summary statement). The Quality Standards Subcommittee of the American Academy of Neurology. *Neurology.* 1995 May;45(5):1012–4.
3. Wijdicks EF, Varelas PN, Gronseth GS, Greer DM; American Academy of Neurology. Evidence-based guideline update: determining brain death in adults: report of the Quality Standards Subcommittee of the American Academy of Neurology. *Neurology.* 2010 Jun 8;74(23):1911–8.
4. Ceccaldi PF, Bazin A, Gomis P, Ducarme G, Chaufer AL, Gabriel R. Persistent vegetative state with encephalitis in a pregnant woman with successful fetal outcome. *BJOG.* 2005 Jun;112(6):843–4.
5. American Academy of Neurology (AAN). Report of the Quality Standards Subcommittee of the American Academy of Neurology Practice parameters: assessment and management of patients in the persistent vegetative state (Summary statement). *Neurology.* 1995;45:1015–18.

CHAPTER 16

1. Demaerschalk BM, Kleindorfer DO, Adeoye OM, et al. Scientific rationale for the inclusion and exclusion criteria for intravenous alteplase in acute ischemic stroke: a statement for healthcare professionals from the American Heart Association/American Stroke Association. *Stroke.* 2016 Feb;47(2):581–641.
2. Madden B, Chebl RB. Hemi orolingual angioedema after tPA administration for acute ischemic stroke. *West J Emerg Med.* 2015 Jan;16(1):175–77.
3. Jauch EC, Saver JL, Adams HP, Jr, et al. on behalf of the American Heart Association Stroke Council, Council on Cardiovascular Nursing, Council on Peripheral Vascular Disease, and Council on Clinical Cardiology. Guidelines for the early management of patients with acute ischemic stroke: a guideline for healthcare professionals from the American Heart Association/American Stroke Association. *Stroke.* 2013;44:870–947; originally published online January 31, 2013.
4. Furie KL, Goldstein LB, Albers GW, et al.; American Heart Association Stroke Council; Council on Quality of Care and Outcomes Research; Council on Cardiovascular Nursing; Council on Clinical Cardiology; Council on Peripheral Vascular Disease. Oral

antithrombotic agents for the prevention of stroke in nonvalvular atrial fibrillation: a science advisory for healthcare professionals from the American Heart Association/American Stroke Association. *Stroke*. 2012 Dec;43(12):3442–53.

5. Messe SR, Gronseth G, Kent DM, et al. Practice advisory: Recurrent stroke with patent foramen ovale (update of practice parameter): Report of the Guideline Development, Dissemination, and Implementation Subcommittee of the American Academy of Neurology. *Neurology*. Published online July 27, 2016.

6. Ferguson GG, Gary G. Ferguson, Michael Eliasziw, Hugh WK Barr, et al. The North American symptomatic carotid endarterectomy trial surgical results in 1415 patients. *Stroke* 1999;30(9):1751–8.

7. Furie KL, Kasner SE, Adams RJ, et al.; American Heart Association Stroke Council, Council on Cardiovascular Nursing, Council on Clinical Cardiology, and Interdisciplinary Council on Quality of Care and Outcomes Research. Guidelines for the prevention of stroke in patients with stroke or transient ischemic attack: a guideline for healthcare professionals from the American Heart Association/American Stroke Association. *Stroke*. 2011 Jan;42(1):227–76.

8. Barnett HJ, Taylor DW, Eliasziw M, et al. North American Symptomatic Carotid Endarterectomy Trial Collaborators: benefit of carotid endarterectomy in patients with symptomatic moderate or severe stenosis. *N Engl J Med*. 1998;339(20):1415–1425

9. Adams HP Jr, Bendixen BH, Kappelle LJ, et al. Classification of subtype of acute ischemic stroke. Definitions for use in a multicenter clinical trial. TOAST. Trial of Org 10172 in Acute Stroke Treatment. *Stroke*. 1993 Jan;24(1):35–41.

10. Sanna T, Diener HC, Passman RS, et al.; CRYSTAL AF Investigators. Cryptogenic stroke and underlying atrial fibrillation. *N Engl J Med*. 2014 Jun 26;370(26):2478–86.

11. Furie KL, Kasner SE, Adams RJ, et al., on behalf of the American Heart Association Stroke Council, Council on Cardiovascular Nursing, Council on Clinical Cardiology, and Interdisciplinary Council on Quality of Care and Outcomes Research. Guidelines for the prevention of stroke in patients with stroke or transient ischemic attack: a guideline for healthcare professionals from the American Heart Association/American Stroke Association. *Stroke*. 2011;42:227–276; originally published online October 21, 2010.

12. Furie KL, Goldstein LB, Albers GW, et al., on behalf of the American Heart Association Stroke Council, Council on Quality of Care and Outcomes Research, Council on Cardiovascular Nursing, Council on Clinical Cardiology, and Council on Peripheral Vascular Disease. Oral antithrombotic agents for the prevention of stroke in nonvalvular atrial fibrillation: a science advisory for healthcare professionals from the American Heart Association/American Stroke Association. *Stroke*. 2012;43:3442–3453; originally published online August 2, 2012.

13. Hemphill JC 3rd. Guidelines for the management of spontaneous intracerebral hemorrhage: a guideline for healthcare professionals from the American Heart Association/American Stroke Association. *Stroke*. 2015 May 28. pii: STR.0000000000000069.

14. CADISS trial investigators, Markus HS, Hayter E, Levi C, Feldman A, Venables G, Norris J. Antiplatelet treatment compared with anticoagulation treatment for cervical artery dissection (CADISS): a randomised trial. *Lancet Neurol*. 2015 Apr;14(4):361–7.

15. Saposnik G, Barinagarrementeria F, Brown RD Jr, et al. Diagnosis and management of cerebral venous thrombosis a statement for healthcare professionals from the American Heart Association/American Stroke Association. *Stroke* 2011;42(4):1158–92.

16. Saposnik G, Barinagarrementeria F, Brown RD Jr, et al.; American Heart Association Stroke Council and the Council on Epidemiology and Prevention. Diagnosis and management of cerebral venous thrombosis: a statement for healthcare professionals from the American Heart Association/American Stroke Association. *Stroke*. 2011 Apr;42(4):1158–92.

CHAPTER 17

1. Chaudhuri A, Martinez-Martin P, Kennedy PG, Andrew Seaton R, Portegies P, Bojar M, Steiner I; EFNS Task Force. EFNS guideline on the management of community-acquired bacterial meningitis: report of an EFNS Task Force on acute bacterial meningitis in older children and adults. *Eur J Neurol.* 2008 Jul;15(7):649–59.

2. Huang HR, Fan LC, Rajbanshi B, Xu JF. Evaluation of a new cryptococcal antigen lateral flow immunoassay in serum, cerebrospinal fluid and urine for the diagnosis of cryptococcosis: a meta-analysis and systematic review. *PLoS One.* 2015 May 14;10(5):e0127117.

3. Pappas PG. Editorial commentary: an expanded role for therapeutic lumbar punctures in newly diagnosed AIDS-associated cryptococcal meningitis? *Clin Infect Dis.* 2014;59;1615–7.

4. Kincaid O, Lipton HL. Viral myelitis: an update. *Curr Neurol Neurosci Rep.* 2006 Nov;6(6):469–74.

5. Mécharles S, Herrmann C, Poullain P, et al. Acute myelitis due to Zika virus infection. *Lancet.* 2016 Apr 2;387(10026):1481.

6. Nakajima H, Furutama D, Kimura F, et al. Herpes simplex virus myelitis: clinical manifestations and diagnosis by the polymerase chain reaction method. *Eur Neurol.* 1998;39(3):163–7.

7. Andrade P, Figueiredo C, Carvalho C, Santos L, Sarmento A. Transverse myelitis and acute HIV infection: a case report. *BMC Infect Dis.* 2014;14:149.

8. Centers for Disease Control (CDC). Available at http://www.cdc.gov/prions/cjd/

9. Gabbai AA, Castelo A, Oliveira AS. HIV peripheral neuropathy. *Handb Clin Neurol.* 2013;115:515–29.

10. Leis AA, Stokic DS. Neuromuscular manifestations of West Nile Virus infection. *Front Neurol.* 2012;3:37.

11. Culjat M, Darling SE, Nerurkar VR, et al. Clinical and imaging findings in an infant with Zika embryopathy. *Clin Infect Dis.* 2016 May 18;pii: ciw324.

12. Centers for Disease Control (CDC). Available at http://www.cdc.gov/zika/index.html

CHAPTER 18

1. Iwashyna TJ, Ely EW, Smith DM, Langa KM. Long-term cognitive impairment and functional disability among survivors of severe sepsis. *JAMA.* 2010 Oct 27;304(16):1787–94.

2. Ehlenbach WJ, Hough CL, Crane PK, et al. Association between acute care and critical illness hospitalization and cognitive function in older adults. *JAMA.* 2010 Feb 24;303(8):763–70.

3. Pandharipande PP, Girard TD, Jackson JC, et al.; BRAIN-ICU Study Investigators. Long-term cognitive impairment after critical illness. *N Engl J Med.* 2013 Oct 3;369(14): 1306–16.

4. Franco JG, Valencia C, Bernal C, et al. Relationship between cognitive status at admission and incident delirium in older medical inpatients. *J Neuropsychiatry Clin Neurosci.* 2010 Summer;22(3):329–37.

5. Reisberg B, Ferris SH, de Leon MJ, Crook T. The global deterioration scale for assessment of primary degenerative dementia. *Am J Psychiatry.* 1982;139:1136–9.

6. Knezvic S; European Pentoxifylline Multi-Infarct Dementia Study Group. European pentoxifylline multi-infarct dementia study. *Eur Neurol.* 1996;36(5):315–21.

7. Jackson TA, MacLullich AM, Gladman JR, Lord JM, Sheehan B. Undiagnosed long-term cognitive impairment in acutely hospitalised older medical patients with delirium: a prospective cohort study. *Age Ageing.* 2016 Apr 13;pii:afw064.

8. Stern TA, Celano CM, Gross AF, et al. The assessment and management of agitation and delirium in the general hospital. *Prim Care Companion J Clin Psychiatry.* 2010;12(1):PCC .09r00938.

CHAPTER 19

1. Torre DL, Falorni A. Pharmacological causes of hyperprolactinemia. *Ther Clin Risk Manag.* 2007 Oct;3(5):929–51.

2. Chen DK, So YT, Fisher RS; Therapeutics and Technology Assessment Subcommittee of the American Academy of Neurology. Use of serum prolactin in diagnosing epileptic seizures: report of the Therapeutics and Technology Assessment Subcommittee of the American Academy of Neurology. *Neurology.* 2005 Sep 13;65(5):668–75.

3. Krumholz A, Wiebe S, Gronseth GS, et al. Evidence-based guideline: Management of an unprovoked first seizure in adults. Report of the Guideline Development Subcommittee of the American Academy of Neurology and the American Epilepsy Society. *Neurology.* 2015;84:1705–13.

4. Chong DJ, Hirsch LJ. Which EEG patterns warrant treatment in the critically ill? Reviewing the evidence for treatment of periodic epileptiform discharges and related patterns. *J Clin Neurophysiol.* 2005 Apr;22(2):79–91.

5. Misulis KE. *Atlas of EEG, Seizure Semiology, and Management.* Oxford: Oxford University Press, 2013.

6. Abou-Khalil BW. Antiepileptic drugs. *Continuum (Minneap Minn).* 2016 Feb;22(1 Epilepsy):132–56.

7. McKee HR, Abou-Khalil B. Outpatient pharmacotherapy and modes of administration for acute repetitive and prolonged seizures. *CNS Drugs.* 2015 Jan;29(1):55–70.

8. Komaragiri A, Detyniecki K, Hirsch LJ. Seizure clusters: a common, understudied and undertreated phenomenon in refractory epilepsy. *Epilepsy Behav.* 2016 Apr 23;59:83–6.

9. Grover EH, Nazzal Y, Hirsch LJ. Treatment of convulsive status epilepticus. *Curr Treat Options Neurol.* 2016 Mar;18(3):11.

10. Grover EH, Nazzal Y, Hirsch LJ. Treatment of convulsive status epilepticus. *Curr Treat Options Neurol.* 2016 Mar;18(3):11.

11. Beniczky S, Hirsch LJ, Kaplan PW, et al. Unified EEG terminology and criteria for nonconvulsive status epilepticus. *Epilepsia.* 2013 Sep;54 Suppl 6:28–9.

12. Sutter R, Semmlack S, Kaplan PW. Nonconvulsive status epilepticus in adults—insights into the invisible. *Nat Rev Neurol.* 2016 May;12(5):281–93.

13. Sutter R, Kaplan PW. Electroencephalographic criteria for nonconvulsive status epilepticus: synopsis and comprehensive survey. *Epilepsia.* 2012 Aug;53 Suppl 3:1–51.

CHAPTER 20

1. Freitag F, Cady R, eds. *The National Headache Foundation Standards of Care.* 3e. Chicago: National Headache Foundation, 2001.

2. Ford RG, Ford KT. Continuous intravenous dihydroergotamine for treatment of intractable headache. *Headache.* 1997;37:129–136.

3. Institute for Clinical Systems Improvement (ICSI). Diagnosis and treatment of headache. Bloomington, MN: Institute for Clinical Systems Improvement (ICSI); 2006 Jan. Available at http://www.guideline.gov/algorithm/4769/NGC-4769_6.pdf

4. Nagy AJ1, Gandhi S, Bhola R, Goadsby PJ. Intravenous dihydroergotamine for inpatient management of refractory primary headaches. Neurology. 2011 Nov 15;77(20):1827–32. http://www.neurology.org/content/suppl/2011/11/02/WNL.0b013e3182377dbb.DC1/WNL203164.appendix-pjg.pdf

5. Orr SL, Friedman BW, Christie S, et al. Management of adults with acute migraine in the emergency department: the American Headache Society Evidence Assessment of Parenteral Pharmacotherapies. *Headache.* 2016 Jun;56(6):911–40.

6. Goadsby PJ, Cohen AS, Matharu MS. Trigeminal autonomic cephalalgias- diagnosis and treatment. *Curr Neurol Neurosci Rep* 2007;7:117–25.

CHAPTER 21

1. Menna AK. Treatment guidelines for Guillian Barre syndrome. *Ann Indian Acad Neurol.* 2011 Jul;14(Suppl1):S73–S81.

2. Anadani M, Katirji B. Acute-onset chronic inflammatory demyelinating polyneuropathy: An electrodiagnostic study. *Muscle Nerve.* 2015 Nov;52(5):900–5. doi: 10.1002/mus.24667. Epub 2015 Aug 31. PMID: 25809534

3. Chan YC, Lo YL, Chan ES. Immunotherapy for diabetic amyotrophy. *Cochrane Database Syst Rev.* 2012 Jun 13;(6):CD006521. doi: 10.1002/14651858.CD006521.pub3.

4. Marinó M, Ricciardi R, Pinchera A, et al. Mild clinical expression of myasthenia gravis associated with autoimmune thyroid diseases. *J Clin Endocrinol Metab.* 1997; 82(2):438–43.

6. Lacomis D. Electrophysiology of neuromuscular disorders in critical illness. *Muscle Nerve.* 2013;47(3):452–63.

7. Goodman BP, Harper CM, Boon AJ. Prolonged compound muscle action potential duration in critical illness myopathy. *Muscle Nerve.* 2009;40(6):1040–2.

8. Rabinstein AA, Wijdicks EF. Warning signs of imminent respiratory failure in neurological patients. *Semin Neurol.* 2003 Mar;23(1):97–104.

CHAPTER 22

1. Filippi M, Rocca MA, Ciccarelli O, et al.; MAGNIMS Study Group. MRI criteria for the diagnosis of multiple sclerosis: MAGNIMS consensus guidelines. *Lancet Neurol.* 2016 Mar;15(3):292–303.

2. Abdoli M, Freedman MS. Neuro-oncology dilemma: tumour or tumefactive demyelinating lesion. *Mult Scler Relat Disord.* 2015 Nov;4(6):555–66.

3. Le Page E, Veillard D, Laplaud DA, et al.; COPOUSEP investigators; West Network for Excellence in Neuroscience. Oral versus intravenous high-dose methylprednisolone for treatment of relapses in patients with multiple sclerosis (COPOUSEP): a randomised, controlled, double-blind, non-inferiority trial. *Lancet.* 2015 Sep 5;386(9997):974–81. doi: 10.1016/S0140-6736(15)61137-0. Epub 2015 Jun 28.

4. Syed YY, McKeage K, Scott LJ. Delta-9-tetrahydrocannabinol/cannabidiol (Sativex®): a review of its use in patients with moderate to severe spasticity due to multiple sclerosis. *Drugs.* 2014 Apr;74(5):563–78.

5. Siegert RJ, Abernethy DA. Depression in multiple sclerosis: a review. *J Neurol Neurosurg Psychiatry.* 2005 Apr;76(4):469–75.

6. Koppel BS, Brust JC, Fife T, et al. Systematic review: efficacy and safety of medical marijuana in selected neurologic disorders: report of the Guideline Development Subcommittee of the American Academy of Neurology. *Neurology.* 2014 Apr 29;82(17):1556–63. doi: 10.1212/WNL.0000000000000363.

7. Foley PL, Vesterinen HM, Laird BJ, et al. Prevalence and natural history of pain in adults with multiple sclerosis: systematic review and meta-analysis. *Pain.* 2013 May;154(5):632–42.

8. Ariai MS, Mallory GW, Pollock BE. Outcomes after microvascular decompression for patients with trigeminal neuralgia and suspected multiple sclerosis. *World Neurosurg.* 2014 Mar–Apr;81(3–4):599–603. doi: 10.1016/j.wneu.2013.09.027. Epub 2013 Sep 19.

9. Rahn EJ, Hohmann AG. Cannabinoids as pharmacotherapies for neuropathic pain: from the bench to the bedside. *Neurotherapeutics.* 2009 Oct;6(4):713–37. doi: 10.1016/j.nurt.2009.08.002.

10. Kelley BJ, Rodriguez M. Seizures in patients with multiple sclerosis: epidemiology, pathophysiology and management. *CNS Drugs.* Author manuscript; available in PMC 2010 January 1.

11. Tan IL, McArthur JC, Clifford DB, Major EO, Nath A. Immune reconstitution inflammatory syndrome in natalizumab-associated PML. *Neurology*. 2011 Sep 13;77(11):1061–1067. doi: 10.1212/WNL.0b013e31822e55e7 PMCID: PMC3174071

12. Goodin DS, Frohman EM, Garmany GP Jr, et al.; Therapeutics and Technology Assessment Subcommittee of the American Academy of Neurology and the MS Council for Clinical Practice Guidelines. Disease modifying therapies in multiple sclerosis: report of the Therapeutics and Technology Assessment Subcommittee of the American Academy of Neurology and the MS Council for Clinical Practice Guidelines. *Neurology*. 2002 Jan 22;58(2):169–78.

CHAPTER 23

1. Walker RH. Differential diagnosis of chorea. *Curr Neurol Neurosci Rep*. 2011 Aug;11(4):385–95. doi: 10.1007/s11910-011-0202-2. Review. PMID: 21465146

2. Patel AB, Bansberg SF, Adler CH, Lott DG, Crujido L. The Mayo Clinic Arizona spasmodic dysphonia experience: a demographic analysis of 718 patients. *Ann Otol Rhinol Laryngol*. 2015 Nov;124(11):859–63. doi: 10.1177/0003489415588557. Epub 2015 May 29.

3. Fahn S, Jankovic J, Hallett M. et al. *Principles and practice of movement disorders*, 2e. New York: Saunders, 2011.

4. Bondon-Guitton E, Perez-Lloret S, Bagheri H, Brefel C, Rascol O, Montastruc JL. Drug-induced parkinsonism: a review of 17 years' experience in a regional pharmacovigilance center in France. *Mov Disord*. 2011 Oct;26(12):2226–31. doi: 10.1002/mds.23828. Epub 2011 Jun 14.

5. Li Y, Hai S, Zhou Y, Dong BR. Cholinesterase inhibitors for rarer dementias associated with neurological conditions. *Cochrane Database Syst Rev*. 2015 Mar 3;3:CD009444.

6. Wei L, Chen Y. Neuroleptic malignant-like syndrome with a slight elevation of creatine-kinase levels and respiratory failure in a patient with Parkinson's disease. *Patient Prefer Adherence*. 2014 Feb 27;8:271–3.

7. Newman EJ, Grosset DG, Kennedy PG. The parkinsonism-hyperpyrexia syndrome. *Neurocrit Care*. 2009;10(1):136–40.

8. Ding W, Ding LJ, Li FF, Han Y, Mu L Neurodegeneration and cognition in Parkinson's disease: a review. *Eur Rev Med Pharmacol Sci*. 2015 Jun;19(12):2275–81.

9. Ehrenpreis ED, Deepak P, Sifuentes H, Devi R, Du H, Leikin JB. The metoclopramide black box warning for tardive dyskinesia: effect on clinical practice, adverse event reporting, and prescription drug lawsuits. *Am J Gastroenterol*. 2013 Jun;108(6):866–72.

10. Kamble N, Prashantha DK, Jha M, Netravathi M, Reddy YC, Pal PK. Gender and age determinants of psychogenic movement disorders: a clinical profile of 73 patients. *Can J Neurol Sci*. 2016 Jan 13:1–10.

11. Shannon KM. Hemiballismus. *Curr Treat Options Neurol*. 2005 May;7(3):203–10.

12. Bhidayasiri R, Fahn S, Weiner WJ, Gronseth GS, Sullivan KL, Zesiewicz TA; American Academy of Neurology. Evidence-based guideline: treatment of tardive syndromes: report of the Guideline Development Subcommittee of the American Academy of Neurology. *Neurology*. 2013 Jul 30;81(5):463–9. doi: 10.

13. Stremmel W, Meyerrose KW, Niederau C, Hefter H, Kreuzpaintner G, Strohmeyer G. Wilson disease: clinical presentation, treatment, and survival. *Ann Intern Med*. 1991 Nov 1;115(9):720–6.

CHAPTER 24

1. Nafissi S, Niknam S, Hosseini SS. Electrophysiological evaluation in lumbosacral radiculopathy. *Iran J Neurol.* 2012;11(3):83–6.
2. American Academy of Neurological Surgeons (AANS). AANS Guidelines for Management of Acute Cervical Spine and Spinal Cord Injuries, 2013. Available at http://www.aans.org/Education%20and%20Meetings/~/media/Files/Education%20and%20Meetingf/Clinical%20Guidelines/TraumaGuidelines.ashx
3. American Spinal Injury Association (ASIA). ASIA International Standards for Neurological Classification of Spinal Cord Injury Worksheet. Available at http://www.asia-spinalinjury.org/elearning/International%20Stds%20Diagram%20Worksheet%2011.2015%20opt.pdf

CHAPTER 25

1. Louis DN, Perry A, Reifenberger G, et al. The 2016 World Health Organization Classification of Tumors of the Central Nervous System: a summary. Acta Neuropathol. 2016 Jun;131(6):803–20. doi: 10.1007/s00401-016-1545-1. Epub 2016 May 9.
2. Blecharz KG, Colla R, Rohde V, Vajkoczy P. Control of the blood-brain barrier function in cancer cell metastasis. *Biol Cell.* 2015 Oct;107(10):342–71.
3. Bochev P, Klisarova A, Kaprelyan A, Chaushev B, Dancheva Z. Brain metastases detectability of routine whole body (18)F-FDG PET and low dose CT scanning in 2502 asymptomatic patients with solid extracranial tumors. *Hell J Nucl Med.* 2012 May–Aug;15(2):125–9.
4. Anderson MD, Colen RR, Tremont-Lukats IW. Imaging mimics of primary malignant tumors of the central nervous system (CNS). *Curr Oncol Rep.* 2014;16(8):399.
5. Graus F, Saiz A, Dalmau J. Antibodies and neuronal autoimmune disorders of the CNS. *J Neurol.* 2010 April;257(4):509–17.
6. Sanders DB, Guptill JT. Myasthenia gravis and Lambert-Eaton myasthenic syndrome. *Continuum (Minneap Minn).* 2014 Oct;20(5 Peripheral Nervous System Disorders):1413–25.
7. Bekircan-Kurt CE, Derle Çiftçi E, Kurne AT, Anlar B. Voltage gated calcium channel antibody-related neurological diseases. *World J Clin Cases.* 2015 Mar 16;3(3):293–300.
8. Vernino S. Paraneoplastic cerebellar degeneration. *Handb Clin Neurol.* 2012;103:215–23.
9. Zhuang H, Yuan X, Zheng Y, et al. A study on the evaluation method and recent clinical efficacy of bevacizumab on the treatment of radiation cerebral necrosis. *Sci Rep.* 2016 Apr 12;6:24364.
10. Navi BB, Singer S, Merkler AE. Cryptogenic subtype predicts reduced survival among cancer patients with ischemic stroke. *Stroke.* 2014 Aug;45(8):2292–7
11. Merkler et al. Diagnostic yield of echocardiography in cancer patients with ischemic stroke. *J Neurooncol.* 2015 May;123(1):115–21.

CHAPTER 27

1. Patenaude Y, Pugash D, Lim K, Morin L; Diagnostic Imaging Committee (Lim K, Bly S, Butt K, et al.); Society of Obstetricians and Gynaecologists of Canada. The use of magnetic resonance imaging in the obstetric patient. *J Obstet Gynaecol Can.* 2014 Apr;36(4):349–63.
2. Leffert LR, Clancy CR, Bateman BT, et al. Treatment patterns and short-term outcomes in ischemic stroke in pregnancy or postpartum period. *Am J Obstet Gynecol.* 2015 Dec 18;pii: S0002-9378(15)02516-8.
3. Sasidharan PK. Cerebral vein thrombosis misdiagnosed and mismanaged. *Thrombosis.* 2012;2012:210676.

4. Marchenko A, Etwel F, Olutunfese O, Nickel C, Koren G, Nulman I. Pregnancy outcome following prenatal exposure to triptan medications: a meta-analysis. *Headache.* 2015 Apr;55(4):490–501.

5. Reisinger TL, Newman M, Loring DW, Pennell PB, Meador KJ. Antiepileptic drug clearance and seizure frequency during pregnancy in women with epilepsy. *Epilepsy Behav.* Author manuscript; available in PMC 2014 October 1.

6. Beach RL, Kaplan PW. Seizures in pregnancy: diagnosis and management. *Int Rev Neurobiol.* 2008;83:259–71.

7. Montouris G. Teratogenicity and antiepileptic drugs. In: Bui E, Klein A, eds. *Women with Epilepsy* (chapter 12). City: Cambridge, 157.

8. Klein A. Peripheral nerve disease in pregnancy. *Clin Obstet Gynecol.* 2013 Jun;56(2):382–8.

9. Cohen Y, Lavie O, Granovsky-Grisaru S, Aboulafia Y, Diamant YZ. Bell palsy complicating pregnancy: a review. *Obstet Gynecol Surv.* 2000 Mar;55(3):184–8.

CHAPTER 28

1. Kaufmann H, Freeman R, Biaggioni I, et al.; NOH301 Investigators. Droxidopa for neurogenic orthostatic hypotension: a randomized, placebo-controlled, phase 3 trial. *Neurology.* 2014 Jul 22;83(4):328–35.

2. Lai EC, Yang YH, Lin SJ, Hsieh CY. Use of antiepileptic drugs and risk of hypothyroidism. *Pharmacoepidemiol Drug Saf.* 2013 Oct;22(10):1071–9.

CHAPTER 29

1. Vidal-Alaball J, Butler CC, Cannings-John R, et al. Oral vitamin B12 versus intramuscular vitamin B12 for vitamin B12 deficiency. *Cochrane Database Syst Rev.* 2005 Jul 20;(3):CD004655.

CHAPTER 30

1. French JA. Seizure exacerbation by antiepileptic drugs. *Epilepsy Curr.* 2005 Sep–Oct; 5(5):192–3.

2. Barton B, Zauber SE, Goetz CG. Movement disorders caused by medical disease. *Semin Neurol.* 2009 Apr;29(2):97–110.

3. Werner EG, Olanow CW. Parkinsonism and amiodarone therapy. *Ann Neurol.* 1989 Jun;25(6):630–2.

4. Jerrell JM, McIntyre RS. Cardiovascular and neurological adverse events associated with antidepressant treatment in children and adolescents. *J Child Neurol.* 2009 Mar;24(3):297–304.

5. Prakash J, Ryali VSSR, Srivastava K, Bhat PS, Shashikumar R, Singal A. Tobacco-alcohol amblyopia: A rare complication of prolonged alcohol abuse. *Ind Psychiatry J.* 2011 Jan–Jun;20(1):66–8.

6. Slaughter RJ, Mason RW, Beasley DM, Vale JA, Schep LJ. Isopropanol poisoning. *Clin Toxicol (Phila).* 2014 Jun;52(5):470–8. doi: 10.3109/15563650.2014.914527. Epub 2014 May 9.

CHAPTER 31

1. Schrag M, Youn T, Schindler J, Kirshner H, Greer D. Intravenous fibrinolytic therapy in central retinal artery occlusion: a patient-level meta-analysis. *JAMA Neurol.* 2015 Oct;72(10):1148–54.

CHAPTER 32

1. Parham K, Kuchel GA. A geriatric perspective on benign paroxysmal positional vertigo. *J Am Geriatr Soc.* 2016 Jan 25;64(2):378–85.

2. Hilton MP, Pinder DK. The Epley (canalith repositioning) manoeuvre for benign paroxysmal positional vertigo. *Cochrane Database Syst Rev.* 2014 Dec 8;12:CD003162.

3. Pollak L, Book M, Smetana Z, Alkin M, Soupayev Z, Mendelson E. Herpes simplex virus type 1 in saliva of patients with vestibular neuronitis: a preliminary study. *Neurologist.* 2011 Nov;17(6):330–2.

4. Lee H. Neuro-otological aspects of cerebellar stroke syndrome. *J Clin Neurol.* 2009 Jun;5(2):65–73. Published online 2009 Jun 30. doi: 10.3988/jcn.2009.5.2.65

5. Westerlaken BO, Stokroos RJ, Dhooge IJ, Wit HP, Albers FW. Treatment of idiopathic sudden sensorineural hearing loss with antiviral therapy: a prospective, randomized, double-blind clinical trial. *Ann Otol Rhinol Laryngol.* 2003 Nov;112(11):993–1000.

6. Pirodda A, Ferri GG, Raimondi MC, Borghi C. Diuretics in Meniere disease: a therapy or a potential cause of harm? *Med Hypotheses.* 2011 Nov;77(5):869–71. doi: 10.1016/j.mehy.2011.07.060. Epub 2011 Aug 23.

7. Seidman MD, Ahsan SF. Current opinion: the management of tinnitus. *Curr Opin Otolaryngol Head Neck Surg.* 2015 Oct;23(5):376–81.

8. Broomfield SJ, O'Donoghue GM. Self-reported symptoms and patient experience: A British Acoustic Neuroma Association survey. *Br J Neurosurg.* 2015 Nov 2:1–8.

CHAPTER 33

1. de Almeida JR, Guyatt GH, Sud S, et al.; Bell Palsy Working Group, Canadian Society of Otolaryngology—Head and Neck Surgery and Canadian Neurological Sciences Federation. Management of Bell palsy: clinical practice guideline. *CMAJ.* 2014 Sep 2;186(12):917–22.

CHAPTER 35

1. Borg J, Holm L, Cassidy JD, et al.; WHO Collaborating Centre Task Force on Mild Traumatic Brain Injury. Diagnostic procedures in mild traumatic brain injury: results of the WHO Collaborating Centre Task Force on Mild Traumatic Brain Injury. *J Rehabil Med.* 2004 Feb;(43 Suppl):61–75.

2. Sharma D, Vavilala MS. Perioperative management of adult traumatic brain injury. *Anesthesiol Clin.* 2012 Jun;30(2):333–46.

3. Thompson K, Pohlmann-Eden B, Campbell LA, Abel H. Pharmacological treatments for preventing epilepsy following traumatic head injury. *Cochrane Database Syst Rev.* 2015 Aug 10;8:CD009900.

4. Giza CC, Kutcher JS, Ashwal S, et al. Summary of evidence-based guideline update: evaluation and management of concussion in sports: report of the Guideline Development Subcommittee of the American Academy of Neurology. *Neurology.* 2013 Jun 11;80(24):2250–7.

CHAPTER 37

1. National Institute of Neurological Disorders and Stroke (NINDS). Available at http://www.ninds.nih.gov/disorders/neuronal_migration/neuronal_migration.htm

2. Cho WH, Seidenwurm D, Barkovich AJ. Adult-onset neurologic dysfunction associated with cortical malformations. *AJNR Am J Neuroradiol.* 1999 Jun–Jul;20(6):1037–43.

3. Mohan M, Carpenter PK, Bennett C. Donepezil for dementia in people with Down syndrome. *Cochrane Database Syst Rev.* 2009 Jan 21;(1):CD007178.

CHAPTER 38

1. Stone J, Smyth R, Carson A, Warlow C, Sharpe M. La belle indifférence in conversion symptoms and hysteria: systematic review. *Br J Psychiatry.* 2006 Mar;188:204–9.

2. American Psychiatric Association. *Diagnostic and Statistical Manual of Mental Disorders, 5e*. New York: American Psychiatric Association, 2013.

CHAPTER 39

1. Teasdale G, Jennett B. Assessment of coma and impaired consciousness. A practical scale. *Lancet*. 1974;2:81–4.
2. MDCalc Medical Calculators and Clinical Scores. Available at http://www.mdcalc.com/nih-stroke-scale-score-nihss/

CHAPTER 40

1. Misulis KE. *Atlas of EEG, Seizure Semiology, and Management*. Oxford: Oxford University Press, 2013.
2. McGrath ER, Paikin JS, Motlagh B, Salehian O, Kapral MK, O'Donnell MJ. Transesophageal echocardiography in patients with cryptogenic ischemic stroke: a systematic review. *Am Heart J*. 2014 Nov;168(5):706–12.

CHAPTER 41

1. Rangel-Castillo L, Gopinath S, Robertson CS. Management of intracranial hypertension. Author manuscript; available in PMC 2009 May 1. Published in final edited form as: *Neurol Clin*. 2008 May;26(2):521–41.
2. Burton JM, O'Connor PW, Hohol M, Beyene J. Oral versus intravenous steroids for treatment of relapses in multiple sclerosis. *Cochrane Database Syst Rev*. 2012 Dec 12;12:CD006921.

Index

ABCD score, 344
Abducens neuropathies, 56
Abducens palsy, 45, 308–9
Abnormal sensations, 19
Accessory neuropathies, 56
ACE inhibitors, 129
Acoustic neuroma, 53, 65, 306
Acute-chronic inflammatory demyelinating
    polyneuropathy (A-CIDP), 200
Acute disseminated encephalomyelitis
    (ADEM), 182, 220–21, 243, 361
Acute inflammatory demyelinating
    polyneuropathy (AIDP)
  axonal variants, 199–200
  as cancer complication, 86
  characterization, 21, 23
  comorbidities, 158, 198
  CSF findings, 355
  diagnosis, 198
  differential diagnosis, 24, 162t
  immunosuppression, 360–63
  management of, 198–99
Acute ischemic stroke (AIS). see
    ischemic stroke
Acute motor and sensory axonal
    neuropathy (AMSAN), 200
Acute myocardial infarction, 91
Acute neural injury, 74
Acute stroke-ready hospital, 12
Addison disease, 278, 282
Advanced directives, 365
Afferent pupillary defect, 48
Aggrenox, 131
Alcohol withdrawal, 235
Alcoholic cerebellar degeneration, 292
Alcoholic myopathy, 293
Alcoholic neuropathy, 292–93
Alzheimer's disease (AD)
  characterization, 30, 166

diagnosis of, 167–68
differential diagnosis, 32, 32f, 51, 169
Global Deterioration scale, 167
management, 168
stages of, 167
Amantadine, PD, 229–30
Amiodarone, 235, 290
Amnesia, 30, 34
Amyloid angiopathy, 143
Amyotropic lateral sclerosis, 24, 25, 94, 212
Analgesics, 77, 192
Anaplastic astrocytoma/
    oligodendroglioma, 252
Anemia, 66
Anesthetic complications, 25–26, 101
Anisocoria, 47–48
Anterior inferior cerebellar artery (AICA)
    occlusion, 57
Antibiotics, differential diagnosis, 178t
Anticholinergics, PD, 229
Anticoagulation agents, 135
Anticonvulsants, 194, 289–90
Antidepressants, 77, 290
Antiepileptic drugs (AEDs)
  chronic pain, 77
  differential diagnosis, 178t
  discontinuation of, 187
  selection of, 107, 181–82, 182t
Antiphospholipid antibody syndrome
    (APS), 93
Antiplatelets, ischemic stroke, 130–31, 135
Aphasia
  anomic, 50
  Broca's (expressive), 49
  conduction, 50
  diagnosis, differential diagnosis, 51
  global, 50, 123
  PPA (see primary progressive aphasia)
  pure-word deafness, 50

Index

Aphasia (*Cont.*)
  pure-word mutism (aphemia), 50
  subcortical, 51
  subtypes of, 49
  tPA and, 130
  transcortical mixed, 50
  transcortical motor, 50
  transcortical sensory, 50
  Wernicke's (receptive), 50
Apraxia of lid opening, 48
Aqueductal stenosis, 263
Arboviruses, 27
Argyll Robertson pupils, 48
Arrhythmia, 36, 38*t*
Arsenic poisoning, 295
Arterial dissections, 142–43, 268, 270
Arterial occlusive disease, 38*t*
Arteriovenous malformations (AVMs),
  140–41, 244
Aspirin, 130
Asterixis, 93, 224, 225
Astrocytoma/oligodendroglioma, 252
Ataxia
  cerebellar, 63–64, 227
  characterization, 227–28
  differential diagnosis, 62, 64, 127, 228
  Friedreich, 228, 240
  gait, 59, 60, 63–64
  hereditary, 240
  limb, 59, 61
  as MS complication, 219, 228
  psychogenic (hysterical) gait, 241
  sensory, 19, 60, 62, 227
  spinocerebellar, 228, 240
  vestibular, 228
  Wilson disease, 228, 240–41
Athetosis, 224, 226–27
Atrial fibrillation, 134
Autonomic neuropathy, 278–79
Avonex, complications of, 220
Azathioprine, 361–62

B₁ deficiency, 286
B₆ deficiency, toxicity, 287–88
B₁₂ deficiency, 31, 244, 285–86
Baclofen, 34, 290, 357
Barbiturate coma, 359
Bariatric surgery, 100–101
Basal ganglia, 21, 22, 138
Basilar invagination, 36
Basilar thrombosis, 23

Becker dystrophy, 211
Bell palsy, 48, 57, 307–8
Benign paroxysmal positional vertigo
  (BPPV), 60, 62, 65, 301–3
Betaseron, complications of, 220
Billing, coding, 13
Binasal hemianopia, 42
Binswanger disease, 170
Bitemporal hemianopia, 42
Bone marrow transplant, 100
Botulinum toxin, 358
Botulism, 24, 95, 206
Bovine spongiform encephalopathy
  (BSE), 154–55
Brachial plexopathy, 258
Brain
  abscess, 91, 155–56
  death, 30, 34, 121–23, 366–67
  injury medicine, 5*t*
Brain tumors
  diagnostic approach to, 26
  differential diagnosis, 51, 60, 178*t*
  metastatic, 253
  mimics, 251
  in pregnancy, 270
  primary, 251–53
Brainstem
  hemorrhage, 138
  infarction, 22–23
  lesions, 21, 57
  stroke, 34, 47, 65
Brainstem tumors, 48
Brudzinski sign, 148
Business of hospital neurology
  billing, coding, 13
  metrics, 13–14
  records, audits, 13
  risk management, 14
  stroke centers, types of, 11–13

CADASIL, 170
Caffeine, 192
Cancers
  cerebrovascular disease, 89
  chemotherapeutics, differential
    diagnosis, 178*t*
  complications related to, 85
  differential diagnosis, 85–86, 178*t*
  lumbosacral plexus, 87
  lung, 87
  metabolic effects, 88

metastases, 87–89, 178*t*

neuropathic pain, 74, 77

orbital tumor, 47

paraspinal, 87

small-cell lung, 26

treatment, neurologic complications of, 89, 256–59

tumor invasion, local, 86–87

Cannabis, 219

Cardiac disease, 90–92

Carotid arteriovenous fistulas, 142

Carotid dissections, 142–43

Carotid duplex sonography (CDS), 38*t*, 39

Carotid occlusive disease, 38*t*

Carotid sinus hypersensitivity, 36, 37, 38*t*

Carotid sinus massage, 37, 38*t*

Carotid stenosis, 134

Carotid ultrasonography, 353

Carpal tunnel syndrome, 21

Caseload, 5–6, 14

Catatonia, 335

Catecholaminergic polymorphic ventricular tachycardia (CPVT), 37

Catheter angiography, 355–56

Cauda equina syndrome, 76, 244, 248–49

Caudate hemorrhage, 138

Cavernous malformations, 141

Cavernous sinus lesions, 47

Cavernous sinus thrombosis, 47, 144, 311

Cefepime, 108

Central pontine myelinolysis, 115

Central retinal vein occlusion, 47, 299

Central vertigo, 60

Cerebellar ataxia, 63–64, 227

Cerebellar degeneration, paraneoplastic, 88, 228, 256

Cerebellar hemorrhage, 137–38

Cerebellar infarction/hemorrhage, 63–64

Cerebellar lesions, 18

Cerebellar tumor, 64

Cerebral amyloid angiopathy, 170

Cerebral aneurysms, 140

Cerebral angiopathy, postpartum, 268

Cerebral edema, 47, 358

Cerebral hemorrhage, 34

Cerebral ischemia, 34, 73

Cerebral mass lesion, 73

Cerebral venous thrombosis

characterization, 143–44

differential diagnosis, 51, 73

in pregnancy, 268, 269, 271–72

Certifications, 5*t*

Cervical dystonia, 238

Cervical radiculopathy, 76, 246–47

Cervical spondylosis, 37

Chemotherapeutics, differential diagnosis, 178*t*

Chemotherapy neuropathy, 89, 257

Chiari malformations, 264, 311, 327–28

Chlorpromazine, for migraine, 192

Cholinergic neuropathy, 26

Cholinesterase inhibitors (ChEI), 296

Chorea, 224, 227

Chronic fatigue syndrome, 93

Chronic inflammatory demyelinating polyneuropathy (CIDP)

as cancer complication, 86

characterization, 24, 200

comorbidities, 158

diagnosis, 200–201

immunosuppression, 360–63

management of, 201

Clopidogrel, 130

Cluster headache

anisocoria, 47

characterization, 44, 193–94

differential diagnosis, 70, 72, 194

management of, 194

preventive therapies, 194

CMV encephalitis, 153

CMV meningitis, 149

CNS

angiitis, primary, 362

focal disorder, 65

infection, 35

lymphoma, primary, 253

vasculitis, 360

Cognitive disorders

delirium (*see* delirium)

dementia (*see* dementia)

syncope (*see* syncope)

transient global amnesia, 34, 62, 164–65

Colloid cysts, 263

Coma, 34–35

Communication in difficult encounters, 365–66

Compensation, 6

Compliance, 8

Comprehensive stroke center, 12–13

Compressive lesion, 47

Compressive neuropathies, 75

COMT inhibitors, PD, 230

Concussion, 317–18

Confusional state
  cardiac disease, 91
  characterization, 29, 33, 59
  differential diagnosis, 33–34, 62

Congestive heart failure, 91

Continuity of care, 7–8, 14

Contusion, 318

Conus medullaris syndrome, 76, 244, 248–49

Conversion disorder, 337–38

Copaxone (glatiramer), 220, 363

Copper deficiency, 244, 288

Cortical deafness, 53

Cortical lesions, 21

Corticobasal degeneration, 31, 32, 32f,
  232–33

Corticobasal syndrome, 169

Corticospinal lesions, 18

Corticospinal tract dysfunction, differential
  diagnosis, 64

Corticosteroids, 359–61

Cough syncope, 36

CPA tumors, 311

Cranial dystonia, 238

Cranial nerve deficits
  abducens palsy, 45, 308–9
  Bell palsy, 48, 57, 307–8
  diabetic ophthalmoplegia, 308
  glossopharyngeal neuralgia, 68, 74, 310
  herpes zoster ophthalmicus, 156, 310
  Horner syndrome, 47, 48, 309
  multiple palsies, 310–11
  overview, 307
  Ramsay Hunt syndrome, 156, 307–8

Cranial nerve pain, 68

Cranial neuropathies, 55–57, 74

Craniectomy, for ICP, 360

Credibility, 368

Creutzfeldt-Jakob disease, 31, 153–55

Critical illness neuromyopathy, 24, 25,
  94–95, 209–10

Crossed sensory deficit, 20t

Cryptogenic stroke, 134–35

CRYSTAL AF trial, 134

CSF circulation
  flow obstruction, 263–64
  increased pressure, 262–63
  low pressure, 264–65
  overview, 261
  persistent leak, 265
  sampling, 353–55

CT angiography, 352

Cushing syndrome, 278, 281–82

Cyclophosphamide, 362

Dantrolene, 358

Decadron, for ICP, 359

Deep brain stimulation, PD, 230

Degenerative spine disease, 246

Delirium
  anesthesia-associated, 101–2
  cardiac disease, 91–92
  characterization, 29, 30, 163–64
  diagnosis, 164
  hospital, 334–35
  incipient, 62
  management, 164
  peri-operative, 97–99

Delirium tremens (DTs), 235

Dementia
  admission, rationales for, 8
  characterization, 29, 30, 165
  degenerative, 30–31
  diagnosis, 165–66
  differential diagnosis, 32, 32f
  evaluation of, 163
  HIV– AIDS, 32, 158
  hospitalization, 166
  infectious, 31–32
  management, 172
  as MS complication, 218
  nondegenerative, 31
  opportunistic infections, 158
  semantic, 32, 32f

Demyelinating neuropathy, 26

Demyelinating polyneuropathy, 26

Depression, 219

Dermatomal distribution of pain, sensory
  loss, 20t

Dermatomyositis, 26, 210–11

Developmental venous anomaly, 142

Dexamethasone, 151, 217

DHE, 192, 194

Diabetes insipidus, 278, 284

Diabetes mellitus
  hypoglycemia, hyperglycemia, 90
  motor, sensory deficits, 26–27
  neurologic complications of,
    89–90, 109–11
  neurology consultation, 278
  neuropathies, 90

Diabetic amyotrophy, 202, 203, 279

Diabetic autonomic insufficiency, 313, 314
Diabetic ketoacidosis (DKA), 90, 110
Diabetic lumbosacral plexopathy, 202, 203
Diabetic neuropathy, 74, 158–59, 277–79
Diabetic ophthalmoplegia, 308
Dialysis disequilibrium, 107
Difficult encounters tools, 365–66
Diffuse axonal injury, 320
Diplopia, 45, 218–19
Disorders of neuronal migration, 329
Dissociated suspended sensory deficit, 20t
Distal sensory deficit localization, 20t
Distal symmetric polyneuropathy, 158
Dizziness, vertigo. see also vertigo
  confusion (see confusional state)
  gait ataxia, 59, 60, 63–64
  generators, 59
  imbalance, falls, 63–65
  limb ataxia, 59, 61
  pre-syncope, 59, 61, 63
  syncope (see syncope)
  syndromes of, 62–63
  terminology, 59
  vertigo, 60
Dopamine agonists, PD, 230
Down syndrome, 331
Driving, seizures and, 187
Drug-induced parkinsonism, 230–31
Duchenne dystrophy, 211
Dural arteriovenous fistulas, 141
Dysarthria
  ataxic, 52
  diagnosis, differential diagnosis, 52–53
  flaccid, 52
  hyperkinetic, 52
  hypokinetic, 52
  rigid, 52
  spastic, 52
  unilateral upper motor neuron, 52
Dysesthesias characterization, 19
Dyskinesia, 224, 227, 237–38
Dystonias, 224, 227, 238–39

Echocardiography, 356
Eclampsia, 271
Electrocardiogram (EKG), 38t, 39
Electroencephalography (EEG),
    39t, 347–49
Electromyography (EMG), 349–51
Electronic medical records (EMRs), 7, 13
Emergency Department evaluation, 24–25

Encephalitis
  characterization, 152
  differential diagnosis, 35, 83, 177t
  ED evaluation, 25
  limbic, 177–78t, 254–55
  paraneoplastic, 254–55
  viral, 152–53
Encephalopathy
  characterization, 29, 30, 82
  differential diagnosis, 33, 83, 123, 127
  Hashimoto, 277, 280–81
  hepatic, 108–9
  hospital, 33
  hypertensive, 35
  hypoxic, 91, 99
  hypoxic-ischemic (see hypoxic-ischemic
      encephalopathy (HIE))
  medications, altered clearance of, 108
  metabolic, 123, 164
  as neurologic complication, 93
  peri-operative, 97–99, 101
  in pregnancy, 269–70
  septic, 82
  studies, 83
  subacute spongiform, 153–55
  toxic/metabolic, 123, 164
End-of-life care, 367–68
Endocarditis, 160
Endocrine, metabolic myopathies, 212
Enhanced physiologic tremor, 23, 234
Ependymoma, 252–53
Epidural abscess, 83, 244
Epidural hematoma, 136, 319
Epilepsy
  absence, EEG findings, 181t
  AED choice, 182, 182t
  classification of, 179f
  differential diagnosis, 174, 175t
  driving, 187
  EEG findings, 181, 181t
  generalized tonic-clonic, AED
      selection, 182t
  juvenile myoclonic, 226
  juvenile myoclonic, AED selection, 182t
  myoclonic, EEG findings, 181t
  myoclonus, 225
  new-onset, 180
  partial, AED selection, 182t
  partial, EEG findings, 181t
  post-traumatic, 320
  in pregnancy, 273–74

Epilepsy (*Cont.*)
  primary generalized absence, AED
    selection, 182*t*
  progressive myoclonus, 226
  sudden unexplained death, 187
  symptomatic, 176, 177–78*t*
  symptoms, signs of, 178–80
Essential tremor, 23, 225, 235
Ethanol
  intoxication, 290–91
  toxicity, 64, 228, 290
  withdrawal, 291–92
Ethylene glycol toxicity, 294
Extrapyramidal lesions, 18
Eye pain, 44

Facial neuropathies, 56, 57
Falls, imbalance, 63–65
Family conflicts, 365–66, 368
Fascioscapulohumeral dystrophy (FSH), 211
Fibromyalgia, 93
Fingolimod, 363
Fluid, electrolyte disorders, 113–15
Focal CNS disorder, 65
Focal deficits
  cardiac disease, 90
  differential diagnosis, 84–85, 87
  in pregnancy, 270
Focal sensory disturbance localization, 19
Folate deficiency, 287
Follow-up appointments, 8
Fosphenytoin, status epilepticus dosage,
    183, 184*t*, 186*t*
Fourth ventricular outflow
    obstruction, 263–64
Friedreich ataxia, 228, 240
Frontotemporal dementia (FTD)
  characterization, 30–31, 170–71
  diagnosis, 171
  differential diagnosis, 32, 32*f*, 51, 169, 171*t*
  management, 171

Gait ataxia, 59, 60, 63–64
Gaze palsy, 45
Gaze preference, 45
Generalized convulsive status epilepticus.
    see status epilepticus
Generalized sensory disturbance
    localization, 19
Glasgow Coma Scale, 341–42
Glatiramer (Copaxone), 220, 363

Glaucoma, 44, 73
Glioblastoma, 252
Global Deterioration scale, 167
Glossopharyngeal neuralgia, 68, 74, 310
Glossopharyngeal neuropathies, 56
Graves disease, 279–80
Guillain-Barré syndrome. *see* acute
    inflammatory demyelinating
    polyneuropathy (AIDP)

Hashimoto encephalopathy, 277, 280–81
Hashimoto thyroiditis, 277, 280–81
Head injuries, 99, 320, 321. *see also*
    traumatic brain injury (TBI)
Headache. *see also* migraine
  admission criteria, 189
  characterization, 70, 189–90
  cluster (*see* cluster headache)
  differential diagnosis, 72–73
  evaluation of, 70
  laboratory testing, 71
  localization, diagnosis of, 69, 69*t*
  low pressure, 264–65
  lumbar puncture, 71
  medication overuse, 193
  MS-associated, 219
  neuroimaging, 71
  pregnancy, 267–68
  primary exertional/sexual, 72
  primary stabbing, 72
  scenarios, 70–71
Health information Exchanges (HIE), 7
Hearing loss, 53, 62
Heart transplant, 100
Heavy metals toxicity, 294–95
Hematoma
  epidural, 136, 319
  spinal cord, 244
  subdural, 136, 319, 358
Hemiballismus, 23, 224, 227, 236–37
Hemifacial spasm, 227, 239
Hemisensory sensory deficit
    localization, 20*t*
Hemorrhage
  basal ganglia (thalamus), 138
  brainstem, 138
  caudate, 138
  cerebellar, 137–38
  cerebellar infarction, 63–64
  cerebral, 34
  intracerebral, 135–40, 268, 318–20

intraocular, 44
intraparenchymal, 318–19
lobar intracerebral, 137
putamen, 138
subarachnoid (*see* subarachnoid hemorrhage)
thalamic, 138
Hemorrhagic stroke
ataxia, vertigo and, 65
brainstem, 34, 47, 65
dural arteriovenous fistulas, 141
gait ataxia, 59, 60, 63–64
hypertensive emergencies, 94
peri-operative, 98
post-cardiovascular surgery, 99
renal failure and, 107–8
renal insufficiency (*see* renal insufficiency)
risk factors, 133
Hepatic failure, 108–9, 225
Hepatic insufficiency, 33, 92–93
Hereditary neuropathy with pressure palsies, 203–4, 329–30
Hereditary sensory and autonomic neuropathies, 313, 315
Hereditary spastic paraparesis, 244, 330
Herpes viruses, 27, 156–57
Herpes zoster, 74, 156–57, 202, 310
Herpes zoster ophthalmicus, 156, 310
Herpes zoster oticus, 308
HIE. *see* hypoxic-ischemic encephalopathy (HIE)
Hip surgery complications, 99
HIV/AIDS, 27, 157–59
HIV/AIDS dementia, 32, 158
HIV meningitis, 149
Holter monitor, 38t, 39
Homonymous hemianopia, 42
Horner syndrome, 47, 48, 309
Hospital admission/discharge, 7–8
Hospital-at-home, 14
Hospital delirium, 334–35
Hospital encephalopathy, 33
Hospital neurologist, 4t
Hospital neurology generally
mid-level providers, 5
models of, 3, 4t
organizational issues, 5–6
terminology, 3
training, subspecialties, 4, 5t
HSV encephalitis, 152–53
HSV meningitis, 149

Huntington disease, 31, 238
Hydrocephalus, 262–66
Hypercalcemia, 114
Hypercapnia, 113
Hyperesthesia characterization, 19
Hyperglycemia, 90
Hyperkalemic periodic paralysis, 211
Hypernatremia, 113
Hyperosmolar hyperglycemic state (HHS), 90, 110
Hyperpathia characterization, 19
Hypertension
with acute intracranial hemorrhage, 105
with acute ischemic stroke, 104–5
characterization, 94
malignant, 47, 94, 105–6
Hypertensive crisis, 47, 94, 105–6
Hypertensive emergencies, 94
Hypertensive encephalopathy, 35
Hyperthyroidism, 279–80
Hypertonic saline, for ICP, 359
Hyperventilation, for ICP, 359–60
Hypocalcemia, 114
Hypoglossal neuropathies, 56
Hypoglycemia, 66, 90, 110–11, 234
Hypokalemia, 25, 212
Hypomagnesemia, 114–15
Hyponatremia, 113–14
Hypophosphatemia, 25
Hypotension, 64, 73
Hypothermia, 123
Hypothyroidism, 31, 33, 280
Hypoxia, 112–13
Hypoxic encephalopathy, 91, 99
Hypoxic-ischemic encephalopathy (HIE)
family, discussion with, 118–19
management, 117–18
neurologic consultation, 118
overview, 117
prognosis, 118
therapeutic hypothermia (TH), 118

Ictal paralysis, 23
ICU evaluation, 25
Idiopathic brachial plexitis, 202
Idiopathic intracranial hypertension (IIH). *see* pseudotumor cerebri
Idiopathic orbital inflammatory syndrome (orbital pseudotumor), 44
Idiopathic orthostatic hypotension, 313–14
Imbalance, falls, 63–65

Immune reconstitution inflammatory syndrome (IRIS), 219, 220
Immunosuppression, 360–63
Implanted loop recorder, 38t, 39
In-coordination, localization of, 18
Incipient delirium, 62
Infectious diseases. *see also specific diseases*
    diagnostic approach to, 27
    ED evaluation, 25
    focal deficits, 84–85, 87
    overview, 147
Infectious meningitis, 57, 76
Inflammatory myopathies, 24–26
Inflammatory neuropathies, 158
Informed consent, 130
Insomnia, 323, 325
Interferons, 220, 361
Internal capsule infarction, 22
Internal capsule lesions, 21
Intoxications
    alcohol withdrawal, 235
    arsenic poisoning, 295
    chemotherapeutics, 178t
    differential diagnosis, 60
    ethanol, 64, 228, 290–92
    ethylene glycol toxicity, 294
    isopropanol toxicity, 293
    lead poisoning, 294–95
    papilledema, 47
Intracerebral hemorrhage, 135–40, 268, 318–20
Intracranial aneurysm, 310
Intracranial catastrophes, 35
Intracranial hemorrhage (ICH), 51, 73, 270
Intracranial hypotension, 73
Intracranial pressure (ICP)
    management, 358–60
Intracranial tumor, 47
Intraocular hemorrhage, 44
Intraparenchymal hemorrhage, 318–19
Ischemic optic neuropathy (ION), 43, 47, 298
Ischemic stroke
    antiplatelets, 130–31, 135
    aphasia and, 51
    ataxia, vertigo and, 65
    brainstem, 34, 47, 65
    cardioembolic source, 133–34
    carotid stenosis, 134
    characterization, 126
    confusion and, 32t, 92

cryptogenic, 134–35
    differential diagnosis, 51
    dural arteriovenous fistulas, 141
    emergent evaluation, management, 126–28, 126f
    endovascular therapies, 129, 130
    gait ataxia, 59, 60, 63–64
    hypertension with, 104–5
    hypertensive emergencies, 94
    IV heparin, 130
    IV thrombolytics, 128–30
    peri-operative, 98
    pharmacotherapy, 135
    post-acute evaluation, 131–32, 132f
    post-cardiovascular surgery, 99
    in pregnancy, 270, 271
    recurrent, 135
    renal failure, insufficiency, 92, 107–8
    (*see also* renal insufficiency)
    risk factors, 133
    statins, 135
    therapy, 135
Isopropanol (isopropyl alcohol) toxicity, 293
IV tPA, 128–30, 337
IVIg, 201, 361

Kernig sign, 148
Ketamine, status epilepticus dosage, 183
Kidney transplant, 100
Korsakoff psychosis, 31

Labyrinthitis, 303–4
Lacosamide, status epilepticus dosage, 186t
Lacunar syndrome, 170
Lambert Eaton myasthenic syndrome, 26, 88, 206, 255–56, 314–15
LAPSS, 343
Lateral medullary syndrome, 22–23
Lead poisoning, 294–95
Lennox-Gastaut syndrome, 225
Leptomeningeal tumors, 253–54
Lethargy, 30. *see also* weakness
Levetiracetam, status epilepticus dosage, 186t
Levodopa, 229
Lewy body dementia
    characterization, 31, 168–69, 231–32
    differential diagnosis, 32, 32f, 169
    management, 169, 232
Lhermitte sign, 219
Lidocaine, cluster headache, 194

Limb ataxia, 59, 61
Limb-girdle dystrophy, 211
Lithium carbonate, cluster headache, 194
Liver transplant, peri-operative
    complications, 100
Lobar intracerebral hemorrhage, 137
Locked-in syndrome, 23, 34, 123
Long bone fracture, surgery
    complications, 99
Lorazepam, status epilepticus dosage, 183,
    184t, 186t
Lumbar epidural abscess, 83
Lumbar puncture, 353–55
Lumbar radiculopathy, 76, 247–48
Lumbar radiculoplexopathy, 202, 203, 279
Lumbosacral plexopathy, 258
Lumbosacral plexus cancer, 87
Lung cancer, 87
Lung transplant, peri-operative
    complications, 100
Lyme disease, 161, 311

Malignant hyperthermia, 25–26, 102
Mannitol, for ICP, 359
MAO-B inhibitors, PD, 230
MCA infarction, 22
Medical decision-making, 123
Medication-induced tremor, 225
Medications
    altered clearance of, 108
    anisocoria, 47
    chemotherapeutics, 178t
    differential diagnosis, 33, 73, 178t
    myoclonus, 225
    neuroleptic malignant syndrome, 336
    overuse headache, 193
    papilledema, 47
    reconciliation, 8
    toxicity, 289–90
    tremor and, 235–36
Medulloblastoma, 252
Meige syndrome, 238
Ménière disease
    characterization, 53, 65, 302, 304
    differential diagnosis, 60, 62, 305
Meningeal metastases, 88
Meningioma, 252
Meningitis
    bacterial, 149–51, 354
    cerebral edema, 151
    characterization, 47, 53, 148

chronic, 311
differential diagnosis, 70, 73, 83,
    177t, 262
fungal, 151–52, 354–55
infectious, 57, 76
neoplastic, 57, 76, 258, 311, 355
pregnancy, 268
seizures, 151
viral, 148–49, 354
Meningovascular neurosyphilis, 157
Mental status changes, 29–30
Mercury poisoning, 295
Metabolic disorders, 25, 177t, 234
Metabolic encephalopathy, 123, 164
Metastases, 87–89, 178t
Methanol toxicity, 293–94
Methotrexate, 362
Methylprednisolone, for MS, 217
Metoclopramide, 236
Micturition syncope, 36
Midazolam, status epilepticus dosage, 184t
Migraine. see also headache
    admission rationales, 8
    anisocoria, 47
    with aura, 190–91
    characterization, 44, 190
    complicated, 191
    differential diagnosis, 62, 70, 72
    equivalent, 191
    hemiplegic, 191
    management of, 192–93
    migrainous infarction, 191 (see also
        ischemic stroke)
    in pregnancy, 268, 272–73
    preventive therapies, 193
    status, 8
    without aura, 191
Mild cognitive impairment, 171
Mistakes, 368–69
Mitochondrial disorders, 25, 26
Mixed office/hospital model, 4t
Mobile cardiac telemetry (MCT), 39
Modified Fisher scale, 345
Mononeuritis multiplex, 26, 203
Mononeuropathies
    characterization, 68, 95, 201, 278, 279
    diabetic amyotrophy, 202, 203, 279
    femoral, 202
    HNPP, 203–4
    idiopathic brachial plexitis, 202
    median, 202

Mononeuropathies (*Cont.*)
  peri-operative, 101
  peroneal, 201–2
  radial, 201
  sciatic, 202
  ulnar, 202
Mononeuropathy multiplex, 56, 159,
  278, 279
Motoneuron lesions, 22
Motor disturbances
  anatomic localization, 19
  diagnosis, approach to, 24–27
  differential diagnosis, 18
  localization by correlation, 21–22
  physiologic localization, 18–19
  types of, 18
Motor nerve lesions, 18
Motor neuron degeneration, 244
Movement disorders
  abnormal movements, localization
    of, 18
  admission, rationales for, 8
  ataxia (*see* ataxia)
  differential diagnosis, 65, 174–76,
    175–76*t*
  overview, 223–24
  seizures (*see* seizures)
  syndromes, 224–28
MRA/MRV, 39*t*, 352
MRI, 351–52
Multi-infarct dementia, 170
Multifocal motor neuropathy (MMN),
  24, 201
Multiorgan dysfunction syndrome
  (MODS), 82
Multiple sclerosis (MS)
  characterization, 23, 65, 215–16
  complications of, 218–19, 228
  CSF findings, 355
  diagnosis, 216
  differential diagnosis, 60, 64
  disease-modifying therapy, 217
  exacerbation of, 218
  first diagnosis, 217–18
  immunosuppression, 360–63
  management of, 216–17
  medication-specific
    complications, 219–20
  myelitis, 217–18
  in pregnancy, 275
  primary progressive, 216

  relapsing-remitting, 216, 217, 363
  secondary progressive, 216
  subdivisions, 216
  tumefactive, 217
Multiple system atrophy, 228, 231, 313, 314
Muscles
  cramps, 68
  lesions, 19
  pain with exertion, 68
  weakness, 26, 207
Muscular dystrophies, 25, 211
Muscular ocular palsy, 45
Musculoskeletal spine pain, 76
Myasthenia gravis (MG)
  admission, rationales for, 8
  anesthetic complications, 26
  characterization, 24, 94, 204
  cholinergic crisis, 206
  diagnosis, 25, 204
  immunosuppression, 360–63
  management of, 205
  medications in exacerbation of, 205
  in pregnancy, 274
  ptosis, 48
  severe exacerbations, 205
Myelopathy
  anesthesia-associated, 102
  characterization, 243
  clinical diagnosis, 245
  compressive, from vertebral disease, 244
  differential diagnosis, 243–45
  necrotizing, 244
  peri-operative, 101
  radiation, 89, 244, 258
  radiculopathy (*see* radiculopathy)
  spondylotic, 248
Myocardial infarction, 129
Myoclonus
  characterization, 223, 236
  common causes of, 225–26
  drug-induced, 236
  epileptic, 225
  essential, 225
  hepatic failure-associated, 109
  palatal, 226
  post-hypoxic, 225
Myoglobinuria, 208
Myopathy, necrotizing, 26
Myotonia congenita, 26
Myotonic dystrophy, 26
Myotonic muscular dystrophy, 25

Narcolepsy, 323, 324
Nasopharyngeal carcinoma, 311
Natalizumab (Tysabri), 219, 363
National Institutes of Health Stroke Scale (NIHSS), 126*f*
Neck rigidity, 148
Necrotizing myopathy, 26
Needle, catheter injuries, 75
Neoplastic meningitis, 57, 76
Nerve conduction study (NCS), 349–51
Nerve injuries, 98, 100, 274–75
Nerve root lesions, 22
Neuro-critical care, 5*t*
Neurocardiogenic syncope, 36, 165
Neurofibromas, 311, 330
Neurofibromatosis, 311, 330
Neurogenic amyotrophy, 202
Neuroleptic malignant syndrome, 336
Neuroleptic toxicity, 290
Neuromuscular blockade/pharmacologic agents, 25, 34
Neuromuscular disorders
  admission, rationales for, 8
  anesthetic complications, 25–26
  characterization, 198
  critical illness neuromyopathy, 94–95
  differential diagnosis, 65
  follow-up appointments, 8
Neuromuscular junction lesions, 19
Neuromuscular paralysis, 102, 123
Neuromuscular respiratory failure, 213–14
Neuromyelitis optica (NMO)
  characterization, 23, 220
  CSF findings, 355
  differential diagnosis, 217–18, 243
  immunosuppression, 361–62
Neuronal migration, disorders of, 329
Neuropathy
  alcoholic, 292–93
  autonomic, 278–79
  chemotherapy, 89, 257
  cholinergic, 26
  compressive, 75
  demyelinating, 26
  diabetic, 74, 158–59, 277–79
  hereditary, 329
  hereditary with pressure palsies, 203–4, 329–30
  optic, 101, 292
  pain, 19, 219
  pain syndromes, 67, 68, 74–75

paraneoplastic autonomic, 313–15
peripheral, 68, 278
sensory, 21
ulnar, 21
Neurosyphilis, 31, 157
Neutropenia, 89
NIHSS, 342–43
NMO. *see* neuromyelitis optica (NMO)
Nonconvulsive seizure, 36
Nonepileptic psychogenic events, 174, 175*t*, 181*t*
Normal pressure hydrocephalus (NPH), 31, 64, 169
NSAIDs, 192
Numbness (sensory loss), 19
Nystagmus
  brainstem lesion associated, 46
  characterization, 45–46
  downbeat, 46
  gaze-evoked, 46
  jerk, 45
  medication associated, 46
  as MS complication, 218–19
  ocular muscle weakness, 46
  pendular, 45
  upbeat, 46
  vestibular, 46

Obstructive sleep apnea, 323–24
Occipital nerve blocks, 193
Occipital neuralgia, 73
Ocular motor palsy, 278
Ocular neuropathies, 55, 57
Oculomotor neuropathies, 55
Oculomotor palsy, 45, 47, 48
Olfactory neuropathies, 55
Optic disc edema, 46
Optic neuritis
  characterization, 43, 44, 46, 221
  differential diagnosis, 217
  immunosuppression, 360–63
Optic neuropathy, 101, 292
Orbital cellulitis, 44
Orbital pseudotumor (idiopathic orbital inflammatory syndrome), 44
Orbital tumor, 47
Organ transplantation
  diagnostic approach to, 26
  differential diagnosis, 51, 60
  failed organ effects, 100
  immune suppression, 100

Organ transplantation (*Cont.*)
neurological complications, 100
opportunistic infection, 100
underlying disease, 100
Organophosphate poisoning, 24
Orthostatic hypotension, 36, 37, 38*t*, 66, 313–14
Osmotic agents, for ICP, 359
Osmotic demyelination syndrome (ODS), 115
Otosclerosis, 302
Outpatient care
admission, rationales for, 8
continuity of care, 7–8, 14
discharge criteria, 9
Oxygen, cluster headache, 194

Pain syndromes
chronic, 70, 76–77
classification, 67–68
compressive neuropathies, 75
headache (*see* headache)
hospital neurologist consultation, 77
limb pain, 69*t*
localization, diagnosis of, 69, 69*t*
as MS complication, 219
muscular, 68
needle, catheter injuries, 75
neuropathic, 67, 68, 74–75
nonorganic, 77
psychology of pain, 69–70
skeletal, 68
spine pain, 69*t*, 76
surgical injuries, 75
vascular, 68
visceral, 68
Pain/temperature vs vibration/ proprioception deficits on opposite sides localization, 20*t*
Papilledema, 46–47, 94
Paramedian branch occlusion/basilar, 57
Paraneoplastic autonomic neuropathy, 313–15
Paraneoplastic cerebellar degeneration, 88, 228, 256
Paraneoplastic disorders, 88
Paraneoplastic encephalomyelitis, 86
Paraneoplastic myelitis, 244
Paraneoplastic neuropathies, 88
Paraneoplastic syndrome, 60
Paraspinal tumors, 87

Parenchymatous neurosyphilis, 157
Paresthesias characterization, 19
Parkinsonian tremor, 225
Parkinsonism
characterization, 23
drug-induced, 230–31
hospital implications of, 233–34
Parkinson's disease
akinesia, acute, 233
characterization, 65, 228–29
delirium, psychosis, 233
with dementia, 31, 32, 32*f*, 231–32
differential diagnosis, 60, 229
exacerbation of, 233
hospital implications of, 233–34
management of, 229–30
med schedule disturbance, 233
medical complications of, 233
medications, inability to take, 233
misdiagnosis of, 233
Paroxysmal hemicrania, 73
Parsonage-Turner syndrome, 202
Patent foramen ovale (PFO), 134
PCA stroke, 22, 57
Pentobarbital, status epilepticus dosage, 185*t*
Periodic limb movement disorder, 237, 323–25
Periodic paralysis, 24, 211–12
Peripheral nerve lesions, 22
Peripheral neuropathy, 68, 278
Peripheral vertigo, 60
Persistent CSF leak, 265
Persistent vegetative state, 30, 34, 122–23, 367
Phenytoin, 108
Pheochromocytoma, 277, 282
Pick disease, 31
Pituitary apoplexy, 268, 278, 283–84
Pituitary tumor, 278, 283
Plasma exchange, 201, 362
Plexopathy, 68
Plexus lesions, 22
Polymyositis, 210
Polyneuropathy
demyelinating, 26
distal symmetric, 158
ICU evaluation of, 25
management of, 279
progressive, 26
small-fiber, 26
vitamin/mineral deficiencies, 101

Post-concussive syndrome, 321
Post-discharge care, 8
Post-herpetic neuralgia, 74, 157, 202
Posterior inferior cerebellar artery (PICA)
    occlusion, 57
Posterior reversible encephalopathy
    syndrome (PRES), 94, 106, 182
Postpartum cerebral angiopathy, 268
Postviral myelitis, 153
Pre-eclampsia, 268, 269, 271
Pre-syncope, 59, 61, 63. *see also* syncope
Prednisone, 194, 201, 217
Pregnancy
    AEDs, management of, 186
    cerebral venous thrombosis in, 268,
        269, 271–72
    characterization, 66
    encephalopathy in, 269–70
    epilepsy in, 273–74
    focal deficits in, 270
    headache, 267–68
    ischemic stroke in, 270, 271
    migraine in, 268, 272–73
    multiple sclerosis in, 275
    myasthenia gravis in, 274
    neurologic consultation, 267
    neurologic disorders in, 270–75
    peripheral nerve injuries in, 274–75
    pseudotumor cerebri, 268, 270–71
    seizures in, 268–69
    subarachnoid hemorrhage, 268
    tPA, 129
Primary CNS angiitis, 362
Primary lateral sclerosis, 244
Primary progressive aphasia, 32, 32*f*, 51,
    171, 171*t*
Primary stroke center, 12
Prion diseases, 153–55, 177*t*
Prognostic indicators, imperfect, 123
Progressive lumbosacral
    plexopathy, 158–59
Progressive multifocal
    leukoencephalopathy (PML),
    159–60, 219
Progressive muscular atrophy, 212–13
Progressive myoclonus epilepsy (PME), 226
Progressive polyneuropathy, 26
Progressive supranuclear palsy (PSP), 31,
    169, 232
Propofol, status epilepticus dosage, 184*t*
Protein-energy malnutrition, 287

Proximal sensory deficit localization, 20*t*
Pseudoseizures, 174, 175*t*, 181*t*, 337
Pseudotumor cerebri
    characterization, 44, 47, 195
    CSF findings, 355
    diagnosis, 195
    differential diagnosis, 73
    management of, 195
    pregnancy, 268, 270–71
Psychogenic (hysterical) gait, 241
Psychogenic tremor, 225, 236
Psychogenic unresponsiveness, 34, 36, 123
Psychosis, 333–34
Ptosis, 48
Pulmonary embolism, 36
Pure word deafness, 53
Putamen hemorrhage, 138

Quality improvement, 6
Quality measures, 13–14
Quality of care concerns, 366
Quality of life assessment, 123

Radiation
    cerebral edema, 89
    injury, to brain, 257
    myelopathy, 89, 244, 258
    plexopathy, 89, 258
    toxicity, in brain, 259
    vasculopathy, 89
Radiculopathy
    cervical, 76, 246–47
    lumbar, 76, 247–48
    thoracic, 76, 248
Ramsay Hunt syndrome, 156, 307–8
Rebif, complications of, 220
Renal insufficiency
    dialysis disequilibrium, 107
    differential diagnosis, 33
    medications, altered clearance of, 108
    movement disorders, 225
    myoclonus, 225
    neurologic consultation, 92
    seizures, 106–7
    stroke, 107–8
Repetitive head injuries, 321
Repetitive nerve stimulation (RNS), 350
Respiratory disorders, complications
    of, 112–13
Restless legs syndrome, 237
Retinal artery/vein occlusion, 47, 298–99

Retinal detachment, 44
Return-to-play criteria, 321
Rheumatoid arthritis (RA), 93, 111–12
Rheumatologic disease, 26, 93–94, 111–12
Rigidity, 18, 224, 226
Risk management, 14
Rituximab, 362

Sacral sparing localization, 20t
Sarcoidosis, 112, 310
Scleroderma, systemic sclerosis, 93–94
Scope of responsibilities, 5
Sedatives, delayed clearance of, 34, 35
Seizures
    anesthesia-associated, 102
    cancer-related, 87
    characterization, 23, 83–84, 224
    clinical, spectrum of, 173–74
    clusters, 183
    conversion disorder, 337–38
    differential diagnosis, 36, 38–39t, 51, 62,
        84, 127, 174–76, 175–76t
    driving, 187
    epileptic, 174, 175t (see also epilepsy)
    focal, 174
    follow-up appointments, 8
    generalized tonic-clonic, 173–74, 181t
    hepatic encephalopathy, 108–9
    ictal paralysis, 23
    MS-associated, 219
    as neurologic complication, 93
    nonconvulsive, 36, 83
    peri-operative, 98, 99
    post-head injury, 320
    in pregnancy, 268–69
    renal insufficiency, 106–7
    studies, 84
    Todd's paralysis, 23
Sellar masses, 252
Semantic dementia, 32, 32f
Sensory ataxia, 19, 60, 62, 227
Sensory disturbances. see also specific
    disorders by name
    diagnosis, approach to, 24–27
    localization, 19, 20t
    localization by correlation, 21–22
    types of, 19
Sensory ganglionopathy, 26
Sensory neuropathy, 21
Sepsis/SIRS
    characterization, 66, 82

differential diagnosis, 177t
    focal deficits, 84–85
Septic shock, 82
Serotonin syndrome, 335–36
Shift duration, 14
Shingles, 74, 156–57
Shoulder surgery complications, 98
Single-fiber EMG (SFEMG), 350–51
Single-infarct dementia, 170
Single-limb sensory deficit localization, 20t
Sjögren syndrome, 94
Skew deviation, 45
Sleep deprivation, 33, 323, 325
Small-cell lung carcinoma, 26
Small-fiber polyneuropathy, 26
Smoking cessation, 77
Spasmodic dysphonia, 227
Spasmodic dystonia, 238
Spasticity
    characterization, 224
    management of, 357–58
    MS-associated, 218, 219
Spinal cord
    degenerative spine disease, 246
    disease characterization, 74
    hematoma, 244
    hemisection (Brown-Sequard), 22
    infarction, 144–45, 244
    lesions, 21, 65, 244
    metastases, 87–88
    surgery complications, 99
    traumatic injury, 249
    tumors, 253–54
Spine pain, 69t, 76
Spinocerebellar ataxia, 228, 240
Spinocerebellar degeneration, differential
    diagnosis, 64
Statins, ischemic stroke, 135
Status epilepticus
    characterization, 183
    convulsive, 183–84
    management of, 184–85t
    nonconvulsive, 185–86, 185–86f
    pregnancy, AED management, 186
Status migraine, 8
Steroid-responsive encephalopathy with
    autoimmune thyroiditis (STREAT),
    277, 280–81
Stiffness, 18, 224, 226
Stroke mimics, 131, 218
Stroke scales, 342–44

Stroke syndromes
   in cancer patients, 259
   cardiac disease, 91
   cerebellar, 65
   with cerebral edema, 105
   clinical scenarios, 22–23
   complications, 86
   cranial nerve palsies, 311
   cryptogenic stroke, 134–35
   as diabetes complication, 89–90
   differential diagnosis, 60, 71
   endovascular therapy, 105
   follow-up appointments, 8
   hemorrhagic (*see* hemorrhagic stroke)
   ischemic (*see* ischemic stroke)
   IV tPA, 105
   peri-operative, 98, 99
   radiation therapy and, 89
   renal insufficiency, 107–8
Structural brain lesion, 38*t*
Structural heart disease, 38*t*
Study follow-up, 8
Subacute bacterial endocarditis
      (SBE), 155
Subarachnoid hemorrhage
   assessment scales, 344–45
   characterization, 136–37, 320
   CSF findings, 355
   differential diagnosis, 36, 70, 262
   management of, 139–40
   pregnancy, 268
Subclavian steal, 36
Subdural hematoma, 136, 319, 358
Sudden unexplained death with epilepsy
      (SUDEP), 187
Sumatriptan, cluster headache, 194
SUNCT, 72–73
Surgery
   ICP, 360
   injuries, 75
   PD, 230
   spasticity, 358
Surgical patient complications
   bariatric surgery, 100–101
   cardiovascular, 99
   nerve injuries, 98, 100
   orthopedic, 98–99
   overview, 97–98
   transplantation, 100
Syncope
   cardiac disease, 91

characterization, 35–36, 35*f*, 59, 165
clonic, 62
convulsive (clonic), 36, 37
cough, 36, 165
diagnostic studies, 37–39, 38–39*t*
differential diagnosis, 36–37, 61–62,
      174–76, 176*t*
micturition, 36, 165
neurocardiogenic/vasovagal, 36, 165
neurologic consultation, 40
Syndrome of inappropriate antidiuretic
      hormone (SIADH), 278, 284
Syringobulbia, 328
Syringomyelia, 21, 244, 264, 328
Systemic lupus erythematosus (SLE),
      93, 111

Tabes dorsalis, 157
Tardive dyskinesia, 237–38
Tardive dystonia, 238
Teleneurology, 4*t*, 13
Temporal arteritis
   characterization, 44, 195–96
   differential diagnosis, 73
   immunosuppression, 360–63
   management of, 196
   as neurologic complication, 93
Thalamic hemorrhage, 138
Thalamic infarction, 21, 22
Thalamic lesions, 21
Thalamic pain syndrome, 21
The Joint Commission (TJC), 11
Thiamine, status epilepticus dosage, 184*t*
Thoracic radiculopathy, 76, 248
Thyroid ophthalmopathy, 277, 281
Thyrotoxicosis, 277
Tick paralysis, 24, 206–7
Tics, 224, 227
Tilt table, 38*t*
Tinnitus, 305–6
Tizanidine, 358
Todd's paralysis, 23
Tolosa-Hunt syndrome, 311
Tonic pupil (Adie), 47, 48
Topiramate, 73
Topiramate, status epilepticus dosage, 183
Torsion dystonia, 238
Toxic myopathies, 24
Toxicity, differential diagnosis, 60
Toxin exposure, 289. *see also specific toxins*
Toxoplasma, 159

Transient global amnesia, 34, 62, 164–65
Transient hypotension, 62
Transient ischemic attack (TIA)
  antiplatelets, 131
  as diabetes complication, 89–90
  differential diagnosis, 36, 37, 73
  follow-up appointments, 8
  psychogenic, 37
Transient loss of consciousness (TLOC).
    see syncope
Transient monocular blindness, 43, 297–98
Transplantation. see organ transplantation
Transthoracic echocardiogram (TTE), 38t, 39
Transverse myelitis, 218, 221–22, 243
Trauma, 34, 71, 99, 177t
Traumatic brain injury (TBI)
  concussion, 317–18
  contusion, 318
  differential diagnosis, 51
  diffuse axonal injury, 320
  epidural hematoma, 136, 319
  intracerebral hemorrhage, 135–40, 268,
    318–20
  overview, 317
  post-concussive syndrome, 321
  repetitive head injuries, 321
  return-to-play criteria, 321
  seizures, post-head injury, 320
  subdural hematoma, 136, 319
Tremor, 219, 223–25, 234–36
Trigeminal neuralgia
  characterization, 21, 68, 195
  differential diagnosis, 74
  management of, 195, 219
Trigeminal neuropathies, 56
Triptans
  cluster headache, 194
  migraine, 192
  in pregnancy, 272
Trochlear neuropathies, 55
Trochlear palsy, 45
Tumor mimics, 251
Tumors. see brain tumors
Tysabri (natalizumab), 219, 363

Ulnar neuropathy, 21
Uveitis/iritis, 44

Vagus neuropathies, 56
Valproate
  migraine, 192

status epilepticus dosage, 183, 186t
  tremor and, 235
Variant CJD, 154–55
Vascular dementia
  characterization, 31, 169–70
  diagnosis, 170
  differential diagnosis, 32, 32f
  management, 170
  subtypes, 170
Vascular neurology, 5t
Vasculitis, 57
Vegetative state, 34
Ventricular drain, for ICP, 360
Verapamil, cluster headache, 194
Vertebral artery dissection, 142–43,
    268, 270
Vertebrobasilar insufficiency, 66
Vertigo. see also dizziness, vertigo
  with appendicular ataxia, 62
  characterization, 60
  with hearing loss, 62
  management of, 302
  post-traumatic, 302
Vestibular neuropathy, 303
Vestibular schwannoma, 53, 65, 306
Vestibulocochlear neuropathies, 56
Vestibulopathy
  acoustic neuroma, 53, 65, 306
  benign paroxysmal positional vertigo,
    60, 62, 65, 301–3
  differential diagnosis, 65
  labyrinthitis, 303–4
  Ménière disease (see Ménière disease)
  neurology consultation, 301
  otosclerosis, 302
  overview, 301–2
  peripheral, 228
  tinnitus, 305–6
Viral myelitis, 153
Visual loss
  anisocoria, 47–48
  diplopia, 45
  localization, diagnosis, 42, 43t
  monocular vs. binocular, 42, 43t
  nystagmus, 45–46
  papilledema, 46–47
  partial-field vs. full-field, 42
  ptosis, 48
  syndromes of, 43–44
  timing of, 42
Vitamin D deficiency, 288

Water intoxication, 115
Weakness
    differential diagnosis, 65
    endocrine, metabolic myopathies,
        212
    inflammatory myopathies, 210–11
    localization of, 18
    muscle, 26, 207
    muscular dystrophies, 211
    myoglobinuria, 208
    periodic paralysis, 24, 211–12
    psychogenic, characterization, 24
    rhabdomyolysis, 208–9
Wegener granulomatosis, 310
Wernicke's encephalopathy
    differential diagnosis, 228

nystagmus in, 46
peri-operative complications, 101
West Nile virus (WNV)
    characterization, 24, 161
    diagnostic approach to, 27
    differential diagnosis, 162t
    ED evaluation, 25
    viral myelitis, 153
WFNS scale, 344–45
Whipple disease, 160–61
Wilson disease, 228, 240–41
Withdrawal states, syndromes, 98, 102
Work, call schedule, 5

Zika virus, 27, 162
Zolmitriptan, cluster headache, 194

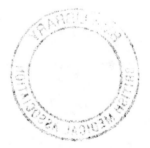

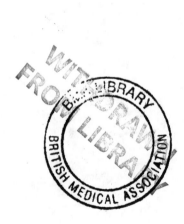